P9-DHR-883

Challenges of an Aging Society

RECENT AND RELATED TITLES IN GERONTOLOGY

Stuart H. Altman and David I. Shactman, eds. *Policies for an Aging Society*

Mary M. Ball, Molly M. Perkins, Frank J. Whittington, Carole Hollingsworth, Sharon V. King, and Bess L. Combs. *Communities of Care: Assisted Living for African American Elders*

Robert H. Binstock, Leighton E. Cluff, and Otto von Mering, eds. *The Future of Long-Term Care: Social and Policy Issues*

Leighton E. Cluff and Robert H. Binstock, eds. *The Lost Art of Caring: A Challenge to Health Professionals, Families, Communities, and Society*

Tom Hickey, Marjorie A. Speers, and Thomas R. Prohaska, eds. *Public Health and Aging*

Robert B. Hudson, ed. *The New Politics of Old Age Policy*

Robert L. Kane, Reinhard Priester, and Annette Totten, *Meeting the Challenge of Chronic Illness*

Nancy Morrow-Howell, James Hinterlong, and Michael Sherraden, eds. *Productive Aging: Concepts and Challenges*

Karl Pillemer, Phyllis Moen, Elaine Wethington, and Nina Glasgow, eds. *Social Integration in the Second Half of Life*

Joseph White. *False Alarm: Why the Greatest Threat to Social Security and Medicare Is the Campaign to "Save" Them*

Robert H. Binstock, Consulting Editor in Gerontology

Challenges of an Aging Society

Ethical Dilemmas, Political Issues

Edited by

Rachel A. Pruchno

and

Michael A. Smyer

The Johns Hopkins University Press
Baltimore

Publication of this volume was supported by the generous gift of Darlene Bookoff, in memory of her father, Morris Bookoff, who devoted much of his life to enhancing quality of care and life for elderly people.

© 2007 The Johns Hopkins University Press
All rights reserved. Published 2007
Printed in the United States of America on acid-free paper
9 8 7 6 5 4 3 2 1

The Johns Hopkins University Press
2715 North Charles Street
Baltimore, Maryland 21218-4363
www.press.jhu.edu

Library of Congress Cataloging-in-Publication Data

Challenges of an aging society : ethical dilemmas, political issues /
edited by Rachel A. Pruchno and Michael A. Smyer.
     p. ; cm.
  Includes bibliographical references and index.
  ISBN-13: 978-0-8018-8648-5 (hardcover : alk. paper)
  ISBN-10: 0-8018-8648-1 (hardcover : alk. paper)
  1. Aging—Moral and ethical aspects. 2. Aging—Moral and ethical
aspects. 3. Aging—Political aspects. 4. Older people—Health and
hygiene—Social aspects. 5. Medical ethics. 6. Medical policy.
I. Pruchno, Rachel. II. Smyer, Michael A.
  [DNLM: 1. Aged. 2. Bioethical Issues. 3. Long-Term Care—ethics.
4. Public Policy. WT 100 C4375 2007]
  RA408.A3C47 2007
  174.2'9897—dc22

                                     2006039066

A catalog record for this book is available from the British Library.

In memory of Howard "Chip" Piper and Martin V. Faletti, Ph.D.,
both of whom cared passionately about philosophy and ethics

Contents

Contributors

W. Andrew Achenbaum, Ph.D., Professor of History and Social Work, University of Houston, Houston, Texas

Vern L. Bengtson, Ph.D., University Professor of Gerontology, AARP Professor of Sociology, and Director, Social and Behavioral Sciences, Andrus Gerontology Center, University of Southern California, Los Angeles, California

Robert H. Binstock, Ph.D., Professor of Aging, Health, and Society, School of Medicine, Case Western Reserve University, Cleveland, Ohio

Christine E. Bishop, Ph.D., Atran Professor of Labor Economics, Heller School for Social Policy and Management, Brandeis University, Waltham, Massachusetts

Thomas R. Cole, Ph.D., Director, McGovern Chair in Medical Humanities, John P. McGovern Center for Health, Humanities, and the Human Spirit, University of Texas–Houston School of Medicine, Houston, Texas

Peter A. Diamond, Ph.D., Institute Professor and Professor of Economics, Massachusetts Institute of Technology, Cambridge, Massachusetts

Nancy Neveloff Dubler, LL.B., Director, Division of Bioethics, Department of Family and Social Medicine, Montefiore Medical Center, and Professor of Bioethics, Albert Einstein College of Medicine, Bronx, New York

Msgr. Charles J. Fahey, Program Officer, Milbank Memorial Fund, and Marie Ward Doty Professor Emeritus, Fordham University, Bronx, New York

Lucy Feild, Ph.D., R.N., Partners Human Research Quality Improvement Program, Boston, Massachusetts

Martha B. Holstein, Ph.D., Adjunct Faculty in Medicine, Ethics, and Society, Department of Religious Studies, DePaul University, Chicago, Illinois

Robert B. Hudson, Ph.D., Professor of Social Policy, Boston University, Boston, Massachusetts

Eric R. Kingson, Ph.D., Professor of Social Work and Public Administration, School of Social Work, College of Human Services and Health Professions, Syracuse University, Syracuse, New York

Ronald J. Manheimer, Ph.D., Executive Director, North Carolina Center for Creative Retirement, University of North Carolina at Asheville, Asheville, North Carolina

Kyriakos S. Markides, Ph.D., Annie and John Gnitzinger Professor of Aging Studies; Editor, *Journal of Aging and Health;* and Director, Division of Socio-medical Sciences, Department of Preventive Medicine and Community Health, University of Texas Medical Branch, Galveston, Texas

Daniel C. Marson, J.D., Ph.D., Professor of Neurology, Director, Division of Neuropsychology, and Director, Alzheimer's Disease Research Center, University of Alabama at Birmingham, Birmingham, Alabama

H. Rick Moody, Ph.D., Director of Academic Affairs, AARP, Washington, D.C.

Peter R. Orszag, Ph.D., Director, Congressional Budget Office, Washington, D.C.

Rachel Pruchno, Ph.D., University Professor, Endowed Professor of Gerontology, and Director of Research, New Jersey Institute for Successful Aging, University of Medicine and Dentistry of New Jersey–School of Osteopathic Medicine, Stratford, New Jersey

Norella M. Putney, Ph.D., Research Associate, Andrus Gerontology Center, University of Southern California, Los Angeles, California

Michael Smyer, Ph.D., Dean, Graduate School of Arts and Sciences, and Associate Vice President for Research, Boston College, Chestnut Hill, Massachusetts

Bruce Stuart, Ph.D., Professor and Director, Peter Lamy Center on Drug Therapy and Aging, School of Pharmacy, University of Maryland, Baltimore, Maryland

Melanie A. Wakeman, Ph.D., Lecturer, California State University, Los Angeles, California

Steven P. Wallace, Ph.D., Professor and Vice-Chair, Department of Community Health Sciences, and Associate Director, Center for Health Policy Research, School of Public Health, University of California at Los Angeles, Los Angeles, California

John B. Williamson, Ph.D., Professor, Department of Sociology, Boston College, Chestnut Hill, Massachusetts

Acknowledgments

The editors gratefully acknowledge funding from the National Institute on Aging (R13 AG20144) and from Boston College's Jesuit Institute, which provided the resources enabling us to convene scientists and ethicists interested in aging. Special thanks to our colleague Patrick Byrne, Ph.D., who brought expertise in ethics to our dialogue during those conferences.

The first conference, entitled "The Science and Ethics of Aging Well: End of Life," was held on March 17–18, 2003. The second conference, entitled "The Science and Ethics of Aging Well: Public Policy and Responsibility across the Generations," was held on March 15–26, 2004. The editors appreciate thoughtful presentations made at these conferences by: Sandra Bertman, Ph.D.; Daniel Callahan, Ph.D.; Emily Chandler, Ph.D., R.N., C.S.; John Cornman; Norman Daniels, Ph.D.; Rose Dobrof, D.S.W.; Terri Fried, M.D.; Sara Fry, Ph.D., R.N., F.A.A.N.; Jerry Gurwitz, M.D.; Carolyn Hayes, Ph.D., R.N.; Laurel Herbst, M.D.; Karla Holloway, Ph.D.; James Lubben, D.S.W., M.P.H; Ray Madoff, J.D.; Kevin Mahoney, Ph.D.; Keith Meador, M.D., Th.M., M.Ph.H.; Douglas Miller, M.D.; Susan Miller, Ph.D., M.B.A.; John Paris, S.J., Ph.D.; Gloria Ramsey, J.D., R.N.; Greg Sachs, M.D.; David Solomon, Ph.D.; and Patricia A. Tabloski, Ph.D.

Finally, the editors are extremely grateful to Mary Cavalieri for her perseverance in tracking down missing details and information, to Bob McBride and his staff for completing all artwork in the book, to Wendy Harris and Bob Binstock for their never-ending confidence and encouragement, to the anonymous reviewers who encouraged us to push the envelop, and to Lois Crum for her fine work as copy editor.

Challenges of an Aging Society

The Science and Ethics of Aging Well

Rachel A. Pruchno, Ph.D., and Michael A. Smyer, Ph.D.

The aging of American society has combined with advances in medical technology to present Americans with difficult decisions that were irrelevant only a generation ago: Should succeeding generations be responsible for one another? How should scarce resources be allocated across generations and populations? Who should make decisions when questions arise about medical care at the end of life? At best, crafting answers to each of these issues requires a tacit understanding of the fields of ethics and aging. Unfortunately, dialogue among philosophers, geriatric practitioners, and gerontologists is rare.

The National Institute on Aging and the Jesuit Institute at Boston College sponsored two conferences under the rubric of the Science and Ethics of Aging Well. Each conference was designed to provide a unique exchange among scientists and ethicists who are committed to understanding the intersection of aging and ethics. Together, the participants helped define the salient unanswered questions and crafted the foundation for the next generation of empirical research in these important areas. Their contributions form the basis of this volume.

Almost 20 years ago, Daniel Callahan's *Setting Limits: Medical Goals in an*

Aging Society (1987) sounded an alarm about what has more recently been labeled the "perfect storm" (Kotlikoff and Burns, 2004) of demographics and entitlements. Callahan noted that the combination of increasing numbers of older adults and increasing costs of their care would require some limitations for access to care in later life. As Callahan (1994, p. 398) has more recently reminded us, we may be victims of our own successes: "It is the success of medicine, not its failures, that has created the problem of sustaining and paying for decent health care for the elderly. It is the success of the campaign against ageism, increasing the expectations of everyone for a medically and socially transformed old age, that has added to that problem. If there is any blame to be apportioned it should be directed at our dreams, some of which have come true. It is just that we did not know what that would mean. Now we are finding out."

Demographics and Ethics

By the year 2030, one-fifth of the U.S. population, or 70 million people, will be age 65 or older. The explosion of the elderly population between 2010 and 2030 is inevitable as the baby boom generation (those 76 million people born between 1946 and 1964) reaches age 65. Demographers today predict that the most dramatic growth in our population will be in those over age 85, with the number of people ages 90–99 expected to rise from just over 8 million today to 60 million in 2050, a sevenfold increase. Comparable figures for centenarians are even more impressive, increasing from today's 190,000 people to 2.5 million, a thirteenfold increase—and this does not take into account possible medical or technological advances in the near future.

This demographic generalization glosses over significant variation in life expectancies across ethnic and racial groups, across genders, and across social classes, however. For example, African American men in the contemporary United States have an average life expectancy at birth of 66.1 years, while their non-Hispanic white counterparts have an average life expectancy at birth of 73.8 years (Ventura et al., 1997). Hayward and Heron (1999, pp. 77–78) summarized the racial differences in life expectancy at the outset of adulthood: "for men aged 20 in 1990, the life expectancy of Native Americans is 54.7 years compared with 47.6 years for blacks, 49 years for white Hispanics, 54.6 years for non-Hispanic whites, and 59.1 for Asian American. By the beginning of adulthood, approximately 11.5 years of life separate black men from Asian American men. There is comparatively less racial disparity among women, although almost eight years of life separate black and Asian American women."

These age norms might shape the expectations of members of an aging society in two ways: first, an earlier disability or death might be considered "off time" and therefore might cause people to be less prepared for encountering the end of life; second, these age norms may well shape the expectations of family members and clinicians alike regarding a sick or dying person—and their assumptions about what is appropriate care and responsibility.

Longer life expectancies carry with them two important implications: compressed morbidity (Fries, 1980, 1989), which will forestall functional decline until older ages; and an increased likelihood that growing numbers of Americans will experience the ravages of dementias such as Alzheimer disease. Currently there are approximately 4.5 million Americans with Alzheimer disease, a number that has more than doubled since 1980. The predictions are that as the baby boomers enter old age, this number will increase to between 11.3 million and 16 million by the year 2050 (Hebert et al., 2003). These trends suggest that we are entering a world in which most elderly Americans may spend their final years with multiple chronic illnesses. The growing number of older people with multiple chronic illnesses will cause demands for health care, including long-term care, to rise, and the costs of this health care will increase significantly.

In this context, the ethical principles of autonomy, responsibility, and distributive justice will become both more salient and more interdependent. Callahan (1987) notes that in early days of the bioethics field, the good of the individual, particularly his or her autonomy, was the dominant theme. As the bioethical movement evolved, ethicists struggled first with questions regarding searches for cures through better biological understanding and technological innovation, and then with debates over issues of equitable access as the costs of health care rose. As our society's demographic changes evolve, ethicists and society as a whole will continue to debate the primacy of autonomy. Policymakers, practitioners, and ethicists will focus greater attention on issues of responsibility and distributive justice and how these ethical principles interrelate.

Balancing autonomy, responsibility, and distributive justice can be likened to balancing the needs of the older person, those of her or his immediate family, and those of society at large. By its nature, autonomy has as its primary goal respect for the individual person. It presumes that people will do what is in their own best interest. One perspective on reaching a balance is that if all people do what is in their own best interest, the needs of others, including the family and society, will not be taken into consideration. For example, 80-year-old Mr. X might decide that he "wants everything done" to keep himself alive. Acting in an autonomous fashion, he could develop an advance directive instructing health care providers and his family to "keep him alive at all costs." With available medical technology, Mr. X could find himself on a ventilator with a feeding tube, requiring 24-hour skilled nursing care.

The next question would be "Whose responsibility is it to care for Mr. X?" Typically, we turn to the family. Yet, by placing this responsibility on a family member, it could be argued, we are removing the opportunity for family members' own autonomous decision making. To carry out the scenario, it is likely that Mr. X's 60-year-old daughter will be in the labor force and will be looking forward to her own retirement. Requiring her to provide care for her father may force her to leave the labor force earlier than she had planned, possibly jeopardizing her future earnings and her own autonomy in later life. An alternative scenario would be for Mr. X to be cared for in a nursing home or by another paid caregiver. The issue of distributive justice would then be raised: Who should pay for this care?—the individual, the family, or society? and would caring for Mr. X be done at the expense of another person who could better benefit from treatment?

A significant issue guiding our understanding of the interrelationship of autonomy, responsibility, and distributive justice is the stability of individuals' decisions over time. Do the treatment decisions that people articulate when they are capable remain constant when impairment occurs? There is good evidence that even in competent persons, treatment preferences change over time. There is also good evidence that as health conditions become more serious, the bar is lowered, and the decisions individuals spurned initially begin to look more appealing.

There is evidence that patients may prefer to have others make end-of-life decisions for them. Research by High (1994), Hines et al. (1999), and Terry et al. (1999) finds that many competent patients defer to the wishes of their family members in making their treatment decisions and may in fact withhold completing an advance directive to give family members greater latitude (High, 1994). These findings suggest that individuals do not act solely with autonomy in mind. Instead, people consider both their own needs and desires and the implications that these may have for others, especially family members.

At a policy level, it is essential to balance patient autonomy with family responsibility and distributive justice. Advocating solely for patient autonomy is not in the best interests of the patient, the family, or society. Instead, an appreciation of the interdependence that is evident at the end of life requires responding to the concerns of all three—the patient, the family, and society—simultaneously.

Improving the care that is available at the end of life would improve the balance between patient autonomy and distributive justice. Again, Callahan (1994, p. 394) outlined the concerns well: "Aging and death in old age are inevitable, and there should be no unlimited claim on public resources to combat them. . . . The first health task of a society is that the young should have the chance to become old. That should always take priority over helping, at great cost, those who are already old from becoming still older. That is exactly what we can look forward to, as we throw more and more money into the fight to cure chronic and degenerative diseases of aging, but not to care well for those who cannot be saved."

These three ethical issues—autonomy, responsibility, and distributive justice—resonate in the individual, family, and policy decisions faced by an aging society. We turn to each ethical issue in the next sections.

Autonomy

Questions about autonomy are central to the problems and prospects of aging. A tradition of patient autonomy has shaped our medical and legal traditions. Increasingly, responsibility for care decisions has shifted from the physician to the patient. However, individual differences and interdependence significantly affect how autonomy is exercised in later life.

The ethnic, social, and religious beliefs of patients, family members, and members of the professional health care team influence the ways in which decisions about autonomy are made. In the absence of patient competence to actually make decisions about care, patient autonomy requires that the preferences of the patient should be honored when treatment decisions are made. Advance directives, in the form of durable power of attorney for health care or health care proxy and living will, are mechanisms by which people with decisional capacity can maintain their voice in health care decisions should they later lose their capacity to make those decisions. Yet, the reality is that most Americans do not have an advance directive (Elpern, Yellen, and Burton, 1993; Singer et al., 1995; Hoefler, 1997), and even when an advance directive exists, it is frequently ignored (Doukas and Hardwig, 2003).

Most people feel that they can rely on close family members to make health care decisions for them (High, 1988, 1994; Hayley et al., 1996). And most health care providers turn to family members when critical decisions need to be made and the patients involved are unable to make them (Keating et al., 1994; High and Rowles, 1995). The President's Commission for the Study of Ethical Problems in Medicine and Biomedical and Behavioral Research (1983) endorsed "substituted judgment" as a means for promoting patient autonomy. Substituted judgment calls for surrogates to make decisions in a manner that approximates the patient's wishes. It assumes that surrogates understand patient preferences and correctly represent the wishes of the patient.

Although the substituted-judgment standard may be ethically sound, it is unclear whether people actually use this standard in practice. Several studies have shown that, when faced with hypothetical decisions about life-sustaining medical care, family members and physicians do not consistently predict a patient's preferences at levels of accuracy beyond those expected by chance alone (Uhlmann, Pearlman, and Cain, 1988; Hare, Pratt, and Nelson, 1992; Druley et al., 1993; Gerety et al., 1993; Suhl et al., 1994; Sulmasy et al., 1998; Fried, Bradley, and Towle, 2003). Rather, family proxies consistently tend to overestimate the frequency with which patients would like to receive treatment (Uhlmann et al., 1988).

A related issue is the limit of individual autonomy or the extent to which ethical decisions, such as withdrawing life support, should best serve the interests of the patient or the family. As Fisher and Raper (2000) acknowledge, when treatment is continued largely for the benefit of the family, the patient is being used to serve the interests of others. While it could be argued that such a decision is not ethical, it could also be argued that because patients have the best interests of their family members at heart, what is good for the family is also good for the patient.

Responsibility

Issues regarding responsibility across generations are equally complex. The changing U.S. demographics also affect our understanding of responsibility. Arno, Levine, and Memmott (1999) estimate that in 1997 there were 25.8 million informal caregivers. For more than three decades, research has documented the primary role played by middle-aged women—the daughters, daughters-in-law, and wives of disabled older people—as primary caregivers. Estimates are that between 55 and 70 percent of primary caregivers are women

(Stone, Cafferata, and Sangl, 1987; National Alliance for Caregiving and the American Association of Retired Persons, 1997) and that the average woman can expect to spend 18 years caring for a parent, comparable to the number of years spent raising and taking care of her children (National Alliance for Caregiving, 1997).

Family members' help given to their disabled older members has been documented since the 1960s. The U.S. Department of Health, Education, and Welfare (1972) revealed that the family provides 80 percent of medically related services (such as bandage changing and injections) needed by older people living in the community. The classic study of the Cleveland area carried out by the U.S. General Accounting Office (Comptroller General, 1977) found that the family provides between 80 and 90 percent of household maintenance and other instrumental services. The 1982 Long-Term Care Survey reported that nearly 75 percent of disabled older people living in the community rely solely on family and friends for the assistance they require; most of the remainder depend on a combination of family care and paid help (Doty, 1986).

Despite a pervasive literature on family caregiving, trends characterizing patterns of family caregiving over the past several decades are difficult to identify. A combination of different ways of defining and operationalizing the term *caregiver,* a literature that is largely based on small samples of convenience, and the use of measures in datasets that are not comparable are responsible for this problem. Nonetheless, work by Wagner (1997) does provide an interesting glimpse of these trends over the 10-year period from 1987 to 1997.

Comparing data from the 1987 study by the American Association of Retired Persons, in collaboration with the Travelers Foundation, with the 1997 study done by the National Alliance for Caregiving and AARP, Wagner finds striking similarities between the studies in terms of the average age of caregivers (45 years in both studies), the average length of time that care is provided (4.5 to 5 years), and the average age of the care recipient (77–78 years).

Now, just as our need for caregivers has begun its exponential growth, there is evidence that our country's supply of these caregivers, both paid and unpaid, is dwindling. Wagner reported significant differences over the 1987–97 period, including the amount of time caregivers spent providing care (in 1987 only 28% of caregivers spent eight hours or less helping their older relative; in 1997 the figure was 48%) and the number of activities of daily living (ADL) tasks with which they helped (32% of caregivers did not provide any ADL assistance in 1987; in 1997 the figure was 49%).

Wagner also noted the increase in the number of caregivers who were employed, a figure that rose from 55 percent in 1987 to 64 percent in 1997. Together, these data suggest that the tendency for women to enter and stay in the labor force during their middle and later years has the potential to severely limit the extent to which they will be able to be involved in traditional family caregiver roles. Moreover, although Wagner reported an increasing trend among the caregivers to use personal care services (22% in 1987; 38% in 1997), the current severe shortage of nurses and nursing aides is likely to severely limit options for older people and their families to purchase care.

These trends are developing, while the costs associated with caring for disabled older people, especially those with dementia, are escalating. Data from Arno et al. (1999) indicate that the economic value of informal caregiving in 1997 was $196 billion, a figure that dwarfs national spending for formal home health care ($32 billion) and nursing home care ($83 billion). The economic value of informal caregiving is equivalent to approximately 18 percent of the total national health care spending ($1,092 billion) budget. Unfortunately, the costs of informal caregiving are not counted as part of national health care spending; if they were, the trillion-dollar figure would rise by nearly $200 billion.

Distributive Justice

Issues grounded in distributive justice include such questions as "How much money should our society spend on curing Alzheimer disease as opposed to curing other serious chronic illnesses that strike younger people, such as multiple sclerosis, cancer, and cystic fibrosis?" Another issue revolves around the question of whether age or health condition should be a factor to consider when making decisions about allocation of scarce resources, such as kidney or heart transplants. A by-product of our society's ability to find cures for ailments such as some cancers and pneumonia is the need to decide when to implement these cures. We are now faced with ethical decisions that make the distinction between "What can be done?" and "What should be done?" more pressing.

Resource issues become paramount in end-of-life decisions when patients or family members request that treatment be continued at all cost, in spite of a minimal chance of survival on the part of the patient. Here compliance with individual requests may conflict with the rights of other patients who have a greater chance of survival, yet who need access to limited resources (e.g., intensive care or organ transplant) in order to survive. A frequent topic of debate in intensive care meetings is the management of the "last ICU bed" (Fisher, 2004). These debates focus on which patient should be offered the one bed available in the intensive care unit. Society has, in general, provided no mandate for doctors to withhold unilaterally or withdraw even marginally beneficial treatment; the result is a projected need for double the current number of intensive care beds during the next 25 years (Fisher, 2004). In the future, our society will be faced with developing mechanisms for justly limiting access to treatment and for deciding how to prioritize the allocation of scare resources.

The family is and has been the bedrock of support for its disabled older members. As we go forward, it is informative to consider programs such as Cash and Counseling Demonstration and Evaluation, funded by the Robert Wood Johnson Foundation and the Office of the Assistant Secretary for Planning and Evaluation of the U.S. Department of Health and Human Services. This program offers persons with disability a cash allowance in place of agency-delivered services. It is part of a larger movement toward consumer-directed, community-based long-term care (Benjamin, 2001). Consumers meeting project eligibility criteria are randomly assigned to participate in the program or serve as a control group and receive services through their state's existing system. The demonstration project was carried out in three states, Arkansas, New Jersey, and Florida (Mahoney et al., 2004). An evaluation (Dale et al., 2003) revealed that Arkansas Medicaid beneficiaries who had the opportunity to direct their personal care services themselves received better care than did the control group. The effects on caregivers were equally dramatic: caregivers for consumers managing the cash allowance experienced less financial, emotional, and physical strain. The Cash and Counseling program suggests practical approaches for addressing the problem of distributive justice across age groups and birth cohorts in our aging society. It shows how a society can make the mechanisms for distributive justice more adjustable to the needs of different segments of society and better address the concerns of multiple generations simultaneously.

The Plan of the Book

Questions raised by the ethical principals of autonomy, responsibility across the generations, and distributive justice are central to this volume. Cross-cutting each of these ethical principles is the question of how the good of the individual fares vis-à-vis that of the family and society. These themes emerge in each of the chapters that follow.

Chapter 1 looks at issues regarding autonomy and end-of-life decisions. Nancy Dubler first examines the legal aspects of end-of-life decision making. She focuses on the importance of involving the family as well as society in these decisions. Her chapter then examines the legal and policy barriers to providing adequate care at the end of life, and she concludes with comments on the future of the legal debate. These are essential issues for an aging society. As Byock (1997, p. xiii) noted: "While death may cast a long shadow upon us as we journey through life, Americans typically refuse to notice. We stride ahead, looking toward a bright future, concentrating on health and living fully. . . . But, then, when death approaches, we are stunned and feel unprepared to deal with the situation we face."

Questions regarding the competence of an individual to make end-of-life decisions are at the intersection of legal, ethical, and clinical issues. Daniel Marson's chapter examines the constructs of competence and autonomy in end-of-life decision making. He notes that even though competence is ultimately a legal status, physician assessments are critical, and he points to the importance of assessing competence for medical decision making in special populations, such as nursing home residents.

Charles Fahey considers the ethical issues raised by our society's increased need for long-term care. Noting that people are interdependent at every moment of life, and that we now have more people alive at every stage of life who have frailties that limit their participation in everyday activities, Fahey raises questions that include "What ethically based demands can those with impairments make on other people?" and "Who should bear the burden in meeting the needs of those with impairment?" Fahey argues that within the framework of striving for a just society, the overall social policy goal is to assure that individuals have what they need to respond effectively to their frailty. He makes suggestions for reform in long-term care that are consistent with this premise.

Salient to end-of-life issues are religiosity and spirituality. Lucy Feild reviews the conceptual and methodological issues characterizing the literature on religiosity and spirituality, highlights relevant research findings, and examines the clinical relevance of religiosity and spirituality in end-of-life care. Religious beliefs in general and belief in an afterlife, in particular, are cultural beliefs that profoundly affect the individual's approach to the end of life (Cicirelli, 2002).

In this area, however, there is debate about the role that physicians can and should play. Post, Puchalski, and Larson (2000) suggest that physicians and other clinicians must attend to the healing roles of spirituality and religion in the lives of their patients. Sloan et al. (2000), in contrast, criticize the empirical studies of the efficacy of religion in healing and coping with anxiety at the end of life. This difference of opinion embodies Byock's assessment (1997, p. 244): "America, as a culture, has no positive vision and no sense of direction with regard to life's end. Without a position on the compass pointing the way, the health care professions' and society's approach to care for the dying has been confused, inconsistent, and frequently ill-considered."

Part 2 of the book explores the future of family responsibility. In their chapter, Putney, Bengtson, and Wakeman present a comprehensive overview of the challenges, stresses, and prospects for American families in the near future using both macrosocial and microsocial perspectives. They identify three issues that will continue to stress families in the next decade: marital instability; the challenges of balancing work and family life; and the increasing need to care for elderly family members. They consider the many ways that families have been responding to these challenges, concluding that families are incredibly adaptable and resilient. Their chapter ends with positive predictions about families and their roles in the next decade, as they highlight the increasing diversity that family forms, structures, and functions will take.

Martha Holstein's chapter makes the point that the need for long-term care touches on the lives of older people who need help with tasks of daily living and on the lives of those who provide this help. The caregivers are most often family members, in particular women, and poorly paid home care aides, also predominantly women. Contending that these individuals are bound together by ties of vulnerability, she cautions that the labor of caregivers is often exploited, thereby rendering it a problem of justice. She argues for greater collective responsibility for caregiving. Her chapter builds on feminist political and legal theorists as she addresses the philosophical and political issues underlying dependency.

H. Rick Moody's chapter begins with a tongue-in-cheek case report that reminds us that ethical dilemmas and struggles between family members are timeless. He identifies broad social-structural trends that are important for thinking about responsibility across the generations in families, and he provides an analytic framework for considering the meaning of conflict, ambivalence, and competition among generations.

Part 3 focuses on policies and politics of generational responsibility. Kyriakos Markides and Steve Wallace, in chapter 8, review literature regarding the changing demographics of African Americans and Hispanics, with a focus on how these trends will affect the health of these populations. They examine differential family and community supports and examine the ways in which autonomy, family responsibility, and distributive justice are experienced in minority communities.

Ronald Manheimer begins his chapter with a personal story that questions who should be responsible for paying for the education of a single retiree. Manheimer asks whether lifelong learning opportunities, a limited resource on which our society spends a great deal of money, should be fairly distributed across the life course. His poignant story personalizes the issue of distributive justice and demonstrates the potential to create win-win solutions.

Andrew Achenbaum and Tom Cole examine the role that age plays in social policy and social programs. Using a framework of "three boxes of life," they discuss the fluidity with which people experience getting an education, going to work and earning a living, and living in retirement. They argue that the three boxes of life are not isolated, indeed that in history they have never been compartmentalized by age. They suggest that lifelong learning should be more available, that there should be greater investment in vocational rehabilitation for disabled persons of all ages, and that Social Security policy should be changed so that individuals can borrow against their retirement accounts to pay for workforce "repotting" and other forms of lifelong learning. They also suggest that people should receive Social Security credits for caring for children and other disabled family members.

Robert Hudson contends that two developments, one economic and one political, have transformed aging policy in American society over the past half century. Citing the dramatic aggregate improvement in well-being experienced by older people over the past 30 years and the rise of conservative thought as tectonic developments, Hudson examines the implications that these trends have had for older people, the relations among the generations, and social welfare.

Robert Binstock argues that the primary goal is to achieve continuity in American society's public policy responsibilities for older Americans, suggesting that the top priorities are to sustain and improve existing old-age benefit programs without radical reforms that abandon present and future cohorts of older Americans. He ponders whether responsibility across generations is politically feasible and addresses the ways in which "intergenerational equity" developed into "intergenerational inequity." He examines the changing political contexts of old-age policies, identifies political obstacles to contemporary action, and asks what might enhance action on policies for the aging of the baby boom generation.

Part 4 takes up issues of responsibility for health and wealth. In his chapter, John Williamson reviews the history of the debate over the Social Security crisis, situates this debate within the more general contest between the right and the left over how to frame discourse about Social Security reform, and presents policy alternatives linked to two of the most important packages used in the debate over Social Security reform. Prominent in Williamson's response are the roles played by "generational equity" and "generational interdependence."

Eric Kingson raises questions about the extent to which the political environment is conducive to the type of reform that many have called for. He points to historical reasons why other reforms moved quickly through Congress with bipartisan support, offering them as providing important insight with regard to moving Social Security reform forward.

Although Social Security is one of the most successful U.S. government programs, Peter Diamond and Peter Orszag remind us that the program now faces two serious problems, including a long-term deficit and questions regarding increasing benefits for particularly needy groups of people. They argue that restoring long-term balance to Social Security is necessary, but it is not necessary to destroy the program in order to save it. They review the financial position of Social Security, present a plan for saving it, and explain why Social Security revenue should not be diverted into individual accounts. Their plan for overhauling Social Security includes a provision for protecting some of its most vulnerable beneficiaries, including low earners, widows and widowers, and disabled workers and survivors. An important feature of this collection of articles in part 4 is their demonstration that the long-term Social Security funding gap can be closed in such a way that the burden is evenly divided between those in the labor force and those who are retired.

Prescription drug coverage under Medicare has long produced angst for economists, policymakers, physicians and other health care providers, the pharmaceutical industry, and society. Thus, it represents a prototypical issue addressing the concerns of public policy and responsibility across the generations. In his chapter, Bruce Stuart examines the economic returns to be expected from the new Medicare drug benefit. Stuart presents the complex effects likely to be experienced by a host of stakeholders. He examines issues including whether the benefit will affect drug use and whether the pharmaceuticals will be able to pay for themselves.

In the final chapter, Christine Bishop considers the ways in which programs to expand the Medicare Prescription Drug Plan have the potential to affect the distribution of well-being in society. She suggests that the goals of such programs should include protection of retirement income, efficient use of inputs in production of health, and improvements in health status. She concludes her chapter with ideas for a research agenda.

Aging in contemporary society requires ethical clarity from individuals, families, and society at large. This volume reflects contemporary thought and practice at the intersection of ethics and aging. Together, these contributions confirm that autonomy, responsibility, and distributive justice are themes that resonate in personal and public life. The collection offers hope in negotiating among individual and collective rights, duties, and responsibilities.

REFERENCES

Arno, P. S., Levine, C., and Memmott, M. M. 1999. The economic value of informal caregiving. *Health Affairs* 18:182–88.
Benjamin, A. E. 2001. Consumer-directed services at home: A new model for persons with disabilities. *Health Affairs* 20(6):80–95.
Byock, I. 1997. *Dying Well.* New York: Riverhead Books.
Callahan, D. 1987. *Setting Limits: Medical Goals in an Aging Society.* New York: Simon & Schuster.
Callahan, D. 1994. Setting limits: A response. *Gerontologist* 34:393–98.
Cicirelli, V. G. 2002. *Older Adults' Views on Death.* New York: Springer Publishing Co.
Comptroller General of the U.S. 1977. Report to Congress: The well-being of older people in Cleveland, Ohio. No. RD-77-70. Washington, DC: U.S. General Accounting Office.
Dale, S., Brown, R., Phillips, B., Schore, J., and Carlson, S. L. 2003. The effects of cash and counseling on personal care services and Medicaid costs in Arkansas. *Health Affairs* (Web exclusive), w3-56-w3-575, http://content.healthaffairs.org/cgi/reprint/hlthaff.w3.566v1.pdf, accessed October 24, 2006.
Doty, P. 1986. Family care of the elderly: The role of public policy. *Milbank Quarterly* 64(1): 34–75.
Doukas, D. J., and Hardwig, J. 2003. Using the family covenant in planning end-of-life care: Obligations and promises of patients, families, and physicians. *American Geriatrics Society* 51:1155–58.
Druley, J. A., Ditto, P. H., Moore, K. A., Danks, J. H., Townsend, A., and Smucker, W. D.

1993. Physicians' predictions of elderly outpatients' preferences for life-sustaining treatment. *Journal of Family Practice* 37:469–75.

Elpern, E. H., Yellen, S., and Burton, L. 1993. A preliminary investigation of opinions and behaviors regarding advance directives for medical care. *American Journal of Critical Care* 2:161–67.

Fisher, M. 2004. Ethical issues in the intensive care unit. *Current Opinions in Critical Care* 10:292–98.

Fisher, M., and Raper, R. F. 2000. Delay in stopping treatment can become unreasonable and unfair. *British Medical Journal* 320:1268–69.

Fried, T. R., Bradley, E. H., and Towle, V. R. 2003. Valuing the outcomes of treatment: Do patients and their caregivers agree? *Archives of Internal Medicine* 163:2073–78.

Fries, J. 1980. Aging, natural death, and the compression of morbidity. *New England Journal of Medicine* 303:130–35.

Fries, J. 1989. The compression of morbidity: Near or far? *Milbank Quarterly* 67:208–32.

Gerety, M. B., Chiodo, L. K., Kanten, D. N., Tuley, M. R., and Cornell, J. E. 1993. Medical treatment preferences of nursing home residents: Relationships to function and concordance with surrogate decision-makers. *Journal of the American Geriatrics Society* 41:953–60.

Hare, J., Pratt, C., and Nelson, C. 1992. Agreement between patients and their self-selected surrogates on difficult medical decisions. *Archives of Internal Medicine* 152:1049–54.

Hayley, D., Cassel, C., Snyder, L., and Rudberg, M. 1996. Ethical and legal issues in nursing home care. *Archives of Internal Medicine* 15:1–9.

Hayward, M. D., and Heron, M. 1999. Racial inequality in active life among adult Americans. *Demography* 36(1):77–91.

Hebert, L. E., Scherr, P. A., Bienias, J. L., Bennett, D. A., and Evans, D. A. 2003. Alzheimer disease in the U.S. population: Prevalence estimates using the 2000 census. *Archives of Neurology* 60(8):1119–22.

High, D. M. 1988. All in the family: Extended autonomy and expectations in surrogate health care decision-making. *Gerontologist* 28:46–51.

High, D. M. 1994. Families' roles in advance directives. *Hastings Center Report* 24:S16–18.

High, D. M., and Rowles, G. D. 1995. Nursing home residents, families, and decision making: Toward an understanding of progressive surrogacy. *Journal of Aging Studies* 9:101–17.

Hines, S. C., Glover, J. J., Holley, J. L., Babrow, A. S., Badzek, L. A., and Moss, A. H. 1999. Dialysis patients' preferences for family-based advance care planning. *Annals of Internal Medicine* 130:825–28.

Hoefler, J. M. 1997. *Managing Death.* Boulder, CO: Westview Publishers.

Keating, R. F., Moss, A. H., Sorkin, M. I., and Paris, J. J. 1994. Stopping dialysis of an incompetent patient over the family's objection: Is it ever ethical and legal? *Journal of the American Society of Nephrology* 4:1879–83.

Kotlikoff, L. J., and Burns, S. 2004. The perfect demographic storm: Entitlements imperil America's future. *Chronicle of Higher Education,* March 19.

Mahoney, K., Simon-Rusinowitz, L., Loughlin, D., Desmond, S., and Squillace, M. 2004. Determining personal care consumers' preferences for a consumer-directed cash and counseling option: Survey results from Arkansas, Florida, New Jersey, and New York elders and adults with physical disabilities. *Health Services Research* 39(3):643–63.

National Alliance for Caregiving and the American Association of Retired Persons. 1997. *Family Caregiving in the U.S.: Findings from a National Survey.* Bethesda, MD: National Alliance for Caregiving.

Post, S. G., Puchalski, C. M., and Larson, D. B. 2000. Physicians and patient spirituality: Professional boundaries, competency, and ethics. *Annals of Internal Medicine* 132(7):578–83.

President's Commission for the Study of Ethical Problems in Medicine and Biomedical and Behavioral Research. 1983. *Deciding to Forego Life-Sustaining Treatment: A Report on the Ethical, Medical, and Legal Issues in Treatment Decisions.* Gov. Doc. No. Pr 40.8: Et 3/L 62/2. Washington, DC: U.S. Government Printing Office.

Singer, P. A., Thiel, E. C., Naylor, C. D., Richardson, R. M. A., Llewellyn-Thomas, H., and Goldstein, M. 1995. Life-sustaining treatment preferences of hemodialysis patients: Implications for advance directives. *Journal of the American Society of Nephrology* 6:1410–17.

Sloan, R. P., Bagiella, E., VandeCreek, L., Hover, M., Casalone, C., Hirsch, T. J., Hasan, Y., and Kreger, R. 2000. *New England Journal of Medicine* 342(25):1913–16.

Stone, R., Cafferata, G. L., and Sangl, J. 1987. Caregivers of the frail elderly: A national profile. *Gerontologist* 27:616–26.

Suhl, J., Simons, P., Reedy, T., and Garrick, T. 1994. Myth of substituted judgment: Surrogate decision making regarding life support is unreliable. *Archives of Internal Medicine* 154:90–94.

Sulmasy, D. P., Terry, P. B., Weisman, C. S., Miller, D. J., Stalling, R. Y., Vettese, M. A., and Haller, K. B. 1998. The accuracy of substituted judgments in patients with terminal diagnoses. *Annals of Internal Medicine* 128:621–29.

Terry, P. B., Vettese, M., Song, J., Forman, J., Haller, K. B., and Miller, D. J. 1999. End-of-life decision making: When patients and surrogates disagree. *Journal of Clinical Ethics* 10:286–93.

Uhlmann, R. F., Pearlman, R. A., and Cain, K. C. 1988. Physicians' and spouses' predictions of elderly patients' resuscitation preferences. *Journal of Gerontology: Medical Sciences* 43:115–21.

U.S. Department of Health, Education, and Welfare. 1972. Home care for persons aged 55 and over in the U.S. July 1966–June 1968. *Vital and Health Statistics,* series 10: 73.

Ventura, S. J., Peters, K. D., Martin, J. A., and Maurer, J. D. 1997. Births and deaths: United States, 1996. *Monthly Vital Statistics Report, vol. 46, no. 1, suppl. 2.* Atlanta, GA: National Center for Health Statistics, CDC, USDHH, 1997.

Wagner, D. L. 1997. *Comparative Analysis of Caregiver Data for Caregivers to the Elderly, 1987 and 1997.* Bethesda, MD: National Alliance for Caregiving.

Part I / Autonomy and End-of-Life Decisions

CHAPTER ONE

The Legal Aspects of End-of-Life Decision Making

Nancy Neveloff Dubler, LL.B.

Framing the Issue

A colleague of mine has coined a phrase that I find particularly descriptive in these times: The patient, he says, is afflicted with "failure to die" (Joseph Fins, M.D., personal communication). This formulation identifies a problem that has emerged over the last two decades. It arises from two sources. First, medical technology has developed interventions that can sustain organ function long after an integrated and reactive personality has disintegrated. Second, these technologies tend to be used rather than withheld at the end of life. These developments reflect both the desire to extend life and the impact of defensive medicine. Furthermore, they demonstrate the inability of medicine to comprehend the limits of technology for the care of dying patients.

Part, but only part, of the etiology of the problem is the law—writ large— as federal and state statutes and judicial opinions. This chapter will present some of the legal reasoning that has either guided or hindered medicine in its pursuit of patient well-being. It will highlight what patients increasingly want at the end of life and how the law responds, or acts as a barrier, to these wishes. It will suggest that the impulse of the law—which is, to the greatest degree possible, to rely on the wishes, preferences, and sentiments of the patient as the "gold standard" of decision making—has, paradoxically, worked to undermine patient choice at the end of life.

There is a "pitch" to this discussion; it is that as physicians, patients, and families are making their voices heard, end-of-life care will change. From the outset of the discussion, lawyers, judges, legislators, and, to some degree, physicians have talked both to and over each other. The agenda has been dominated by matters of defensive medicine and conservative legislative and judicial practice. But this must change as conversations among all the players increase in frequency and velocity and as palliative and hospice care continue to make their marks.

How did we arrive at this moment? An answer to the question must invoke a brief historical narrative, which begins with the exponential growth of medical technology at the end of World War II. The war itself is the beginning, as it spurred the founding of the National Institutes of Health and supported the development of that first effective battlefield technology, resuscitation of injured soldiers, which then crept into the nonmilitary arsenal of medical interventions. The 1960s produced the development of dialysis, the creation of ventilators (which were vastly more effective than the iron lungs that had sustained patients with breathing problems during the polio epidemics), and the discovery of therapeutics that made the machines viable in fragile human bodies. This was the good news. The growing problem, as the 1986 PBS television series produced by Fred Friendly Seminars Inc. stated, was not producing new technologies but rather *Managing Our Miracles*.[1] New technologies made nuanced moral choices necessary. Whereas before the middle of the twentieth century, medicine could diagnose and comfort, it could now cure; more importantly to some, it could extend life. Whether that extended life was merely a simulacrum was the basic ethical question raised. At least it could focus on and restore organ function. The questions then immediately arose: who should authorize or refuse these interventions, on what legal basis, with what oversight and review?

In this process, to present a ludicrous example of linked legal and medical reasoning, resuscitation developed into the standard intervention for all patients in the hospital, including the 97-year-old woman with widely disseminated breast cancer. Why, the rational person would ask? Because, the puzzled spectator would reply, the shared opinion among liability experts was that not to resuscitate was murder.

As a result, when I first stumbled into medicine out of the juvenile justice system in 1976, I found a "Alice-down-the-rabbit-hole" universe in which purple dots and pink stars pasted on charts, or names written on a blackboard, indicated patients for whom resuscitation was not appropriate. No discussions were held either with patients or with families. My favorite example of this ludicrous system was the "blackboard war" in which a patient was DNR (Do Not Resuscitate) from 8:00 a.m. to 4:00 p.m. and from 4:00 p.m. to midnight but not from midnight to 8:00 a.m.—ridiculous, unethical, medically unsupportable, and just plain silly. It was the product of risk-averse hospital administrators talking to risk-averse outside counsel with no regard for the wishes and interests of patients and family. By now, the open conversations among all players preclude these inadequate secret decisions by staff.

New technologies, it was soon agreed, needed solid scientific bases, guidelines for medical and nursing supervision, and, most importantly, moral agreement on when it was justified to use these interventions and when it was permissible to forgo their use. This moral consensus has been slow in materializing; the law has reflected this fact in the increasingly specific decisions that were crafted by courts to protect the rights, as the court perceived them, of patients and families.

The pendulum, some would argue, has begun to swing not back to those days when pneumonia was the "old man's friend," but to an ethically new time when the abilities of medicine to ward off death are balanced against the wishes of patient and family, the ability to control pain, and a realistic assessment of the possible success of the medical intervention. Medicine can provide almost limitless extensions of organ function, but this ability is being challenged by the growing number of patients struggling to escape high-tech dying. One reason we know about this changing picture of medicine is that the conversation is changing. Whereas medicine and law have engaged in a lively debate over the years from the 1970s until now, the discussion is gradually being joined by the public.[2]

Some forces have been particularly helpful in opening the debate to the public. The Robert Wood Johnson Foundation and the Soros Foundation through its Project on Death and Dying have both fostered a growing debate on the process of dying, supported the growth of palliative-care medicine, and encouraged public discussion.[3] The debate on physician-assisted suicide in the courts and the legislation in Oregon permitting this physician action under particular circumstances have encouraged patients and families to consider the range of alternatives. The growth of hospice care has also helped underscore the notion that patients can be cared for and not abandoned as they die. The choice is not whether to permit death or oppose it—as if it were ever possible to defeat death. The question is how to accommodate changing patterns of medical care and how to support the growing awareness of the limitations of medical interventions in an era when the independence of medicine, in managed care arrangements, is under growing scrutiny. Law, in all of its facets, legal analyses, opinions, and statutes, has been enmeshed in this attempt to tame and control medical interventions if they would merely prolong the process of dying.[4]

This openness to new approaches is a multifaceted creation of the newly expanded dialogue among patients, families, medical providers, organizations, and the courts. Some of the themes have been articulated by new players such as the foundations that have come into the debate. The *Robert Wood Johnson Quarterly Newsletter* stated: "People want to die at home, but most don't. They want to die free from pain, but too many don't. At the same time, most people don't want to talk about their wishes—or about dying at all—and they either don't know about options for end-of-life care or they don't ask for them."[5]

The facts about our dying are gradually emerging: 2.5 million Americans die each year, of whom 80 percent are Medicare beneficiaries. Approximately $262 billion is spent each year on Medicare, of which 27 percent is spent in the last year of life.[6] That is the usual statistic. What it does not reveal is the quality of the care that patients received at the end of life. Some decisions are guided by wisdom and clarity. Some are not.

It is difficult to move behind the statistics to the lives of the patients that the statistics reflect. Surveys show the following:

- 25 percent of deaths occur at home although, when asked, 70 percent of patients state that they prefer this option;
- Experts agree that 95 percent of pain can be treated, but one-half of dying people experience pain at the end of life;
- Less than 60 percent of hospitals offer hospice or palliative care services.[7]

These statistics reveal the slowly growing pace of the services that are needed to manage the process of dying in ways that are supportive for the patient and the family. In addition, these statistics demonstrate the total failure of advance directives, our primary public policy intervention into matters of patient death. They have clearly failed; a pitifully small percentage of patients have advance directives, and that percentage likely correlates with patients who are clients of trust and estate lawyers or board-certified geriatricians. When I structured a research project and reviewed patients over the age of 65 coming into a hospital, only 1.5 percent had advance directives.[8] All scholarship indicates that this is failed policy; let us move on to robust notions of family decision making with procedural protections as the next best alternative to the gold standard of patient choice.

In addition to how little they are used by patients, there are other confounding aspects of advance directives as "death-managing" interventions. Advance directives vary state by state, and people, those few who do want to think about issues of dying and future care, are often unsure how to go about protecting themselves from unwanted care in different locations. There is also a shift in focus for some advance directives. It is a given that patients can consent to or refuse care but cannot demand care. In the past, advance directives were generally used to prospectively limit care despite the fact that they are value-neutral. Today, some advance directives are formulated to request care rather than prospectively refusing care. This seems a reasonable, even prudent, response to a health care system whose incentives have been totally reordered in the last years. As hospitals now increase income by limiting rather than extending length of stay, patients and families could reasonably become convinced that the danger to individual interests is the curtailment rather than the extension of care in the dying process.

Legal and Policy Barriers to Providing Adequate End-of-Life Care

In an ideal system of care, which this society's system does not approach, there would be universal access to care and a care system that engaged in wide public health programs to increase health status, addressed acute medical problems as they arose, treated pain as a medical and ethical emergency, and provided choices at the end of life that permitted patients and families to opt for supported services in a comfortable location. Whereas this describes some of the care that patients with unfettered access to care might receive, data presented previously indicate that, even for these patients, access to appropriate services may be limited by structural barriers. Patients cannot access what hospitals have not created. Palliative care is not a real option in many hospitals that have not created palliative care programs and acquired sufficient numbers of trained staff members. Hospice is not an option where it does not exist. The hegemony of acute care medicine is challenged only slowly by those who see support and comfort as appropriate goals of medicine and nursing.

There are structural deficiencies in health care coverage that explain additional gaps in actual care that is offered to patients. Hospitals are struggling with Medicare and Medicaid payments that fail to cover the computed costs of care. (Economists can argue whether these costs are actual losses or the artifacts of inefficient management.) Drug costs have increased 1,500 percent over the last 20 years, and it remains to be seen, as experience with the Medicare drug benefit accumulates, how much of the drug bill of the dying will be covered. Medicare continues to limit its hospice benefit to six months, and physicians and institutions fear that a more extended dying will subject them to penalties and charges of fraud. Financing for long-term care has never been debated successfully by the nation and its legislators, and the vast majority of seniors have no long-term-care insurance; most depend on Medicaid to cover the costs of care. In the absence of either long-term-care insurance or Medicaid, the costs of long-term care make it an unaffordable option for many.[9]

The courts entered the arena of death and dying rather slowly. The first bright line and well-publicized decision of a court was that in the New Jersey case of Karen Ann Quinlan.[10] Karen, a previously healthy 21-year-old, was brought into the hospital in respiratory distress and placed on a ventilator. When it was determined that Karen was in a persistent vegetative state, her parents, devout Catholics, with the advice and support of the church, asked that her ventilator be removed. The hospital, in the increasingly risk-averse universe of medicine and with genuine puzzlement over what to do legally and morally in the case, went to court to ask for guidance. The court in *Quinlan* broke new legal ground. It stated that the hospital should have an ethics (prognosis) committee to declare the situation hopeless. If the committee made this finding, then, stated the court, a guardian for Karen could exercise her "right to privacy" and, if it found that she would have "wanted" the ventilator turned off, could do so.

The importance of this case is that it courageously broke new ground and held that treatment could be withdrawn and care stopped based on the intellectual calculus of a surrogate. The problem with the case is that it began the dependence of the law on the fiction of individual choice—what would Karen want if she could tell us—which has addicted courts in this arena, committed them to the search for prior articulated preference, and prevented the development of clear medical, moral, and social rules for considering what the valid components of decisions at the end of life are and who should exercise this choice. But note in this case and in others that followed, whereas the court seemed to rely on the patient's preference—whether explicitly stated or recovered through the additional fiction of substituted judgment—it went on to provide a formula that could accompany or actually supplant the indicia of individual choosing.

In the category of fiction, consider the following paragraph from the Quinlan court: "We have no doubt, in these unhappy circumstances, that if Karen were herself miraculously lucid for an interval (not altering the existing prognosis or the condition to which she would soon return), and perceptive of her irreversible condition, she could effectively decide upon the discontinuance of the life-support apparatus, even if it meant the prospect of natural death."[11]

Following that rather exalted exercise in narrative fiction, consider the simple formula that the court proposes for deciding when care can properly be withdrawn: "We think that the state's interest contra weakens and the individual's right to privacy grows as the degree of bodily invasion increases and the prognosis dims. Ultimately there comes a point at which the individual's rights overcome the state interests."[12]

Quinlan and other subsequent cases established the rule that courts should, in the first instance, search out the wishes of the patient for guidance. Some courts were satisfied to seek patterns of behavior and extrapolate from them, whereas others insisted on the "prior explicit statement of the patient." When this last standard was linked with a required high degree of evidence, it led to the morally suspect result that patients were maintained in slow patterns of extended dying. The fact remains, and the endless experience with the failure of advance directives demonstrates, that most patients do not prepare for death by telling others what they want. Most patients slip slowly into the process of dying depending on family and medical providers to act for them and in their best interest.[13]

Gradually physicians have begun to grapple with the problem and professional societies have started to articulate when care is appropriate and when not. Some state legislatures have crafted rules governing care at the end of life. All of this activity is well-meaning and is designed to protect patients at the end of life when they cannot make their own decisions—when they are incompetent beings who need the protection of the courts and government to ensure that their rights and interests are identified and pursued. But the net result is still the imposition, in many settings, of lengthened stretches of dying during which the quality of the patient's life is compromised by untreated pain in unfamiliar settings. As the next sections show, however, new perspectives and procedures are emerging that may assist in redressing the unbalanced tip to treatment.

As noted above, since the *Quinlan* decision, state courts have struggled to develop guidance for physicians, patients, and families regarding decisions to treat or withhold acute care treatment at the end of life. *Quinlan* set the formula and tried to develop a rule that would provide direction and leadership to the medical profession and to medical institutions without usurping the professional mantle of power. Many of the courts, in early decisions, followed the *Quinlan* path and tried to fashion roles that depended on the "fiction" of patient decision. The struggle to make it seem as if the patient had made the decision was necessary because of the feeling of many courts that for them, or even for medical providers or the family, to make this decision was somehow inappropriate. It had been settled case law for many years that patients who are capable of making decisions have the right to consent to or refuse care even if the result of the decision is death. As that principle was well accepted, many courts, uncomfortable with the decisions of others to permit death, attempted to shoehorn all circumstances into this accepted mold.

Thus, in the *Saikewicz* case, the court attempted to elicit from the history some notion of the wishes of the patient—although in the case of Mr. Saikewicz, a profoundly retarded man, that was clearly beyond the demands of the usual fiction.[14] That court, like the *Quinlan* court, provided a formula for the somewhat objective and abstract decisions that were faced.

> The "best interests" of an incompetent person are not necessarily served by imposing on such persons results not mandated as to competent persons similarly situated. It does not advance the interest of the state or the ward to treat the ward as a person of lesser status or dignity than others. To protect the incompetent person within its power, the State must recognize the dignity and worth of such a person and afford to that person the same panoply of rights and choices it recognizes in competent persons. If a competent person faced with death may choose to decline treatment which not only will not cure the person but which substantially may increase suffering in exchange for a possible yet brief prolongation of life, then it cannot be said that it is always in the "best interests" of the ward to require submission to such treatment. Nor do statistical factors indicat-

ing that a majority of competent persons similarly situated choose treatment resolve the issue. The significant decisions of life are more complex than statistical
determinations. Individual choice is determined not by the vote of the majority
but by the complexities of the singular situation viewed from the unique perspective of the person called on to make the decision. To presume that the incompetent person must always be subjected to what many rational and intelli-
gent persons may decline is to downgrade the status of the incompetent person
by placing a lesser value of his intrinsic human worth and vitality.[15]

In this way, both of these key early cases provided two streams of decision making: the first ostensibly from the voice of the patient and the second according
to some formula that attempts to weigh the potential benefits of care against
the likely burdens.

The apotheosis of this mixed-logic reasoning—fictionalized patient preference in the light of objective formulas—was articulated again by the New Jersey Supreme Court in the matter of Clair Conroy. In this case, the court provided guidance for patients with and without patient directives, taking into
account patient suffering and the burdens of continued care. It also provided
for a process (by reference to a state agency) to oversee the decisions for these
most vulnerable and needy of patients.[16]

A few courts, New York and Missouri most prominent among them, es-
chewed this path and situated themselves only in the realm of clearly documented patient decision according to explicitly articulated wishes. This sort of
law, which required that the previously competent patient leave an explicit directive by clear and convincing evidence, has been an increasing barrier to delivering appropriate care at the end of life. As noted above, many people do not
want to think about these issues and fail to establish the sorts of statement in
formal advance directives or in less formal but yet focused discussions with
medical providers, physicians, or friends. As the choices for end-of-life care
have multiplied, the fact that explicit choices need to be made before incapacity has intervened has left many family members and physicians scrambling to
make decisions in a potentially hostile legal climate. In the absence of objective
formulas and without even permitting an expanded notion of substituted
judgment—that is, extrapolating from the actions of the patient what his or
her wishes might be—New York and Missouri provide no real guidance for
providers and family at the end of life.

As one based in New York, I can attest to the results. Many decisions are simply negotiated between providers and family in the space "under the radar." There are a few reasons why this is not a desirable solution. Secrecy is the worst possible nonprocess, as it shields these decisions from scrutiny and oversight. Death is the ultimate absolute; there is no redoing the care plan. As dying patients are, by definition, a vulnerable class, and as such persons are always at risk for abuse, from both undertreatment and overtreatment, such decisions should be more, rather than less, visible. The second result of this policy is the reality that far more aggressive care is delivered than the physicians think is appropriate or than the family wants. Finally, because most providers and institutions would like to avoid overly aggressive and "futile" care, they tend to send hints to families about the sorts of statement the patient would have to have made for care to be limited or withdrawn. The result is that savvy families will likely get the hint, while less sophisticated families will not. This exercise in what I have called "benign collusion" is unfair to all of the parties involved and is a guilt-inducing exercise for family and care providers.

The U.S. Supreme Court has waded into these waters only twice, first in 1990 in the *Cruzan* case and then in 1997 with *Washington v. Glucksberg*.[17] The first case established that it was not unconstitutional under the U.S. Constitution for states to have these very rigorous rules that required the prior explicit statement of a previously competent patient as a basis for withdrawing or withholding care from an incompetent patient. The court stated that "the principle that a *competent* person has a constitutionally protected liberty interest in refusing unwanted medical treatment may be inferred from our prior decisions. . . . We believe that Missouri may legitimately seek to safeguard the personal element of this choice through the imposition of heightened evidentiary requirements. It cannot be disputed that the Due Process Clause protects an interest in life as well as an interest in refusing life-sustaining medical treatment."[18]

The second Supreme Court foray, in *Glucksberg*, established that there was no constitutional right, based either on a theory of equal protection or on a theory of a fundamental right to privacy, to physician-assisted suicide (PAS).[19] That was of course before the 2003 case of *Lawrence v. Texas* (a case establishing the right of same-sex couples to intimate relationships) reinvigorated the fundamental rights of individual choice based on notions of liberty and privacy; although candor requires the concession that the same decision would still be likely.[20] *Glucksberg* held, however, that where there was not a constitutionally protected federal right, the states were free to experiment with solutions to the problem of terminally ill patients who want help in ending their lives.[21]

The court stated, in failing to find a constitutionally protected right to PAS, that "at the heart of liberty is the right to define one's own concept of existence, of meaning of the universe, and of the mystery of human life. Beliefs about these matters could not define the attributes of personhood were they formed under the compulsion of the state."[22] The court went on to emphasize that its holding permitted the debate to continue as appropriate in a democratic society, clearly not anticipating *Oregon v. Ashcroft* (see below).[23] It went out of its way to emphasize that there are no legal barriers to providing adequate pain relief even if it hastens death.

But most remarkable about the Glucksberg case was the debate that it engendered in the world of medicine and biomedical ethics. Whereas in the Quinlan case and later state cases there were a few briefs filed by a limited number of interested parties, the PAS case was the catalyst for expanded discussion. This heartening new element in the discussion of end-of-life care is the creation of a wide circle of discussants whose voices all enrich the debate.

Balancing the benefits of this expanded discussion are the burdens of new legal obstacles. Whereas there is a new openness to voices of patients, providers, and organizations, there is a new willingness to impose one position on all of the disputants.[24] As an example, consider the impediment to decent end-of-life care as presented by the recent attempt by the U.S. attorney general to prevent physicians in Oregon from using appropriate analgesia when engaging in the legal activity of physician-assisted suicide. In the case of *Oregon v. Ashcroft*, the U.S. attorney general has intervened to overturn the Oregon PAS law by forbidding physicians to provide pain relief using any substance that could be considered a narcotic under the Controlled Substances Act.[25]

The Future of the Legal Debate

This chapter is being written at a particularly interesting legal juncture. The U.S. Supreme Court recently decided the case of *Lawrence v. Texas*, which declared that gay persons are "entitled to respect for their private lives."[26] This case, which has single-handedly rescued the notions of the right to privacy and substantive due process from the dust heap, might provide the basis for a renewed willingness in the Court to consider individually desired plans of care at the end of life.

But whether or not that is the case, the issues have gained a public persona over the last decade that will not fade away. People are engaged, foundations are committed, and physicians have regained a hold on the discussion and on patterns of practice. That last is, perhaps, the most important. Consider two case examples to support this last point.

The first example involves a law case. In August 2001 the California Supreme Court decided the case of the Conservatorship of the Person of Robert Wendland. In that case the court considered the proper interpretation of the California conservatorship law. But more importantly, it articulated its understandings of the rules that should govern end-of-life care.[27]

The case involved the person of one Robert Wendland, who when he was 42 and drunk, rolled his truck over when driving at a high speed and crashed into a coma. His wife, after authorizing the placement of three feeding tubes, refused permission for the fourth replacement. By that point, two years after the accident, she had become convinced that he would not improve and that his prior wishes would direct them to let him die. She, her children, and her brother stated that he had said, in reference to a case very similar to his: "Don't let them do that to me."[28] The case went to court as an attempt to define the powers of a conservator—a person appointed by the court to decide for an incompetent person. The patient's mother and sister opposed powers for the conservator that would let her refuse treatment for the patient.

In its holding, the court stated, "only when the patient's prior statements clearly illustrate a serious, well thought out, consistent decision to refuse treatment under these exact circumstances, or circumstances highly similar to the current situation, should treatment be refused or withdrawn."[29]

Here we have articulated, in 2001, the "clear and convincing standard" that has acted as a barrier to decent and humane end-of-life care in New York since 1981. But this time the physicians were not silent. In a well-reasoned article in the *New England Journal of Medicine,* Dr. Bernard Lo argued that the case was very troubling and should not be well received in the world of medicine. Indeed, Dr. Lo argued that "physicians should promote legal reforms that both safeguard incompetent patients and avoid imposing undue burdens on close family members who could appropriately make decisions about life-sustaining interventions. . . . The scope of oral advance directives to physicians should be broadened. . . . Spouses should be given more explicit authority to make decisions on behalf of incompetent patients."[30]

In 1981, when the New York court articulated the same sort of rule, the medical profession was silent. It did not occur to the medical community that its role was to fight against legally imposed rules that affected the practice of medical care in ways that would be harmful to patients. Now the importance of that sort of action is clear. It is clear from more than two decades of writing of legal scholars, medical experts, moral philosophers, political commentators, and religious advisers that these are individual issues of great religious, personal, and political significance. But it is also clear that physicians who care for patients have an obligation not to be cowed by the law when it is wrong, according to the ethics of medicine. Here the issue has been joined. Physicians know that, except for a few patients who choose to execute advance directives, most people do not approach the issue of future possible morbidity with such clarity and direction. There are times when the default position of providing care makes no medical or moral sense. We cannot and should not limit aggressive interventions depending only on a patient's choosing that precise and particular death.

The second example of a development that could be very important is the new statute in Texas that addresses the issues of futility in end-of-life decisions. In the new law there is crafted a legislatively sanctioned, extrajudicial, due process mechanism for resolving medical futility disputes and other end-of-life disagreements. This is an extremely important development because it puts legal-statutory authority behind a well-reasoned and fair process for resolving end-of-life care disagreements and disputes. The law provides that if there is disagreement between the family and the care providers on the issue of whether care is "futile" and can be stopped, a lengthy process is triggered with notice, the involvement of the ethics committee, possible transfer of the patient to another institution, and final appeal to a court. If the process reaches its end and the disagreement remains, however, then the hospital may stop treatment over the family's objection. This new, open, transparent, and engaged process will be of interest to scholars and providers as it gathers data on its effectiveness and acceptance.[31]

Conclusion

There are times when the moral and medically responsible decision is to stop treatment and provide palliative care measures to ensure comfort. Most legal and medical scholars agree that these times are characterized by circumstances when the burdens of providing care clearly outweigh the benefits; when the person has given some sense of the nature of her or his wishes, so that strong religious or philosophical positions can be factored into the discussion; when the person's statements would lend support to the decision; when the process of dying has been extended and no improvement has been realized or can be expected; when the family has engaged in anticipatory grieving and is ready for the moment of death; and when the medical debate about appropriate care has consulted a wide range of persons from a variety of disciplines and has included, when appropriate, clergy and the ethics committee. When all of these conditions and attributes of good and responsible care have been engaged in and there seems to be a legal doctrine that would preclude the medical decision, then that law needs to be interpreted narrowly and contested broadly.

These are not easy times in which to talk about emotionally and ideologically loaded issues. This is a society increasingly polarized by politics, religion, and lack of agreement on socially and morally appropriate behavior. Medicine stands in the midst of this maelstrom as it struggles to do the best for individual patients. Its voice in the discussion is a necessary component of the development of good legal statutes and opinions governing end-of-life care.

NOTES

1. *Managing Our Miracles: Health Care in America,* a ten-part series, Fred Friendly Seminars, Inc., broadcast on PBS, 1986.

2. Janny Scott, An Onassis Legacy: Facing Death on One's Own Terms, *New York Times,* June 4, 1994; Tamar Lewin, Ignoring "Right to Die" Directives, Medical Community Is Being Sued, *New York Times,* June 2, 1996.

3. See the Soros Foundation Web site, www.soros.org/initiatives/pdia.

4. Ann Alpers and Bernard Lo, Avoiding Family Feuds: Responding to Surrogate Demands for Life-Sustaining Interventions, 27 *Journal of Law, Medicine and Ethics* 74 (1999); American Medical Association Council on Ethics and Judicial Affairs, Advance Directive Instruments for End-of-Life and Health Care Decision Making: Optimal Use of Orders not to Intervene and Advance Directives, 4 *Psychology, Public Policy, and Law* 668 (1998); Kenneth W. Goodman, End-of-Life Algorithms, 4 *Psychology, Public Policy, and Law* 719 (1998).

5. Nancy Volkers, No Best Place to Die in the United States, 4 *Advances: The Robert Wood Johnson Quarterly Newsletter* 1 (2002). Available at www.rwjf.org/files/publications/newsletter/Advances4_2002.pdf.

6. Elizabeth Austin, Q&A with Judith R. Perez, L.C.S.W.; Creating a Good Death, 4 *Advances: The Robert Wood Johnson Quarterly Newsletter* 1, 4 (2002). Available at www.rwjf.org/files/publications/newsletter/Advances4_2002.pdf.

7. Nancy Volkers, No Best Place to Die in the United States, 4 *Advances: The Robert Wood Johnson Quarterly Newsletter* 1, 2 (2002). Available at www.rwjf.org/ files/publications/newsletter/Advances4_2002.pdf.

8. Jomarie Zeleznick, Linda Farber Post, Michael Mulvihill, Laurie G. Jacobs, William B. Burton, and Nancy Neveloff Dubler, The Doctor-Proxy Relationship: Perception and Communication, 27 *Journal of Law, Medicine and Ethics* 13, 17 (1999).

9. The costs of long-term care for elderly people range from $50,000 to 120,000 annually, depending on geographical location. See BestWire, *HIAA Survey: Growth in LTC Insurance Exceeds Tenfold since 1987,* February 4, 2003; see also Reality Check: Long Term Care Insurance Covers Costs, Preserves Assets, 86 *ABA Journal* 62 (2000). Currently, among the estimated 82 million Americans over the age of 45, the demographic for whom long-term care insurance is recommended, only 6.5 million carry it. Mergers and Acquisitions: Long Term Care Group Acquired for $130M, *Physician Business Week,* May 4, 2004.

10. *In re Quinlan,* 355 A.2d 647 (NJ 1976).

11. *In re Quinlan,* 70 NJ 10 at 39 (1976).

12. Id. at 41.

13. Bart J. Collopy, The Moral Underpinnings of the Proxy-Provider Relationship: Issues of Trust and Distrust, 27 *Journal of Law, Medicine and Ethics* 37 (1999).

14. *Superintendent of Belchertown State Sch. v. Saikewicz,* 370 N.E.2d 417 (Mass. 1977).

15. Id. at 428.

16. *In re Conroy,* 486 A.2d.1209 (N.J. 1985).

17. *Cruzan v. Missouri,* 497 U.S. 261 (1990), *Washington v. Glucksberg,* 521 U.S. 702 (1997).

18. *Cruzan v. Missouri,* 497 U.S. 261, 287, 281 (1990).

19. *Washington v. Glucksberg,* 521 U.S. 702 (1997).

20. *Lawrence v. Texas* 539 U.S. 558 (2003).

21. *Washington v. Glucksberg,* 521 U.S. 702 (1997).

22. Id. at 727, quoting *Planned Parenthood v. Casey,* 505 U.S. 833, 851 (1992).

23. *Oregon v. Ashcroft* 368 F.3d.1118 (9th Cir. 2004).

24. See Compassion in Dying at www.compassionindying.org/index.php and the Soros Foundation Project on Death in America at www.soros.org/initiatives.pdia.

25. *Oregon v. Ashcroft* 368 F.3d.1118 (9th Cir. 2004).

26. *Lawrence v. Texas* 539 U.S. 558, 578 (2003).

27. *In re Conservatorship of Wendland,* 28 P.3d 151 (Calif., 2001).

28. Id. at 157.

29. Id. at 549, quoting *In re Martin,* 539 N.W. 2d 399, 411 (1995).

30. Bernard Lo, Laurie Dorrnbrand, Leslie E. Wolf, and Michelle Groman. The Wendland Case: Withdrawing Life Support from Incompetent Patients Who Are Not Terminally Ill, 346 *New England Journal of Medicine* 1489, 1492 (2002).

31. Health and Safety Code, Title 2, Subtitle J. Public Health Provisions, Chapter 166 Advance Directives, Subchapter B, Directive to Physicians. Tex. Health and Safety Code Ann. §166.039 (2004).

CHAPTER TWO

Assessing Competency to Make Medical Decisions at the End of Life

Clinician and Patient Issues

Daniel C. Marson, J.D., Ph.D.

Competency and Autonomy in End-of-Life Decision Making

In the past century, medical technology and science have increased human longevity and prolonged survival from chronic diseases and trauma to a degree that would astonish our nineteenth-century counterparts. Large numbers of people are now for the first time living into the far reaches of human old age—into the ninth, tenth, and even the eleventh decades. This longevity often comes at a cost for patients and families, as it is frequently accompanied by chronic disease, cognitive decline, and dementia (Marson and Zebley, 2001). Cognitive changes and dementia threaten patients' quality of life, their capacity to live independently, and their competency to make medical, financial, and other decisions.

In response to the ongoing revolution in longevity, a complex body of medical-legal case law, ethical principles, and clinical care guidelines has emerged regarding care at the end of life. These rules and principles seek to provide legal regulation and moral and therapeutic guidance to patients, families, and clinicians as they negotiate end-of-life issues. Nancy Dubler discusses these and their various legal and political implications in Chapter 1. Key legal and clinical distinctions that define this area include *competent* versus *incompetent, conscious* versus *unconscious, terminally ill* versus *chronically ill, life sustaining medical treatment* (LSMT) versus *futile medical care, palliative care* versus *assisted suicide,* and *legally authorized representative* versus *no surrogate decision maker.*

Of these distinctions, competency versus incompetency (specifically, to make medical treatment decisions) is arguably the most fundamental. Competency is the conceptual fulcrum for understanding end-of-life case law (Marson, 2003), which, viewed broadly, has served (1) to support the decisions of competent individuals and (2) to protect the rights and interests of incompetent persons (see Chapter 1). A patient's decisional competency is thus the starting point for analyzing most end-of-life medical-legal issues. If competent, a patient can elect or refuse LSMT at the end of life. If competent, a patient can execute an advance directive indicating preferences regarding LSMT (a living will) or indicating the selection and scope of activities of a health care proxy (a durable power of attorney for health care). If competent, a terminally ill patient can decide whether to seek palliative care and whether additional pain medication is needed. If competent and terminally ill, a patient in the state of Oregon can seek assisted suicide under the Death with Dignity Act (Angell, 1997). Competency thus reflects an individual's autonomy to make a range of treatment and care choices at the end of life.

Incompetency, in contrast, represents loss of autonomy and results in more limited options in end-of-life decision making (Marson, 2003). If incompetent, a patient can no longer make medical decisions for himself or herself—a proxy or surrogate decision maker must step forward to make these decisions. The proxy cannot rely on current patient indications (if any) regarding LSMT but must seek other, less direct and usually prior, indications of patient wishes. Written advance directives are the best evidence of patient intentions other than current statements of a competent patient. However, written advance directives are still infrequently executed in many settings, including nursing homes; a recent study indicated that only 51 percent of nursing home residents nationally have an advance directive (Mezey et al., 2000). Written advance directives are also not uniformly accepted in all situations (Lens and Pollack, 2000), key examples being nursing home placement of feeding tubes and involuntary psychiatric commitments (Ely et al., 1992; Teno et al., 1997; Miller, 1998; Sbrenik and Brodoff, 2003). Oral advance directives are less well accepted, as they often are not specific to subsequent circumstances and can be hard to verify.

When there is no advance directive, a surrogate decision maker usually has far less information to guide decision making. If the patient's prior wishes regarding LSMT were generally known and sufficiently documented, the surrogate can make a "substituted judgment" and act in accordance with this knowledge (Kapp, 1992). However, it has been shown that substituted judgments by family members are often not congruent with the patient's previously expressed wishes (Sachs, 1994). In a few states, surrogates are permitted to make decisions based on the "best interests" of the patient (Kapp, 1992). While certainly a practical and workable approach in many instances, the "best interests" standard permits even greater surrogate subjectivity in end-of-life decisions and corresponding risk of discrepancy with what the patient, if competent, might have chosen. Thus, compared to situations of competency, incompetency involves a different and more restricted set of choices for a patient and her or his surrogate and takes the patient and the family down a distinctly different path at the end of life.

Competency status at end of life thus is linked inextricably to patient autonomy and to the fidelity and quality of the medical decisions made at end of life. It is therefore important to support and enhance decisional competency at the end of life. Interestingly, however, this topic has received relatively little attention from legal professionals, bioethicists, and clinicians (Allen et al., 2003). While a body of empirical literature has emerged regarding assessment of competency in psychiatric and dementia populations (Grisso and Appelbaum, 1991; Appelbaum and Grisso, 1995; Marson et al., 1995; Marson, Sawrie, et al. 2000; Dymek et al., 2001; Kim et al., 2001), to date there has been little published about such assessments in the context of end-of-life care (Allen et al., 2003).

This chapter focuses on two aspects of competency assessment at the end of life: (1) the real challenges for physicians and other clinicians in assessing competency in cognitively impaired older adults; and (2) the competency of nursing home residents (Allen et al., 2003)—a group for whom decisional capacity at the end of life is highly relevant—to execute advance directives. The research discussed will, I hope, serve as an initial platform and guide for future investigations into competency at the end of life.

Physician/Clinician Assessment of Competency

Although competency is ultimately a legal status, the realities of clinical practice compel physicians and other health care professionals to make competency judgments on a daily basis (Appelbaum and Gutheil, 1991). Physician judgments currently represent the accepted criterion in medical and legal practice for determining capacity to consent to treatment (Grisso, 1986; Appelbaum and Gutheil, 1991; Marson et al., 1994). Yet physicians and other clinicians have generally not been well prepared to make competency decisions. Medical schools and residency programs, and also clinical psychology programs, have not traditionally offered formal training in competency assessment (Marson, Earnst, et al., 2000). Widely accepted and well-standardized assessment instruments are currently still not available (Marson et al., 1994, 1995). As a result, physicians assessing competency have had to rely almost exclusively on subjective clinical impressions and brief mental status testing. Prior studies have suggested that physicians have difficulty assessing decision-making capacity in older adults (Fitten et al., 1989; Fitten and Waite, 1990) and distinguishing between mental status and competency status in older patients (McKinnon et al., 1989).

The Consistency of Physicians' Judgments of Competency

Our research group previously engaged these issues in a study of physicians' consistency of judgment in a population with Alzheimer disease (AD) (Marson et al., 1997). We posed the following research question: "How consistent are experienced physicians in judging the medical decision-making capacity of dementia patients?" Participants (n = 45) consisted of 16 normal older controls and 29 patients with mild AD who were part of a longitudinal study of competency. All subjects were videotaped responding to a standardized consent capacity interview (SCCI) (Marson et al., 1997) consisting of three parts: (1) a set of standardized clinical history questions, (2) the Mini-Mental State Examination (MMSE) (Folstein et al., 1975), and (3) a brief clinical vignette with follow-up questions testing capacity to consent under different standards. The vignette set forth a hypothetical medical problem (atherosclerotic heart disease/ "heart blockage"), in which only two treatment options, medication and open heart surgery, were available. The SCCI vignette text reads as follows:

MEDICAL DECISION-MAKING CAPACITY VIGNETTE

Mr./Mrs./Ms. _____, on this next task I want you to suppose that I am your personal doctor and that you are my patient.

We are going to suppose that you have a medical problem, which I as the doctor am going to tell you about. I want you to listen carefully to the medical problem, and then decide what you would do if you really had such a problem.

Do you understand? Good. Now let me describe the supposed medical problem.

Let us suppose that last night you had sharp heart pains while sleeping. Today you have come to see me, your doctor. I run some medical tests and find out that you have two blocked blood vessels in your heart.

As your doctor, I tell you that you have a serious heart problem. I also tell you that you have only two choices for treatment. The first choice is to take medication for the heart problem. The second choice is to have open heart surgery and have the blocked blood vessels replaced.

If you decide to take the heart medication, you will not need to have a painful and potentially life threatening surgery. There will be no side effects from the medication. However, you will need to take the medication on a daily basis the rest of your life. In addition, you will have to live a somewhat restricted life at home. You will no longer be able to do some of the activities you currently enjoy doing.

If you decide to have open heart surgery, you will not need to take any heart medication. You will be able to live an unrestricted life and do all of the activities you currently enjoy doing. However, you will feel a great deal of pain in your chest and leg for many weeks after the operation. In addition, the heart operation carries a risk of failure: you have an 80% chance of doing well after the operation, but also a 20% chance of dying during the operation. The operation also carries a small risk of stroke.

That is the end of the story. Now try to answer some questions about this story. (Marson et al., 1997)

After presentation of the vignette, subjects were asked a standardized series of questions that tested their capacity to evidence a choice for treatment, to appreciate personal consequences of the treatment choice, to provide rational reasons for the treatment choice, and to understand the medical situation and respective treatment choices (Roth et al., 1977; Appelbaum and Grisso, 1988; Grisso and Appelbaum, 1995; Marson et al., 1995). (These capacity standards are discussed in more detail below.) Five physicians (two neurologists, one geriatric psychiatrist, and two geriatricians) from the University of Alabama at Birmingham tertiary care medical center were then recruited as competency decision makers. All the physicians had extensive clinical experience with both dementia and competency assessment. Physicians were blinded to subject diagnosis and neuropsychological test performance. Each physician individually

Table 2.1. Physicians' Judgments of Competency, by Subject Group

Physician	Controls (n = 16)		Patients with AD (n = 29)		All Subjects (n = 45)	
	Competent	Incompetent	Competent	Incompetent	Competent	Incompetent
Physician 1	15 (94%)	1 (6%)	3 (10%)	26 (90%)	18 (40%)	27 (60%)
Physician 2	16 (100%)	0 (0%)	14 (48%)	15 (52%)	30 (67%)	15 (33%)
Physician 3	16 (100%)	0 (0%)	22 (76%)	7 (24%)	38 (84%)	7 (16%)
Physician 4	16 (100%)	0 (0%)	25 (86%)	4 (14%)	41 (91%)	4 (9%)
Physician 5	16 (100%)	0 (0%)	29 (100%)	0 (0%)	45 (100%)	0 (0%)
All physicians	79 (99%)	1 (1%)	93 (64%)	52 (36%)	172 (76%)	53 (24%)

Source: Adapted from Marson et al., 1997, p. 455, copyright 1997, American Geriatrics Society. Reprinted by permission.

Table 2.2. Judgment Agreement, by Physician Pair and Subject Group

Physician Pair	Controls (n = 16)	Patients with Mild AD (n = 29)	K	*p*
Physicians 1 and 2	94% (15/16)	62% (18/29)	.22	.24
Physicians 1 and 3	94 (15/16)	35 (10/29)	.07	.58
Physicians 1 and 4	94 (15/16)	24 (7/29)	.04	.70
Physicians 1 and 5	94 (15/16)	10 (3/29)	.00	.99
Physicians 2 and 3	100 (16/16)	72 (21/29)	.45	.005
Physicians 2 and 4	100 (16/16)	62 (18/29)	.26	.15
Physicians 2 and 5	100 (16/16)	48 (14/29)	.00	.99
Physicians 3 and 4	100 (16/16)	83 (24/29)	.45	.04
Physicians 3 and 5	100 (16/16)	76 (22/29)	.00	.99
Physicians 4 and 5	100 (16/16)	86 (25/29)	.00	.99
All physicians	98 (156/160)	56 (161/290)	.14	.44

Source: Data from Marson et al., 1997.
Note: Kappa and associated *p* values relate only to the group with mild AD.

viewed each of the 45 SCCI videotapes. At the completion of each videotape, a physician made a judgment of competent or incompetent to consent to medical treatment (Marson et al., 1997).

As shown in Table 2.1, physician judgment outcomes differed markedly for patients with mild AD but not for control subjects. Physicians as a group achieved 98 percent judgment agreement for the controls, but only 56 percent judgment agreement for the patients with mild AD (Table 2.2). Physicians as a group demonstrated significant judgment agreement not attributable to chance for the controls ($k = 1.00$, $p < .0001$), but not for the patients with AD ($k = .14$, $p = .44$) (Table 2.2). The difference between these two overall kappa coefficients was significant ($z > 4.0$, $p < .0001$), indicative of a real difference in the physicians' capacity consistently to judge competency across the control and mild AD groups (Marson et al., 1997).

The dramatic difference in physician judgment agreement across control and dementia groups represented an important finding. Although blinded to subject diagnostic and neuropsychological status, the study physicians consistently recognized normative subject responses and behaviors in the SCCI interviews and assigned the appropriate competency status to older control subjects. In contrast, physicians appeared to differ dramatically in the clinical significance they attached to the impaired responses and performance of the subjects with mild AD on the SCCI (such as memory loss, factual confusion, strained reasoning, disorientation to task). Specifically, individual physicians appeared to apply, consciously or unconsciously, different standards or thresholds in judging the competency of the subjects with dementia (Marson et al., 1997).

The study findings substantiated a long-standing clinical concern—namely, that physicians' assessment of competency is currently a subjective, inconsistent, and arguably idiosyncratic process (Marson et al., 1994; Marson and Harrell, 1996). While good reasons for this subjectivity exist (lack of an external criterion or gold standard, lack of standardized assessment instruments, lack of formal competency assessment training), the study findings raised troubling concerns about the conceptual and ultimately the moral basis currently of competency judgments in cognitively impaired elderly people (Marson and Harrell, 1996). Physicians (and other health care professionals) seem to differ widely in their conceptual understanding of competency, in their clinical approach to competency assessment, and in the different standards or thresholds they consciously or unconsciously apply in deciding competency (Marson et al., 1997).

The Value of Education and Training in Competency Assessment

A follow-up study provided more encouraging results and a clearer direction for practice (Marson, Earnst, et al., 2000). We asked the following research question: "If they first receive training in competency assessment, how consistent are experienced physicians in judging the medical decision-making capacity of dementia patients?" The impetus for the study was the belief that the consistency of physicians' judgments of competency may be enhanced if those judgments are guided by knowledge of specific capacity standards. Participants (n = 31) consisted of 10 normal older controls and 21 patients with probable AD. The mean MMSE (Folstein et al., 1975) score for controls was 29.3 (sd = 1.1) and for patients with AD was 19.1 (sd = 4.8). All patients had either mild dementia (MMSE score ≥ 20; n = 10) or moderate dementia (MMSE score ≥ 10 and < 20; n = 11). Participants were videotaped being administered a psychometric measure of capacity to consent to medical treatment (Capacity to Consent to Treatment Instrument [CCTI]) (Marson et al., 1995) The CCTI comprises two clinical vignettes (A, neoplasm; B, cardiac) that assess competency under five standards (vignette A) or four standards (vignette B). Each vignette presents a hypothetical medical problem and associated symptoms, along with two treatment alternatives that have associated risks and benefits. After reading and listening to each vignette, participants answered questions designed to assess competency under five established (Roth et al., 1977; Appelbaum and Grisso, 1988) and increasingly stringent standards (Marson et al., 1995):

1. the capacity to evidence a treatment choice (S1);
2. the capacity to make the reasonable treatment choice (when the alternative is manifestly unreasonable) (vignette A only) [S2]. (This standard is not well accepted but is used to evaluate participants' decision-making preferences.) (Dymek et al., 2001);
3. the capacity to appreciate the consequences of a treatment choice (S3);
4. the capacity to provide rational reasons for a treatment choice (S4); and
5. the capacity to understand the treatment situation and choices (S5).

Five physicians (two neurologists, one geriatric psychiatrist, and two geriatricians) from the University of Alabama at Birmingham tertiary care medical center were again recruited as competency decision makers (Marson, Earnst, et al., 2000). Four of the five physicians had participated in the previous decision-making study discussed above. All physicians had extensive clinical experience with both dementia and competency assessment. Each physician was board certified in his or her specialty, had an average of 8 years postresidency (range 5 to 11 years), had geriatric patients comprising an average of 75 percent of her or his clinical practice (range 25% to 100%), and had handled an average of 118 competency cases (range 20 to 200). Before commencing the study, each physician received information and orientation to the study and to the five capacity

Table 2.3. Outcomes of Competency Judgments, by Physician, Capacity Standard, and Group

| Physician | Controls (n = 10)[a] | | | | | | | Pateints with AD (n = 21)[b] | | | | | | |
| | Percentage Competent/Incompetent | | | | | | | Percentage Competent/Incompetent | | | | | | |
	S1	[S2]	S3	S4	S5	PJ	Overall	S1	[S2]	S3	S4	S5	PJ	Overall
Physician 1	95/5	90/10	60/40	75/25	90/10	85/15	82/18	83/17	81/19	21/79	38/68	33/67	33/67	45/55
Physician 2	100/0	90/10	100/0	100/0	100/0	100/0	99/1	91/9	76/24	21/79	38/62	33/67	33/67	46/54
Physician 3	100/0	90/10	100/0	95/5	100/0	100/0	98/2	95/5	86/14	62/38	17/83	24/76	24/76	48/52
Physician 4	100/0	100/0	85/15	100/0	95/5	100/0	96/4	76/24	33/67	26/74	36/64	36/64	36/64	41/59
Physician 5	100/0	90/10	100/0	95/5	100/0	100/0	99/1	88/12	81/19	48/52	48/52	45/55	48/52	58/42
All physicians	99/1	92/8	89/11	93/7	97/3	97/3	95/5	87/13	71/29	36/64	35/65	34/66	36/64	48/52

Source: Marson, Earnst, et al., 2000, p. 914. Copyright 2000, American Geriatrics Society. Reprinted by permission.

Notes: S = capacity standard; S1 = evidencing choice; [S2] = reasonable choice; S3 = appreciating consequences; S4 = reasoning; S5 = understanding treatment; PJ = personal competency judgment; overall = average for all judgments (S1–S5 and PJ).

[a] For each physician, judgments of each of S1, S3, S4, and S5 = 10, and for overall = 110.

[b] For each physician, judgments of each of S1, S3, S4, and S5 = 21, and for overall = 231.

standards (S's) and their operational definitions. Each physician also reviewed a training videotape and made practice competency judgments under the different standards. In the formal study, each physician individually viewed each of 62 CCTI videotapes (videotapes of vignettes A and B for each of 31 participants). Physicians were blinded to a videotaped participant's diagnosis and neuropsychological test performance. In reviewing a competency videotape, physicians could see and hear administration of the vignette and the standard (S) questions to a participant and also follow along with a written transcript. Following examiner questions and participant responses for each standard, the videotape was stopped, and physicians were provided with a definition of the standard in question. A physician then made a competency judgment (competent or incompetent) for that standard and was also given the opportunity to make qualitative comments about the competency judgment. Physician judgments on the standards mirrored the administration of the CCTI vignettes and were made in the following order: S5 (understanding), S1 (evidencing choice), S2 (reasonable choice), S4 (reasoning), S3 (appreciating consequences). At the conclusion of the videotape, and after all five capacity standard judgments had been made, a physician then made a personal judgment of competency (competent or incompetent) (Marson, Earnst, et al., 2000).

Table 2.3 presents competency judgment outcomes (percentage competent and incompetent) for each physician across standards and within group. For controls, physicians individually and as a group generally had a high number of "competent" outcomes, with the overall percentage of the five physicians' judgments being 95 percent competent and only 5 percent incompetent. As expected, physicians had far lower numbers of competent outcomes for AD patients across the standards. Overall, physicians found AD patients competent in only 48 percent of cases, with the rates across S varying from a high of 87 percent competent on S1 (evidencing choice) to a low of 34 percent competent on S5 (understanding treatment and choices) (Marson, Earnst, et al., 2000).

Table 2.4 shows overall and pairwise judgment agreement among physicians for the group with AD. For physicians as a group, the highest percentage agreement was for S1 (84%), followed by S5 (80%), S4 (74%), S2 (71%), and S3 (67%). This pattern of results for patients with AD showed that physicians had the highest levels of judgment agreement for the empirically least stringent standard of competency (S1) and the two most stringent standards (S4, S5); they had somewhat lower levels of agreement for a moderately stringent standard (S3). Physicians as a group showed 76 percent agreement on their personal

Table 2.4. Percentage and Kappa Estimates of Judgment Agreement, by Capacity Standard (S) for the Group with Alzheimer Disease

Physician Pair	S1 Evidencing Choice %	K	[S2] Reasonable Choice %	K	S3 Appreciation %	K	S4 Reasoning %	K	S5 Understanding %	K	PJ Personal Judgment %	K
Physicians 1 and 2	83	.28	76	.30	69	.23	69	.26[a]	74	.42[b]	78	.54[c]
Physicians 1 and 3	88	.40[c]	86	.49[a]	55	.20	74	.38[b]	81	.54[c]	81	.54[c]
Physicians 1 and 4	81	.44[b]	52	.21[a]	80	.48[b]	83	.64[c]	93	.84[c]	83	.63[c]
Physicians 1 and 5	90	.61[c]	90	.69[b]	60	.17	71	.42[b]	79	.56[c]	76	.52[c]
Physicians 2 and 3	90	.29[a]	81	.69	67	.38[b]	86	.47[b]	79	.50[c]	74	.42[b]
Physicians 2 and 4	79	.30[a]	38	-.05	74	.38[a]	76	.41[b]	76	.48[b]	71	.40[b]
Physicians 2 and 5	88	.38[a]	86	.58[b]	62	.23	60	.16	76	.51[c]	74	.47[c]
Physicians 3 and 4	77	.08	52	.15	59	.27[a]	76	.41[b]	79	.55[c]	79	.50[c]
Physicians 3 and 5	93	.54[c]	95	.83[c]	76	.53[c]	69	.36[b]	79	.55[c]	67	.32[a]
Physicians 4 and 5	81	.40[b]	52	.21	69	.37[b]	79	.57[c]	86	.71[c]	74	.47[b]
All Physicians	84	.33	71	.35	67	.31	74	.39[a]	80	.57[c]	76	.48[b]

Source: Marson, Earnst, et al., 2000, p. 915. Copyright 2000, American Geriatrics Society. Reprinted with permission.

Notes: n = 21. For each physician, judgments for each of S1, S3, S4, S5, and PJ = 42, and for [S2] = 21.

PJ = personal compentency judgment; K = kappa; % = percentage agreement.

[a]$p \leq .05$; [b]$p \leq .01$; [c]$p \leq .001$

competency judgments for patients with AD. This level of agreement for patients with AD was substantially higher than the agreement (56%) found in our prior study of personal physician competency judgments in AD (Marson et al., 1997). In addition, we found that the overall kappa value for physicians' personal judgment within the AD subsample was .48 ($p = $ .01, one-tailed), compared to a kappa value of only .14 ($p = $ .22, one-tailed) in our prior study (Marson et al., 1997; Marson, Earnst, et al., 2000).

However, our prior study's sample included only patients with mild AD, who may have represented a more ambiguous and challenging sample for competency assessment than did the current study's sample of patients with mild and moderate AD. Accordingly, in the current study we also examined personal competency judgment agreement for the mild AD subsample itself (n = 10), to permit a more direct comparison between the two studies. Physicians as a group overall achieved 73 percent agreement on their personal competency judgments for this subsample. These pairwise and overall findings were considerably higher than those obtained in the prior study (56% overall agreement; pairwise agreement range from 10% to 86%) (Marson et al., 1997).

The follow-up study showed that competency judgment agreement is enhanced by training and education (Karlawish and Schmitt, 2000). Judgment consistency increased significantly when physicians' judgments were based on and guided by application of specific capacity standards (Marson, Earnst, et al., 2000). The findings supported the assessment value of standardized competency instruments like the CCTI, which incorporate specific capacity standards. The findings also suggested the value of formal training in competency assessment for physicians, clinical psychologists, and other health care professionals (Marson, Earnst, et al., 2000). It should be noted that although our physician assessors were already experienced in competency assessment, the CCTI training format had a substantial and positive impact on their judgment consistency.

Implications for End-of-Life Issues

These two studies have implications for clinician competency assessment of patients at the end of life. The findings of judgment inconsistency from the initial 1997 study (Marson et al., 1997) have obvious and troubling implications for clinician assessment of competency of nursing home patients and other individuals at the end of life. Because the range and quality of choices will turn on a patient's competency status at the end of life, how can one be assured that an accurate competency judgment has been made for a terminally ill loved one? As discussed below, research is needed that focuses specifically on clinician competency assessments of patients at the end of life. The findings from the follow-up 2000 study (Marson, Earnst, et al., 2000) provide encouragement that improved consistency and quality of competency decision making can be made possible in the end-of-life context. However, competency assessment training formats will need to be tailored for end-of-life issues. For example, instruments and research approaches will need to incorporate end-of-life issues such as execution of advance directives and election/rejection of LSMT (Allen et al., 2003).

The Competency of Nursing Home Residents to Execute Advance Directives

In addition to clinician research, there need to be studies of competency in different groups at the end of life. For example, nursing home residents are an important population for study. More than 1.5 million individuals older than 65 reside in nursing homes (American Health Care Association, 1999), and nursing homes together with hospitals represent 54 percent of places where death occurs (Gage and Dao, 2000; Allen et al., 2003). In addition, the cognitive capacity of elderly persons in hospices or nursing homes may be considerably lower than that of community-dwelling persons with dementia (Allen et al., 2003)—such as the patients with AD who participated in the two decision-making studies described above (Marson et al., 1997; Marson, Earnst, et al., 2000). These circumstances raise concerns about the general end-of-life decisional capacity of nursing home residents. For these reasons, Allen and colleagues stated that "the identification of nursing home residents who can continue to participate in advance care planning about end-of-life care is a critical clinical and bioethical issue" (Allen et al., 2003, p. 309).

Allen and colleagues carried out one of the first empirical studies of decisional capacity in nursing home residents (Allen et al., 2003). A sample of 78 nursing home residents with a mean age of 84 (sd = 8.2) and their proxies were recruited from five different nursing homes. Mean MMSE for the group was 14.0 (sd = 6.5). A decisional capacity measure evaluating the capacity to execute an advance directive regarding potential future placement of a feeding tube (Allen et al., 2003) was developed using vignette methodology previously developed by Marson and colleagues (Marson et al., 1995, 1996). Follow-up questions then tapped the subject's capacity under four of the capacity standards previously discussed (evidencing choice, appreciating consequences, reasoning, and understanding).

The feeding-tube vignette text is as follows:

ADVANCE CARE PLANNING—RESIDENT FEEDING TUBE VIGNETTE

I want you to pretend that I am the nursing home social worker, ____. We are going to talk about medical care you may want in the future. We need to talk about this now because you may get too sick to tell us what you want in the future, when a decision has to be made about your medical care.

I want you to listen closely to this situation. We will talk about your plans regarding having a feeding tube placed in your side. You will have to decide whether or not to get a feeding tube in the future. Tell me what you would decide to do if you knew you would have this problem later. Are you ready?

Suppose over the next three years you have several small strokes in your brain. As a result, you have trouble remembering things and thinking clearly. The strokes also make it difficult for you to swallow food, and you have been losing weight. Sometimes when you eat, some of the food seems "to go down the wrong pipe" and you choke. You get pneumonia and have to go to the hospital. The doctor recommends that you have a feeding tube placed in your side. You are too sick and confused at this point to tell the doctor what you want.

The doctor tells you that if you receive the feeding tube, you will not be allowed to eat or drink anything. All of your food and liquids will go in through the tube. The doctor says that the feeding tube will help you stop losing weight. But the doctor also says you will need this feeding tube for the rest of your life. You will never again be able to eat on your own. If you do not receive the feeding tube, you will continue to choke when you eat and will get pneumonia again and again. You will eventually die from the pneumonia.

If you knew this problem would occur in the next 3 years, what decision would you make NOW for the feeding tube? It may be: you want the feeding tube placed in your side in 3 years when you become sick. You will then have to be fed through your side for the rest of your life.

OR, it may be that you do not want the feeding tube in your side in 3 years. Without this treatment, you will probably continue to get pneumonia and would eventually die. (Allen et al., 2003)

Although an older control group was not available, study results suggested significant impairment of advance-directive decisional capacity among the nursing home residents (Allen et al., 2003). On the capacity standard of evidencing a choice, the most elementary capacity standard tested, approximately 40 percent of the residents demonstrated some level of impairment (scores of 0 or 1 out of 2). On the capacity standard of appreciating consequences, 35.1 percent of residents earned a score of 0 out of 5, with another 20 percent earning a score of only 1 out of 5. Thus, upon initial inspection, at least 50 percent of the residents demonstrated probable significant impairment in their capacity to appreciate the consequences of a decision regarding future placement of a feeding tube (mean score = 1.2 [sd = 1.1]). Finally, on the capacity standard of understanding, a factually and memory intensive standard (Marson et al., 1996), 27 percent of nursing home residents earned a score of 0 out of 30, with another 40–50 percent earning scores of 2 or 3 out of 30 (mean score = 2.15 [sd = 2.5]). Thus, on inspection, approximately 70 percent or more of the nursing home residents demonstrated probable significant impairment in their capacity to understand the circumstances of the hypothetical feeding-tube situation and the decision alternatives available. Performance on the reasoning standard could not be evaluated because of low levels of inter-rater scoring reliability. Overall cognitive ability as measured by the MMSE correlated significantly with performance on appreciation (r = .24, p = .04) and understanding (r = .24, p = .04) but not with evidencing a choice (Allen et al., 2003).

The results of this initial study have a number of implications for competency assessment at the end of life. First, many nursing home and terminally ill older patients are likely to suffer significant cognitive impairment and dementia that will adversely affect their decisional capacity. The study sample's mean MMSE score of 14.0 is equivalent to a moderate to severe dementia stage in patients with Alzheimer disease. Thus it is not surprising that the residents' performance on the two complex capacity standards available (appreciation and understanding) was substantially impaired. Second, advance-directive and care planning at the end of life is by nature abstract and complex. In everyday treatment-consent situations, patients are evaluated with respect to existing medical symptoms and problems that are concrete and relatively easy for patients to relate to. In contrast, with advance-care planning, cognitively impaired and often chronically ill older adults are asked to mentally project themselves forward in time regarding potential and often vague future circumstances, when some form of LSMT, such as placement of a feeding tube, may become necessary. This task requires a level of abstraction that may well be beyond the abilities of many older adult patients at the end of life, although additional research is needed to bear out this inference. Third, assuming that the capacity to plan advance care is substantially impaired in many people at the end of life, the importance of early and ongoing family involvement in advance-care planning is underscored. Clinicians and nursing home administrators and staff should also be involved early on in such advance-care planning, and they may need to be proactive to ensure that key issues regarding a patient's competency status are addressed and documented and that proxy decision makers for the patient are available.

Conclusion

Competency at the end of life reflects the autonomy to make a range of treatment and care choices. Incompetency, in contrast, represents loss of autonomy and results in more limited options in end-of-life decision making. Competency status thus is linked closely to patient autonomy and likely to the fidelity and quality of medical decisions available at the end of life.

This chapter has considered, in an initial way, both clinician and patient aspects of competency assessments at the end of life. Specifically, it examined clinician judgments in assessing competency in cognitively impaired older adults and identified both disturbing inconsistencies as well as the value of competency assessment education and training. I also reviewed a recent study of decisional capacity for advance directives in nursing home residents and identified patterns of substantial capacity (and cognitive) impairment in these patients and the need for early involvement of family members, as well as nursing home administrators and staff, in care planning. However, competency at the end of life remains a largely unexamined area, and clearly more clinician- and patient-oriented empirical work is needed in order to enhance and support end-of-life planning and decision making. I hope this chapter, and the volume as a whole, will serve as a stimulus for future investigations into competency at the end of life.

Acknowledgments

The author gratefully acknowledges the assistance of Rebecca S. Allen, Ph.D., in reviewing and commenting on the manuscript and in permitting publication of a clinical vignette developed by her group.

This research was supported by (1) an Alzheimer disease Center Core Grant

(NIH, NIA 1 P30 AG10163–1) (Harrell, PI); (2) an Alzheimer disease Center Grant (NIH, NIA P50 AG16582-04) (Harrell, PI); and (3) the Alzheimer's Disease Cooperative Study (NIH, NIA AG 10483-12) (Thal, PI).

REFERENCES

Allen, R., DeLaine, S., et al. 2003. Advance care planning in nursing homes: Correlates of capacity and possession of advance directives. *Gerontologist* 43(3):309–17.

American Health Care Association. 1999. *Facts and Trends, 1999: The Nursing Facility Sourcebook*. Washington, DC: American Health Care Association.

Angell, M. 1997. The Supreme Court and physician-assisted suicide: The ultimate right. *New England Journal of Medicine* 336(1):50–53.

Appelbaum, P., and Grisso, T. 1988. Assessing patients' capacities to consent to treatment. *New England Journal of Medicine* 319:1635–38.

Appelbaum, P., and Grisso, T. 1995. The MacArthur Treatment Competence Study. I. Mental illness and competence to consent to treatment. *Law and Human Behavior* 19:105–26.

Appelbaum, P., and Gutheil, T. 1991. *Clinical Handbook of Psychiatry and the Law*. Baltimore: Williams & Wilkins.

Dymek, M., Atchison, P., et al. 2001. Competency to consent to treatment in cognitively impaired patients with Parkinson's disease. *Neurology* 56:17–24.

Ely, J., Peters, P. J., et al. 1992. The physician's decision to use tube feedings: The role of the family, the living will, and the Cruzan decision. *Journal of the American Geriatrics Society* 40(5):533–34.

Fitten, L., Lusky, R., et al. 1989. Assessing treatment decision-making capacity in elderly nursing home residents. *Journal of the American Geriatric Society* 38:1097–1104.

Fitten, L. J., and Waite, M. S. 1990. Impact of medical hospitalization on treatment decision-making capacity in the elderly. *Archives of Internal Medicine* 150:1717–21.

Folstein, M., Folstein, S., et al. 1975. Mini-Mental State: A practical guide for grading the cognitive state of the patient for the physician. *Journal of Psychiatry Research* 12:189–98.

Gage, B., and Dao, T. 2000. *Medicare's Hospice Benefit: Use and Expenditures*. Washington, DC: U.S. Department of Health and Human Services.

Grisso, T. 1986. *Evaluating Competencies: Forensic Assessments and Instruments*. New York: Plenum Press.

Grisso, T., and Appelbaum, P. 1991. Mentally ill and non-mentally ill patients' abilities to understand informed consent disclosure for medication. *Law and Human Behavior* 15:377–88.

Grisso, T., and Appelbaum, P. 1995. A comparison of standards for assessing patients' capacities to make treatment decisions. *American Journal of Psychiatry* 19:149–66.

Kapp, M. 1992. *Geriatrics and the Law: Patient Rights and Professional Responsibilities*. New York: Springer Publishing Co.

Karlawish, J., and Schmitt, F. 2000. Why physicians need to become more proficient in assessing their patients' competency and how they can achieve this. *Journal of the American Geriatrics Society* 48:1014–16.

Kim, S., Caine, E., et al. 2001. Assessing the competence of persons with Alzheimer's disease in providing informed consent for participation in research. *American Journal of Psychiatry* 158:712–17.

Lens, V., and Pollack, D. 2000. Advanced directives: Legal remedies and psychosocial interventions. *Death Studies* 24:377–99.

Marson, D. 2003. Competency for end-of-life decision-making. End of Life Conference, Boston College, Boston, MA.

Marson, D. C., Chatterjee, A., et al. 1996. Toward a neurologic model of competency: Cognitive predictors of capacity to consent in Alzheimer's disease using three different legal standards. *Neurology* 46:666–72.

Marson, D., Earnst, K., et al. 2000. Consistency of physicians' legal standard and personal judgments of competency in patients with Alzheimer's disease. *Journal of the American Geriatrics Society* 48:911–18.

Marson, D. C., and L. E. Harrell. 1996. Decision making capacity: In reply. *Archives of Neurology* 53:589–90.

Marson, D. C., Ingram, K. K., et al. 1995. Assessing the competency of patients with Alzheimer's disease under different legal standards. *Archives of Neurology* 52:949–54.

Marson, D. C., McInturff, B., et al. 1997. Consistency of physician judgments of capacity to consent in mild Alzheimer's disease. *Journal of the American Geriatrics Society* 45:453–57.

Marson, D., Sawrie, S., et al. 2000. Assessing financial capacity in patients with Alzheimer's disease: A conceptual model and prototype instrument. *Archives of Neurology* 57:877–84.

Marson, D. C., Schmitt, F., et al. 1994. Determining the competency of Alzheimer's patients to consent to treatment and research. *Alzheimer's Disease and Associated Disorders* 8 (suppl. 4): 5–18.

Marson, D., and Zebley, L. 2001. The other side of the retirement years: Cognitive decline, dementia, and loss of financial capacity. *Journal of Retirement Planning* 4(1):30–39.

McKinnon, K., Cournos, F., et al. 1989. Rivers in practice: Clinicians' assessments of patients' decision-making capacity. *Hospital and Community Psychiatry* 40:1159–62.

Mezey, M., Mitty, E., et al. 2000. Advance directives: Older adults with dementia. *Clinics in Geriatric Medicine* 16:255–68.

Miller, R. 1998. Advance directives for psychiatric treatment: A view from the trenches. *Psychology and Public Policy Law* 4(3):728–45.

Roth, L., Meisel, A., et al. 1977. Tests of competency to consent to treatment. *American Journal of Psychiatry* 134:279–84.

Sachs, G. 1994. Advanced consent for dementia research. *Alzheimer Disease and Associated Disorders* 8 (suppl. 4): 19–27.

Sbrenik, D., and Brodoff, L. 2003. Implementing psychiatric advance directives: Service provider issues and answers. *Journal of Behavioral Health Services and Research* 30(3):253–68.

Teno, J., Licks, S., et al. 1997. Do advance directives provide instructions that direct care? SUPPORT Investigators. Study to Understand Prognoses and Preferences for Outcomes and Risks of Treatment. *Journal of the American Geriatrics Society* 45(4):519–20.

CHAPTER THREE

The Ethics of Long-Term Care

Recasting the Policy Discourse

Charles J. Fahey

The demographic and epidemiological revolution that has marked the close of the twentieth and opening of the twenty-first centuries poses challenges to individuals and society. This is particularly true of the way we deal with the vulnerabilities, dependencies, and illnesses that inevitably accompany the Third Age, the last period of the life journey after the time of reproduction and physical parenting. This chapter forwards the following propositions:

1. The Third Age is now a normal part of the life journey.
2. The Third Age inevitably involves progressive intermittent frailty (i.e., disequilibrium between a person's internal capacity and external demands).
3. People attempt to address this disequilibrium with the support of others and the utilization of various medical interventions, pharmacological agents, prosthetic devices, and modifications in their living space.
4. Frailty entails costs—psychological, monetary, and opportunity.
5. Frailty imposes itself not only on the individual but also on others who supply support or the materials necessary to ease its effects.

6. Frailty is a personal, interpersonal, and societal event evoking value-laden responses, the arenas of personal and social ethics.

In addition, I assert that current long-term-care policy fails to identify and respond to frailty as a key area of social concern and, in so doing, supports a system that is unduly institutionally and medically oriented. Furthermore, current policy inadequately supports the primary care (informal) systems where most care is desired and given. I suggest ethical perspectives that should undergird individual and societal approaches to frailty and concomitant dependency. Finally, I recommend a policy perspective and approach consonant with both the new reality and sound ethics.

Social Solidarity: The Heart of Social Ethics

People are interdependent at every moment of life. This interdependence has contemporary, historical, and futuristic elements. It existed for those who have gone before us and will continue after all of us are gone. We have inherited much of what contributes to the good life that we enjoy. Current structures and goods are the result of the interplay of informal—or, better, primary—interactions, commercial transactions, and public policy activities that have evolved within different eras. Whether it is our democratic institutions, wealth, security, educational opportunities, and commercial prowess or, as particularly significant to this discussion, our health care interventions, each has its beginnings, and in some instances its maturity, in prior generations. In turn, the well-being of future generations is dependent on our stewardship of the social and physical environment within which we live.

Society and culture are rooted in this reality. We are always in need of *the other*. We are engaged in a continuing struggle to find a balance between self and the other(s) in which we abandon neither individual initiative and responsibility nor communities. Intergenerational equilibrium is constantly evolving and challenged but especially so in our current demographic and epidemiologic revolution, fueled by scientific discoveries and their application to the human condition. It has never been this way before. As illustrated in Figure 3.1, the United States had approximately 11.36 times as many people alive at age 65 or older in 2000 as in 1900. This increase in life span is a striking accomplishment, but one with bewildering challenges for individuals, families, and public policy. To help people age well, we need to find a way to manage our miracles. Yesterday's social structures and public policies will no longer do. We

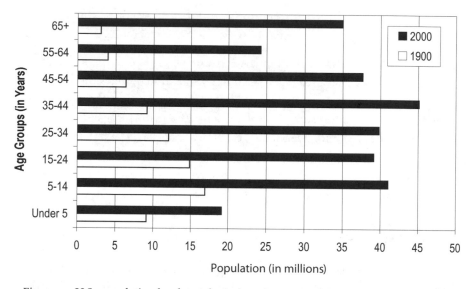

Figure 3.1. U.S. population by chronological age in 1900 and 2000 *Source:* Data from U.S. Census Bureau, 2003

cannot put new wine in old wineskins or patch old cloth with new (Luke 5:36–37, New American Bible).

Simply stated, many more people are alive today at every stage of life who have impairments and consequent disabilities that limit participation in everyday activities than at any previous moment in history. The disabilities can be assuaged to some degree and in some instances with interventions assisting the individuals and modifying their milieu. We are confronted with two fundamental questions. First, what ethically based demands can those with impairments make on others? and second, who should bear the burden in meeting the needs of those with impairments?

In considering these questions, we note that in the latter part of the twentieth century, we developed a new, normal part of the life journey, the *Third Age.* The normalcy of this new facet of life's journey raises issues for all. Individuals in the Third Age are more likely to be consumers than producers in an economic sense, dependent not only on past earnings and wealth but on the support of current participants in the workforce. Concomitantly, they are likely to experience progressive intermittent frailty. Furthermore, most living persons will experience the Third Age as part of their life journey; persons in this segment constitute an ever-larger portion of the overall population. The challenge is exacerbated by the development of a four- and five-generational society, resulting in still more layers of ethical relationships and responsibilities within primary groupings, even as the population characteristics within the generations have changed.

This phenomenon is occurring within the context of an increasingly more interdependent world in which inequalities become ever more painfully evident and cultures clash in more dramatic and dangerous ways. In virtually every arena, we see conflicts between and among the self, *the other,* and *the others;* these conflicts are the stuff of ethical reflection, decisions, and actions.

The New Demands of Shared Decision Making

One of the blessings of being human and of living in community is that we have some control over evolutionary trends, especially as embodied in culture and social structures. The burden is that we must make individual and shared decisions that have personal and societal rewards and costs. The capacity of human beings to think and make contributions to both the "personal" and "common" good frees us from blind, internally determining forces that underlie natural selection and the survival of the fittest. The ability is a burden to the degree that it forces us to make determinations that may involve conflict and cause us inconvenience or narrow our ability to pursue other goods.

The ordering and reordering that is constantly occurring within and among individuals and societies ideally should be rooted in a shared vision about the world, giving rise to shared values. In reality, this ordering and reordering is often driven by self-interest, market forces, and political power, whatever the costs to the other or the others.

Ethical insights should influence the transactions involving frail and apparently nonfrail people. Our common task is to examine, modify, or strengthen when necessary the "ties that bind" to assure dignity for all, especially the most vulnerable among us. These ties are the bonds of love and guilt, wealth and income, and the power of the state in influencing human relationships.

Frailty

Because the goal of long-term care is to maximize a person's capacity and minimize the disequilibrium between internal capacity and external demands, it may be useful to consider frailty as the overarching concept in long-term care. Frailty is not easily defined but is easily recognized. Using it as an organizing concept can help us better understand the challenge and discern how to address the programmatic and financial implications of long-term care.

Used in this context, frailty is both a state and a process. It involves functional, social, intellectual, emotional, and economic considerations. Central to the concept is a person's ability to deal with activities of daily living over an extended period of time after losses both minor and major. In some instances, especially in the First Age (conception to adulthood) and the Second Age (adulthood), frailty is transient and remediable. In the Third Age, it is likely to be progressive with some periods of remission but will ultimately result in the need for care and, finally, in death. Paradoxically, frailty is both predictable and idiosyncratic. All in the Third Age suffer losses but at different times, in differing ways, and with differing severity. We may describe the etiology of frailty as stemming from various causes: genetics; trauma; chronic illness, both physical and emotional; dementia; and aging-related loss of physiological capacity. In addition to physical causes, the person's social relationships and physical environment either ease or exacerbate frailty.

Frailty can be seen as potential or actual (i.e., a person is vulnerable to various internal or external threats to self-sufficiency or is actually experiencing them). It may be relatively benign in the beginning, or it may be devastating. For example, older people are likely to have cataracts and some hearing loss, relatively modest impairments that may be ameliorated by various means, cosmetic or medical. Some major impairments may be reduced by rehabilitation. Some chronic conditions can be controlled to a degree by various pharmacological agents. In addition, frailty's effects can also be diminished by lifestyle choices, prosthetic devices, environmental modifications, and social supports. Many medical interventions, prosthetic devices, and even cultural expectations that moderate frailty have been introduced only in the latter part of the twentieth century, enabling persons who heretofore would have been unable to carry out activities of daily living to continue to live full lives until the frailty progresses significantly.

Frailty is hard to objectify. It involves endogenous and exogenous factors. Culture, values, psychological strength, and personal financial assets have impacts on a person's ability to cope with decreased capacity. Where one lives, the configuration of one's home, and the willingness of others to help are also significant. Whatever the cause, the frail person has difficulty dealing with the basics of life. To compensate for or mitigate frailty entails significant costs.

Frailty manifests itself in many diverse ways that ultimately often coalesce into substantial dependence. It may occur as a result of a cataclysmic physical event such as a stroke, a social event such as the loss of a significant other, or an economic event such as the loss of personal savings. Sometimes frailty occurs over time with various individual physical events and at other times occurs with a sudden cascading of events that can best be characterized as system degradation or failure. The common characteristic of frailty is the loss of capacity to manage without the assistance of people, devices, interventions, drugs, or even supportive physical environments. The financial capacity of the frail person is often the key element in the ability or inability to deal with the demands of everyday life, because these various compensatory aids, both human and material, involve new costs.

Whether the incidence and prevalence of actual dependency are decreasing is still a matter of conflicting views. However, it is clear that many medical advances are warding off premature death, and numerous pharmacological, prosthetic, and lifestyle interventions are currently available that can lessen the possibility of dependency but not the underlying potential for frailty, current or future. The variety of coping mechanisms available can modify frailty but ultimately cannot reverse its trajectory.

Disability

Although birth defects, trauma, and mental illness affect many in the First and Second Ages, these events and their consequences are abnormal. Similarly, persons with episodic frailty/disability at every age have periods of sickness or accidents that render them incapable of full participation. However, these are seen as aberrations. Such episodes and the costs entailed are especially amenable to insurance approaches, in which we pay a certain premium against the possibility of a costly event, and also may be relieved by ordinary resources developed for the rainy day.

Typically, increased frailty occurs in the latter part of life. Economically, two negative forces act synergistically: the material and social assets of the frail person may be diminished by a limited or nonexistent earning capacity for all but the more affluent, and physiological, social, and economic demands require ever-increasing expenditures. As people grow older, they are dependent on past earnings, contributions by others, wealth accumulated over time, and public benefit programs. In addition to the physiological and economic changes, social changes occur. A spouse may die, children may move, the neighborhood may change, and the living environment both internal and external may be less congenial.

A Demographic Framework

It is useful to consider the structure of the population as well as its dynamics. As previously discussed, it is helpful to think of the population as composed of persons in any one of three ages based on biological development and social status. Each age has its particular characteristics in regard to relative physical, emotional, and financial self-sufficiency.

The delineation of three ages is based on the following biological realities that in turn influence physical capacities:

1. The First Age is the period from the first moment of existence to physical maturity; this age is characterized by orderly molecular development.
2. The Second Age is the time of maximum physiological capacity and molecular orderliness with an advantage to continuing the species.
3. The Third Age, relatively new to the human experience, is beyond the ordinary time of physical parenting. This age is marked by random molecular disorganization.

The First Age: From Conception to Adulthood

The First Age is a period of decreasing frailty, or, conversely, a time of progression toward self-sufficiency. Individuals are in need of physical, emotional, intellectual, economic, and spiritual support as they move through a series of stages toward caring for themselves.

No one is frailer than a child. From the moment of conception until maturity is achieved, the child is in need of a supportive environment. However, the vulnerability (read frailty) decreases as the child grows. Granted different genetic endowments, the progression to maturity is generally inexorable and predictable. Because the First Age has been a normal part of the life cycle, different cultures, including that of the United States, have developed various social structures, including governmental programs, to assist in the maturing process both for the benefit of the child and the society in which he or she will become an ever more active participant and contributor. We have an implicit societal agreement reinforced by various informal and formal mechanisms that those who beget children have a responsibility to care for their development. It is expected that the primary, though not sole, responsibility for nurturing those in the First Age belongs to the parent(s), with society in general and government in particular playing a necessary but subsidiary role. Parents cannot do the job alone. We support an extensive educational system and various public health interventions such as immunization programs and well-baby clinics. In the instance of poor families and children abandoned by their parents, we have various social welfare programs. When parents are absent, government stands in loco parentis. Government provides special assistance, and at times programs, for young people with special needs.

The Second Age: Adulthood

The Second Age is the period with maximum capacity for production and reproduction. There is a cultural presumption that individuals are responsible for themselves, including earning income sufficient to meet both current and future needs. We have expectancies in regard to people's contribution to the common good through taxation and service in the armed forces in time of national peril. We have various welfare schemes for the poor such as tax credits, Supplementary Security Income, and Medicaid.

The Third Age: After Reproduction

The Third Age is relatively new as an expected period for a majority of persons in the life journey. Cultural expectations, social values, and public policy, including that touching on the progressive intermittent frailty often associated with this age, are in a period of development. This age is marked by random molecular disarray. In his book *How and Why We Age,* Leonard Hayflick makes this observation in a chapter on theories of aging: "Random changes or errors appear in previously well-ordered molecules, resulting in the normal physiological losses that we call age changes" (p. 260). Some of these changes are relatively nonthreatening, such as hair loss or change of hair color to gray or white. Some changes are more dramatic and physically and emotionally difficult (e.g., menopause, a decrease in sight and hearing, general physiological deterioration with a shrinkage in size and thinning of the bones, and aging-related conditions and illnesses). Table 3.1 compares the life journey at the beginning of the twentieth and twenty-first centuries. At the beginning of the twentieth century, with an average life expectancy of 47.3 years, once reproduction and con-

Table 3.1. The Life Journey

Beginning of the Twentieth Century	Beginning of the Twenty-first Century
First Age: moment of existence until reproductive capacity developed	First Age: moment of existence until reproductive capacity developed
Second Age: reproduction and contribution to the species	Second Age: reproduction and contribution to the species
	Third Age: reproduction accomplished; major consumption in society rather than production; gradual but inexorable system decline
Average life expectancy: 47.3 years	Average life expectancy: 77.0 years

Source: Data from U.S. Department of Health and Human Services, 2003.

tribution to the species had been accomplished, the life journey ended for the majority of people. The 30 years in average life expectancy gained during the twentieth century added a Third Age to the life journey for most people. This age is characterized by gradual but inexorable system decline.

The biologically driven changes of the Third Age entail vulnerability of the population with concomitant increases in both the incidence and the prevalence of frailty and its demands on individuals and society as a whole. While it is part of every individual's life from time to time and for some throughout the life course, persistent progressive episodic frailty is characteristic of the Third Age for everyone. This is different from the first two ages, in which frailty is *accidental* and *incidental*. In the Third Age, it is normative. It may be mild at first or quite debilitating. Inevitably, the last stage is death.

For most people, the Third Age is a period spent outside the workforce. It is a time of consumption rather than production in an economic sense. Random molecular disorganization renders an individual's various systems more amenable to weakness and failure and the total person more vulnerable to external assaults, to frailty that is likely to progress.

A Third Age is now the norm. It has significant consequences for both individuals and society because it involves commitments of others to maintain decency for those experiencing vulnerability and disability. The "others" in this event are those with moral/psychological/professional bonds, such as the family members, friends, and neighbors who are the primary caregivers, the professional caregivers, and the taxpayers.

This analysis of the three ages in the journey of life is incomplete unless we situate it in time amid preceding and succeeding generations. It should be further noted that while these three age categories remain relatively stable in developmental terms, individuals move through the ages with their individual life experiences. People also move as members of cohorts with similar social and cultural experiences, for example, the Depression, wars, and the sexual revolution. Even the generational makeup of society has great significance as we move to a four- and even five-generational structure with family patterns changing within each generation.

The Intersection of Long-Term Care and Ethics

American society is ambivalent about a "public ethic." Respectful of pluralism, emphasizing autonomy and freedom, we nonetheless can express outrage at some behaviors and rise to high degrees of compassion when faced with individual harm (e.g., the "child trapped in the well" phenomenon or massive human suffering from the tsunami in Southeast Asia). But along with our ambivalence, there are strong currents in our culture that recognize the importance of responsible behavior, shared sacrifice for the common good, and recognition of our solidarity. It is these instincts, rather than formal moral/ethical theory, that inform American society. The development of the Third Age as normal challenges the societal structures and current public policies developed at a time when older persons were the exception rather than a significant part of the population.

Managing the Human Household: The Four Economies

A way of analyzing the "frailty challenge" is to consider humans as living in a household with limited resources. The management of these resources can be characterized as the economy or, perhaps better, as several economies in which the goods to be distributed differ and the mode of distribution varies as well. Ethics is an important mediating force in each of these economies. The distributional dynamic should result in decency for the individual and the promotion of the common good both for current and future generations.

The fundamental meaning of the word *economy* is management of a household. The Greek word *oikonomia* is a combination of *oikos* meaning house and *nemein* meaning to manage (according to *Merriam Webster's Collegiate Dictionary*, 10th ed.). We live in several households that can be represented by the following four overlapping but asymmetrical circles:

1.   the family and those who are related to it psychologically or by physical propinquity (the primary household);
2.   the mercantile community;
3.   the civic community, especially as defined by governments; and
4.   the environmental community, both physical and cultural.

All facets of life, including frailty, are influenced by and influence these "households." Only when there is harmony in the interactions within and among the households or economies can personal and community well-being, the goal of ethics, be achieved and maintained. Each household makes use of different instruments to bring about desired exchanges and outcomes. In the instance of the primary community, the instruments include love, fear, guilt, duty, and perceived utility. The desire for the accumulation and spending of income and wealth is the instrument fueling the mercantile community. The instrument of government is public policy enforced by incentives, usually monetary, and sanctions in the case of "bad behavior." The physical aspect of the environmental community functions within its own internal laws (its instruments), with humans using or misusing it within the context of these natural interactions and capacities. The cultural facet of the environment embodies the values and aspirations, for better or worse, of individuals and the communities of the world. The instruments through which it functions are memories, aspirations, social expectancies, and various media of communication within and among generations.

The glue that could bring about some harmonization of these various households is ethics, that is, a world vision and basic values found in various formal declarations such as the U.S. Constitution, the Universal Declaration of Human Rights, the Ten Commandments, and the Sermon on the Mount. In a less formal way, this vision and these values are communicated preeminently in families.

Ethical issues (issues concerning doing the right thing) arise in three domains: personal, corporate, and societal.

Personal

The personal domain involves individuals and their choices throughout the life course, when well and when frail, and all those others with whom they have interactions. These interactions are marked with a variety of moral values and disvalues—love, concern, respect, and prudence or, conversely, selfishness, thoughtlessness, harshness, and profligacy. Others with whom there is a moral/ psychological bond can also evidence such values in their behaviors. We live in moral space with its particular moral field; that is to say, our behavior and well-being both influence and are influenced by others. The "others" may be proximate and individually identifiable such as in the instance of family members, co-workers, and neighbors. Other "others," as in the case of those in the same political jurisdictions, are not individually identifiable, except for public leaders. However, presence in civic "collectivities" (the moral spaces of the citizen) and each person's interaction with the collectivities influences and is influenced to the degree this person participates in the civic dialogue and in turn benefits (or not) from public decisions. Last but not least, we live in a human community upon which each of our individual decisions has an impact. The ethical flow in these relationships is proportionate to the influence of the relationship on another's or the others' well-being. To the degree a person has power over others, certain obligations are generated. To the degree that a person is lacking in power but her or his situation can be ameliorated by another or others, an obligation is generated by the moral tie for the other(s) to make up for that lack in power.

In the light of the potential frailty that all people face, personal responsibility includes making good economic choices throughout life. Saving money, using assets wisely, and caring for one's health are examples of good choices that can positively affect potential frailty. Personal responsibility is not fulfilled by taking care of the self alone, though. Reaching out with physical and emotional assistance to family members, neighbors, co-workers, and people in the community who are frail is a value-laden response to the personal, interpersonal, and societal event of frailty. Reaching out in this way may result in reciprocal action if one then becomes frail. However, that is not the prime reason for doing so. From an ethical perspective, it is the right response in an interdependent world.

The Long-Term-Care Provider (Corporate)

Ethics should have an influence on the long-term-care provider's behavior both in terms of its mission and in terms of the mode of its encounter with the frail person. Often frail persons are agency dependent whether the provider is an institution or a home care provider. Such agencies have a responsibility for the care of the frail person and for the moral space within which care is given and decisions are made that affect the well-being of the frail person. The greater the frailty and the more dependent the frail person is on the agency, the greater the ethical responsibility of the agency.

Ethics, Public Policy, and Long-Term Care (Societal)

Public policy is based on people's perception of *the good* for themselves or for all. Because of the economic vulnerability of frail people, government is an actor in assuring access to needed services and in overseeing quality. A fundamental ethical issue is whether and for whom government should perform these functions. A second, but nonetheless morally significant, question is how and under what circumstances government should be involved in preventing or ameliorating frailty. A third consideration is the standing of the ethical/moral warrant of frailty in the light of other demands for governmental action. In fact, these quandaries are decided in the political realm, in which ethics/morals may play little more than a justifying rationale for actions taken, though one would hope they would play a more significant role.

The concept of a just society is a fundamental element in the ethical discourse about government and frailty. Every person is involved in continual transactions with persons, institutions, and, indeed, the environment in the quest for a satisfying life. Power is an essential in all these interactions—the power of a person to influence others and the power of others to influence the person. In transactions, power can be moral and/or psychological; economic (because money moves people to do things they would otherwise not do); and civil (when government action and public policy order, promote, or inhibit individual and group behaviors).

Frail people have needs. Those with modest or no financial assets are dually compromised. The fundamental issue is how society generally, and government specifically, responds to these needs. Frailty involves the diminution of power even as the ability to negotiate the challenges of everyday life decreases. The frail person's "needs" generate an ethical warrant for resources that may entail some cost or dislocation on the part of another or all others. Note the term *ethical warrant*, a demand rooted in the concept of fundamental human dignity and respect for the person.

Social Justice

Social justice is a phrase that evokes many reactions. For some, its meaning is clear and its pursuit compelling; for others, it is less clear and even generates concern.

Justice is a concept deeply imbedded in the world's sacred writings and philosophical literature. Fundamentally, it means rendering to a person his or her due. It involves both equity and adequacy. With the word *social* is added a dimension of rendering what is due in the variety of relationships that constitute a community.

A tentative working definition or description might characterize a just society as a milieu in which all people have the opportunity for decency (i.e., a life that befits a human being) and in which fairness prevails. Thus, striving for social justice is pursuing strategies and tactics to promote values and structures that afford such decency. Borg (2001, p. 139) explains social justice this way in *Reading the Bible Again for the First Time:* "More comprehensive than criminal justice and procedural justice, social justice is concerned with the structures of society and their results. Because it is results-oriented, it discerns whether the structures of society—in other words, the social system as a whole—are just in their effects. Do they produce a large impoverished class or result in a more equitable distribution of resources?"

Striving for social justice connotes a conscious effort to encourage relationships between and among individuals that respect and implement what is owed. Understanding the significance of social justice begins with an understanding of the fundamental interdependence of all people. Each of us lives at a particular time and place, in relationship with the past and the future, as well as with others in families, neighborhoods, local communities, and even the world community. We live in social, political, cultural, and physical environments that we have inherited, interact with in the present, and will pass on to subsequent generations. We are the beneficiaries of those who have gone before us and who have enabled us to have the opportunity for decency. Generations will follow us to whom we have the responsibility to bequeath the things necessary for the good life, such as a sustainable physical environment, enabling social structures, and an ennobling set of cultural values.

For some persons, the inheritance has not been benign. By accident of birth or social upheaval, some find themselves in oppressive poverty and political regimes. Some squander their inheritance. Some, individuals and groups, become resigned to their diminished state; others struggle for a better, more congenial life, occasionally by peaceful means and at other times through violence. Pragmatism and self-interest would dictate that the *haves* make efforts that work toward assuaging the hurts of the *have-nots*. Harlan Cleveland wrote in the October 23, 2003, issue of the *WorldPaper* that "the swamp of poverty, unemployment and desperation in which terrorism thrives can be drained by getting much more serious about economic and social development" (p. 2).

Well-being is realized within the context of a sense of personal self-worth and responsibility, of people who care for us and for whom we care. It involves nurturing families and neighborhoods; good schools and health services; and recreational and cultural activities. It also involves a safe and stimulating milieu and, for many, a religious community. The interactions of all these factors contribute to and are necessary prerequisites for a just society. Moving in this direction is to some degree countercultural, because it is contrary to the celebration of autonomy, rights, and freedom, all important values, but expressions that can easily become code words for self-centeredness and a lack of concern for others.

Each of the major world religions has its own version of the Golden Rule, saying that people should treat others the way they would like others to treat them. Thus, justice involves responsibilities as well as rights. It entails individual and shared ingenuity, creativity, and industry. Social justice includes not only relationships between and among individuals but also relationships of individuals with society and society with individuals. As taught by Aristotle more than 2,300 years ago, a just society is one in which burdens and benefits are shared equally by equals and unequally by unequals in accord with capacity and need. In his pamphlet *Introduction to Social Justice* (1997, p. 27), William Ferree devotes a chapter to the common good, which he refers to as the "object of social justice."

Values and structures underpinning a just society are embodied in culture. Justice is furthered through mediating structures, such as family, voluntary associations, nongovernmental organizations, churches, synagogues, mosques, and temples. Government plays an indispensable, albeit subsidiary, role in promoting and ensuring justice. An educated, politically engaged people sharing at least fundamental values is an essential element in a democratic society striving to be just. The work of justice is carried on (or not carried on) at all levels of human interactions. Social justice requires responsiveness to the most vulnerable, the "unequals" in Aristotle's teachings.

As others become engaged with the frail person, there are difficult transactions to negotiate both with formal and informal (primary) helpers. These transactions include addressing questions such as these: How long should one be able to drive, and who makes the decision? Is home care adequate in light of the person's needs? How long should autonomy prevail over legitimate caring and the legitimate interests of the common good? Are need and dependency artificially induced by good-willed helpers?

In analyzing the response of public policy to the hurts that frailty entails, it can be helpful to consider two species of justice. The first is equity or fairness, which calls for equals to be treated equally and unequals to be treated differentially in accord with capacity and need. The second is adequacy, which calls for provision of what is necessary for decency. These two overriding concepts help frame an ethical approach to public policy.

Ethics, Frailty, and Policy

Within the framework of "striving for a just society," the overall social policy goal is to assure that individuals have what they need to deal with their frailty. The goal is best reached with the appropriate blending of personal effort and interpersonal relationships, commercial activities, and public policy (the primary, mercantile, and civic economies or households).

The universality of frailty—actual or potential, full-blown or mild—in the Third Age, an age to which all aspire and which most will achieve, and the fact that a significant number of people do not have personal means to address its debilitating sequelae have resulted in major public activity in this area, especially since the mid-1960s. Issues that frailty entails are matters of concern for all levels of government, but especially the states as they face mounting Medicaid expenditures for long-term care. However, despite this considerable activity, current policies do not address in a coordinated manner the multiple elements that contribute to frailty, largely because of an undue reliance on nursing homes and a corresponding underdevelopment of home- and community-based services.

No one expression of public policy (i.e., a particular statute) can bring about adequacy or reflect equity, and public policy alone cannot achieve the social policy goal of the amelioration of frailty. Public policy is built on personal and interpersonal values and behaviors. It assumes, and in some instances encourages or even requires, certain personal choices because these choices have consequences for the common good. Public policy also assumes and even encourages voluntary interactions that can contribute to the goal and are a function of the principle of subsidiarity. In his article "Ten Building Blocks of Catholic Social Teaching," in *America* (1998, p. 4), William J. Byron explained this principle as follows: "The principle of subsidiarity puts a proper limit on government by insisting that no higher level of organization should perform any function that can be handled efficiently and effectively at a lower level of organization by human persons who, individually or in groups, are closer to the problems and closer to the ground."

Each person should have the physical and nonphysical materials for a decent life, especially in frailty. Each individual bears a primary, though not an exclusive, responsibility for developing the resources for decency. However, there is substantial inequality in the ability of individuals to do so. Although everyone bears a responsibility for preserving her or his health, to a greater or lesser degree, frailty is beyond individual control, as are sickness and, ultimately, death.

Adequacy and equity, solidarity and reciprocity, as well as the principles of subsidiarity and the common good, are concepts that help frame an ethical approach to public policy. For public policies to pass ethical muster, they should collectively evidence these values in the real world. Current or proposed policies need to meet the test of appropriately contributing to adequacy. These policies should constitute an equitable burden on those who will contribute to the adequacy. The policies need to reflect our essential oneness as a community with both rights and responsibilities. They ought to encourage individual and community initiatives and cultural diversity.

Adequacy trumps equity, though the latter is a value to be observed to the degree possible. Redistributional schemes may offend against vertical equity but should reflect horizontal equity. As a group, those who do not have adequate resources for decency have a moral claim on society to be treated unequally to compensate for their need. However, those who will contribute to meeting these needs should contribute in a fair and equitable fashion.

To achieve adequacy for some will require burdens on others. The *haves* must help the *have-nots*. Government should strive for adequacy but cannot (and should not) assure sameness of lifestyle, which is the product of personal opportunities, initiatives, choices, and luck. In evaluating the public policy efforts, we must take into consideration the effect of individual behavior before frailty occurs, the impact of voluntary associations, and the effect of statutes, individually and collectively, on frail persons.

There are structural ethical tensions that permeate the policy arena, each of which is value laden. Examples of these tensions include determining the appropriate (a) blend of personal and public responsibilities; (b) role of family vis-à-vis public responsibilities; (c) proportion of social insurance and/or welfare approaches; (d) role of voluntary and philanthropic activities vis-à-vis government activities; (e) mix of cash, vouchers, or direct services; (f) use of an income and/or service approach; (g) blend of medical and/or social support services; and (h) relative responsibilities of federal, state, and local governments. The latter is particularly significant given their differing taxing capacities and approaches to eligibility.

Public Policy and Personal Behavior before Frailty

One way governments at both federal and state levels are attempting to minimize their actual and potential liability in meeting the needs of frail people is by enacting incentives in the tax code to encourage saving and voluntary risk sharing. One example is a tax incentive for long-term-care insurance. Unfortunately, those most at risk financially are those in low-paying jobs with modest benefit programs. They are the least likely to be able to save, because they need their earnings to meet current expenses.

Public Policy and Voluntary Activities to Meet the Needs of Frail People

Historically, the voluntary sector has offered programs to care for frail people. Religiously and ethnically based housing and nursing facilities have long been part of communities. Older Americans Act funds have enabled many neighborhood organizations to provide food and social programs for frail elders. These voluntary associations and activities give evidence of both personal and civic virtues of caring for those in need. Though no substitute for broad governmental actions, they are an important expression of civic solidarity and concern for others, ideals in an ethically sensitive society.

The growing need has generated response from entrepreneurs in the private sector who provide specialized housing, nursing care, and support services for the private-pay market. They are engaged in *doing good* (i.e., meeting the needs of frail people) and simultaneously *doing well* (i.e., making a profit on the provision of services). Such efforts are an important source of capital and offer alternatives to those who can afford them.

Governments have responded to real or potential exploitation of frail people in the private sector with consumer protection techniques, such as licensure, survey and certification of service providers, and consumer hotlines. Governments have encouraged private initiatives in both the for-profit and nonprofit sectors with both capital and operating funds in housing and social services. Furthermore, governments have allowed entitlements in Medicare and Medicaid to be used in nonpublic institutions.

Public Policy in Support of Frail People

Public policy addresses the economic needs of persons who are out of the workforce through broad entitlement programs of social insurance and welfare. As such, both kinds of programs attend to the adequacy needs of the general population, including frail people. However, the programs are not designed to meet all such needs, either alone or in tandem. When it comes to retirement economic security, Social Security is one leg of a three-legged stool, the others being personal savings and retirement programs. Supplemental Security Income, a means-tested program, provides a modest income, but it is hardly sufficient to meet all the needs of many frail persons.

Medicare and Medicaid are analogues to Social Security and Supplemental Security Income. Medicare serves as a base of payments for acute services but does not address the social support often needed by frail people. Medicaid offers comprehensive medical and support services, but only after personal resources are greatly diminished. Additionally, the range of services and the degree of frailty triggering them may be quite limiting. In short, for the most frail there is virtual universal access only to a narrow range of services and only at substantial cost, even to the point of personal impoverishment.

Two overlapping but often diverging approaches have yet to be fully resolved in public policy. One is largely market driven, in which individuals are assumed to have personal financial resources to develop various strategies to deal with their frailty. The other is a public-policy-driven approach, in which government helps to alleviate the disparities through programs that it will subsidize for those who do not have the means to cobble together their own support systems.

This seemingly dichotomous approach is not altogether distinct because the financial capacity to develop one's own program in most instances includes Medicare and Social Security, as well as private savings and pension programs. Even for people with low income and assets, there is some movement toward providing cash and sometimes counseling to enable individuals to develop their own support systems.

Public Policy and the Future

Long-term-care policy is on the front burner both in Washington and in state capitals. One issue in the civic discussion is how to pay for services that mitigate frailty. Another is the concern about changing family patterns and the status of women, changes that are likely to shrink the number of primary care-givers and concomitantly increase the demands on the formal care sector. Currently long-term care is dependent on poorly paid and mostly female frontline personnel. Costs in long-term care are likely to increase with a shortage of all personnel and increased unionization of such workers. Medicaid expenditures of the states for long-term care are a heavy burden. Although frail people have a preference to remain at home as long as possible, the lack of sufficient home- and community-based services leads to an overuse of the more costly institutional care. Only a portion of the frail elderly people living their last days in the more costly nursing homes are living in the homelike and resident-centered institutions they desire.

Conclusion

The virtual universality in the human journey of greater or lesser frailty, with its associated costs to individuals, families, and society, makes it a matter of public concern. Using frailty as a basis for policy helps to better understand what is to be addressed in policy: economic security, protective and supportive environments, services, and medical care.

Public policies such as found in the Americans with Disabilities Act, Medicare, Medicaid, Social Security, and Supplemental Security Income all have great significance in how frailty plays itself out for individuals and populations. However, the idiosyncratic elements in frailty make it difficult to design programs and support that meet the needs of all.

In summary, the virtual universality of progressive, if intermittent, frailty in the Third Age, with its costs to individuals, families, and society in general, should mean and likely will mean changes in current approaches. Key considerations need recognition in building an ethically sound frailty policy. Frailty is idiosyncratic in both when and how it develops, as well as in the personal and environmental factors that can either ameliorate or exacerbate it. These realities make it difficult to develop programs that will match need and capacity with precision. There are costs involved in ameliorating frailty, but they will be incurred in different ways by different people with diverse needs and resources. It is in the public interest to develop equitable means to support frail people and to reduce the burden on state governments. Equity and social solidarity dictate that government benefits be dependent on need rather than geography;

that is, benefits need to be national in scope rather than on a state-by-state basis. Equity would further suggest that the tax base for benefits would be founded in "capacity to pay" and be similarly structured for all Americans. Adequacy should take into account individual effort over a lifetime, as well as the ability or, better, the inability, of persons to provide for their future needs during their work lives. Such a life-span approach suggests a combination of social insurance, personal savings, and private insurance. Social insurance has the advantages of risk sharing and a degree of prefunding, while the individual savings and insurances allow for personal responsibility. Adequacy and subsidiarity supply the moral perspective both for maximizing choice in the type of benefit available in a social insurance approach and for a residual needs-based program for those with inadequate financial resources for needed help.

To respond to these observations and assertions, I suggest consideration of a social insurance approach to establish a resource floor for frailty through which the economic burden and risks would be widely shared. The triggering mechanism for a benefit under this approach would be disability. The benefit would be tied to the degree of disability, and the individual would be able to use the benefit in accord with his or her needs and resources in a setting of his or her choice, whether in a residential setting or in the home.

Because this would be a basic benefit, a residual means-tested program would be necessary for the poor. By the same token, there would continue to be an incentive for persons to save and/or participate in voluntary supplemental risk sharing, such as long-term-care insurance.

This approach, with its equitable funding base, would reflect social solidarity, contribute to adequacy, and relieve economic and psychological burdens while encouraging individual prudence and a responsive marketplace.

I think the most meaningful issues for further research and inquiry are these:

1. The concept of the Third Age, with inevitable diminution of physiological capacity, should be subject to continued testing, because it has such significant social consequences.
2. The social, psychological, political, and financial implications of a four- or in some instances five-generational society deserve study from a variety of perspectives and disciplines.
3. The needs of retirees for adequate and assured income in relationship to the needs of current workers for decency while they transfer some

of the fruits of their labors to the retirees are in need of constant evaluation.

4. The multifactorial description and utility of *frailty* as used in this chapter should be subjected to scrutiny.

5. The possibility and desirability of a "public ethic" in an era of autonomy, independence, and private ownership are worthy of reflection.

REFERENCES

Borg, M. J. 2001. *Reading the Bible Again for the First Time: Taking the Bible Seriously but Not Literally.* San Francisco: HarperSanFrancisco.

Byron, W. J. 1998. Ten building blocks of Catholic social teaching. *America,* October 31. Available at www.americamagazine.org/articles/Byron.htm.

Cleveland, H. 2003. Assaying the Bush team's logic. *WorldPaper.* www.worldpaper.com/archive/2003/october_23/october1.html (page now discontinued).

Ferree, W. J. 1997. *Introduction to Social Justice.* Arlington, VA: Center for Economic and Social Justice; St. Louis: Social Justice Review of the Central Bureau, CCVA. Available at www.cesj.org/thirdway/socialjustice/introtosocialjustice.pdf.

Hayflick, L. 1996. *How and Why We Age.* New York: Ballantine Books.

U.S. Census Bureau. 2003. Population by age, 1900 to 2002. In *Statistical Abstract of the United States, 2003.* No. HS-3. Available at www.census.gov/statab/hist/HS-03.pdf.

U.S. Department of Health and Human Services, Centers for Disease Control and Prevention, National Center for Health Statistics. 2003. Table 27. Available at www.cdc.gov/nchs/data/hus/tables/2003/03hus027.pdf.

CHAPTER FOUR

Religiosity and Spirituality at the End of Life

Challenges and Opportunities

Lucy Feild, Ph.D., R.N.

The vast majority of Americans consider themselves to be spiritual beings, regardless of their membership in an organized religion. In a Gallup poll (2004) of adults in this country, 90 percent professed a belief in God, 84 percent considered religion to be at least a fairly important part of their lives, and 56 percent reported attending a worship service at least once a month. Only 8 percent of this group were convinced that heaven did not exist.

Despite the pervasive influence of religiosity and spirituality in American culture, as well as their importance to people who are coping with advancing age or life-limiting illness (Ainlay and Smith, 1984; Koenig, Moberg, and Kvale, 1988; Stefanek, McDonald, and Hess, 2005), this dimension has until recently received less attention than biophysical issues such as pain and symptom management in end-of-life research (George, 2002). Studies of religious and spiritual matters are also recent additions to the gerontological literature, with scholarly interest accelerating only since the mid-1990s (Atchley, 2005).

We wish for ourselves and our loved ones that the end of life be a time marked by comfort and peace. Yet we know that too many of those who are dying still experience varying degrees of physical, psychological, or existential suffering that is insufficiently recognized or treated (Teno et al., 2004). In an effort to correct these shortcomings, the focus of attention has expanded to include the quality of dying and achievement of a "good death" (e.g., Field and Cassel, 1997; Steinhauser et al., 2000b). A consistent finding in such research is that people who are dying consider religious/spiritual well-being to be as important as physical comfort at this stage of their lives.

This chapter provides an overview of the current status of knowledge development on religiosity and spirituality at the end of life, with an emphasis on recent advances. It begins with a review of the conceptual and methodological challenges that investigators are currently facing and that have affected the quality of work accomplished so far. Then, relevant findings regarding religiosity and spirituality are considered in three areas: life-threatening illness, the time near the end of life, and bereavement. A section on the relevance of these constructs in clinical care includes discussions of research concerning patient preferences, clinician involvement, and care practices. A set of recommendations for future inquiry is also offered.

Conceptual Issues

This section considers the meanings of religiosity and spirituality, examines theoretical perspectives that provide the framework for discovery of new knowledge, and discusses the influence of cultural backgrounds in the study of religiosity and spirituality.

Definitional Inconsistencies

Conceptual clarity is an essential first step in knowledge development. The lack of consensus regarding definitions of religiosity and spirituality results in these terms being operationally defined in sometimes disparate ways. Such inconsistency interferes with comparisons across studies and slows both scientific progress and clinical application.

The meanings of religiosity and spirituality are still evolving. Although the terms are frequently used interchangeably, most scholars agree that *religiosity* and *spirituality* apply to distinct but related constructs that are each complex, latent, culture-bound, and multidimensional, with consensus on their individual dimensions yet to be achieved (Miller and Thoresen, 2003). The lay public, however, usually makes few distinctions between the two terms. Qualitative work with elders and patients describes tendencies to define *spirituality* primarily in religious terms or inclusive of core religious beliefs, but nonreligious aspects are also relevant (Daaleman, Cobb, and Frey, 2001; Hermann, 2001).

Religiosity is rooted in religion and reflects one's affiliation with an organized set of beliefs, doctrines, values, traditions, and rituals, the primary function of which is usually to know God (Hill and Pargament, 2003; Sulmasy, 2002). At the end of life, religion provides both a structural framework for comprehending life events and a foundation for ethical decision making regarding end-of-life care (Clarfield, Gordon, Markwell, and Alihhai, 2003; Daaleman and VandeCreek, 2000). For those who anticipate an afterlife, faith-based religiosity can serve to draw one closer to God while preparing to leave this world for the one to come, but it may also engender distress in those who fear divine judgment or punishment (Koenig, 2002).

Spirituality is generally more broadly defined, often conceived as more personal, individual, and subjective than religiosity. While it frequently encompasses one's religious beliefs, it may also be nonreligious. Typical definitions include a search to understand the meaning, purpose, and value of one's life (McClain, Rosenfeld, and Breitbart, 2003; Tanyi, 2002) as well as that which is transcendent or sacred (Hill and Pargament, 2003; Sulmasy, 2002) and links one to the larger universe, including connections with others and with nature (Daaleman et al., 2001; Hermann, 2001). Miller and Thoresen (2003) contend that current conceptions of spirituality reflect the strong influence of Western culture and Protestant Christianity.

Spirituality may gain added significance as the end of life draws near. For example, Hall (1997, 1998) portrayed spirituality in terminal illness based on more than a decade of research and practice with patients who have advanced HIV. She described a process of self-discovery as persons nearing the end of life searched for meaning within the contexts of their own lives. Such self-discovery involved accepting, loving, and valuing what people found when they looked within themselves. They *became* themselves—authentically and confidently. When this occurred, the consequences were renewal of hope, discovery of meaning, strengthened relationships, and, for some, deepened religious faith.

Religiosity and spirituality have been pictured as overlapping circles with both shared and separate characteristics (Miller and Thoresen, 2003), and also as opposing ends of a continuum ranging from the religious/theistic to the spiritual/secular, with recent movement trending toward the spiritual end of the spectrum (McSherry and Cash, 2004). Hill and Pargament (2003), however, caution against polarizing religion and spirituality. They argue that (1) both of these constructs have social and personal aspects, (2) polarizing implies a good-bad dichotomy, with spirituality cast as better than religion, (3) polarizing ignores the fact that most people experience spirituality within the context of their religious traditions, and (4) polarizing could lead to duplication of effort in conceptual and measurement work among investigators.

Theoretical Perspectives

In her critique of the status of research design in end-of-life studies, George (2002) noted that work to this point has been largely atheoretical. This situation persists despite the existence of at least six categories of frameworks that seek to describe and explain the dying process. These models have so far been subjected to little testing. Copp's (1998) review of these theoretical groups labels them stage theories, context-of-awareness theories, dying trajectories, living-dying phase theories, task-based approaches to dying, and readiness-to-die theories. Few of the extant models explicitly attend to religious or spiritual issues encountered as individuals prepare for the end of their lives. The exceptions include Kübler-Ross's (1969) stage theory, which describes bargaining as a stage in which the dying may attempt to negotiate with God for a longer survival; other spiritual issues are not overtly addressed. In addition, Corr's (1992) task-based approach specifically identifies physical, psychological, social, and spiritual dimensions of coping with dying. In this model, those with terminal illness face the task of harnessing spiritual energy in an effort to maintain hope.

Conceptions of the person are particularly influential in determining whether, and to what extent, religious and spiritual dimensions of human existence are considered in end-of-life research. Most contemporary models of end-of-life care, which are person- rather than process-oriented, incorporate spirituality, broadly defined, as a unique and core aspect of humanity (Daaleman and VandeCreek, 2000; Field and Cassel, 1997; Lunney, Foley, Smith, and Gelband, 2003).

Sulmasy's (2002) biopsychosocial-spiritual model of end-of-life care is premised on views of the human person as a "being-in-relationship" that is intrinsically spiritual. Illness disrupts not only the homeostatic balance of relationships within the body, but also the person's relationships with the physical environment, with other persons, and with the transcendent. From this holistic perspective, healing of the person encompasses attention to all relationships, both intrinsic and extrinsic. At the end of life, when hope for cure of illness is relinquished, the person's relationship with the transcendent may be the most important, and perhaps the only, dimension that is amenable to healing. Spiritual healing occurs when issues regarding meaning, value, and relationships are resolved, giving rise to hope, dignity, and forgiveness.

Similarly, Nolan and Mock (2004) propose a conceptual framework for end-of-life care in which the integrity of the person is the organizing concept, with spirituality being the core domain. In this perspective, the spiritual domain predominates at the end of life because of its importance to the person and its utility in transcending the physical and psychological suffering that may accompany the dying process. And in Chochinov's (2002) model of palliative care, finding comfort within the context of one's personal religious or spiritual beliefs contributes to the conservation of dignity as death approaches.

Cultural Influences

The United States is an increasingly multicultural society, with its residents representing all corners of the globe. Considerable regional variations in perspectives are also evident, even when racial and ethnic backgrounds are similar. The wide variety of religious belief systems present within the population adds to the complexity. Cultural, ethnic, and religious diversity enriches life but also raises the potential for misunderstanding whenever persons with differing backgrounds interact. This can be of special concern at the end of life if meaningful personal cultural/spiritual values, beliefs, and traditions that are part of the patient's and family's heritage are unknown to caregivers. Mazanec and Tyler (2003) provide several examples of significant faith-based practices at the end of life, including (1) the importance to many Catholics of receiving the Sacrament of the Sick, a spiritual blessing that incorporates forgiveness of sins, before death; (2) the desire among some Muslims for the bed of the deceased to be turned east toward Mecca at the time of death; and (3) the significance for some Pacific Islanders of leaving a window open for the soul of the dying to escape.

Becoming culturally competent can present an enormous challenge when the sheer number of cultures, ethnicities, and religions in this country is considered. While it may be impossible to master the intricacies of all traditions, cultural sensitivity through careful *individual* assessment can help to minimize barriers that interfere with valued religious practices and rituals at the end of life.

Virtually every author of culturally relevant end-of-life literature stresses the importance of understanding culture and ethnicity from the perspective of each individual, indicating that widely divergent values, beliefs, and customs within groups may be just as pronounced as those found between groups (e.g., Werth, Blevins, Toussaint, and Durham, 2002). Kagawa-Singer and Blackhall (2001, p. 2994) noted the complexities associated with providing culturally sensitive care at the end of life: Failure to take cultural values and beliefs into account is "culturally destructive"; generalizing cultural patterns to all members of a group is "cultural stereotyping"; and insisting that everyone conform to the norms of the dominant culture is "cultural imperialism." To avoid these pitfalls, the best strategy remains careful individual assessment. Understanding cultural patterns, though, can help to discern important factors to assess at the individual and family level.

African American Perspectives

Most of the research so far that pertains to cultural differences at the end of life addresses African American versus Euro-American perspectives (Tennstedt, 2002). Work specifically related to religious and spiritual beliefs primarily concerns African American viewpoints about advance directives and life-sustaining treatment preferences. A considerable body of work has shown that, compared with Euro-Americans, African Americans, who until recently were the largest minority group in this country (Clemetson, 2003), are less likely to complete advance directives, appoint health care proxies, discuss treatment preferences with relatives, and withhold or withdraw life-prolonging treatment, even when hope for recovery is futile (e.g., Eleazer et al., 1996; Blackhall et al., 1999; Hopp and Duffy, 2000). In a sample representative of the southeastern United States, African Americans were twice as likely as Euro-Americans to attribute recovery from illness to God rather than to doctors (Mansfield, Mitchell, and King, 2002). Belief in God's healing power was strongest among evangelical Christians, women, and those who were older, sicker, poorer, and less well-educated.

Several reports (McAuley, Pecchioni, and Grant, 2000; Mouton, 2000; Waters, 2001) provide insight into prevalent African American religious and spiritual beliefs. Embedded in history and tradition, these perspectives may influence patterns manifested near the end of life. Most African Americans are Christian, with strong connections to the Baptist faith. Against a shared background of slavery, poverty, and racial discrimination, they have come to view God as an all-powerful savior who will ultimately rescue believers from suffering and adversity. God does not cause illness, but allows it to occur as a test of faith or as a consequence of sin. He comforts the sick by limiting pain and suffering and sending others to help the sick to cope. Those who remain steadfast in their faith in God's power are willing to wait patiently for his will to manifest itself, sometimes through miracles. God acts through doctors to heal, and prayer can contribute to this outcome, but only God knows and decides when it is "time to die." When death does come, it is accepted as the fulfillment of the promise of everlasting salvation and peace, a belief that offers comfort and hope to both the dying and the bereaved. Advance planning is difficult, not only because death is painful to discuss, but also because it contradicts a belief that one's fate is in God's hands rather than within one's own control. Leaving future care decisions to trusted loved ones or ministers is preferable to documenting one's wishes in writing.

African Americans also use hospice and palliative care services less frequently than do Euro-Americans. One explanation for this difference, shared by some Christians as well as American Muslims, again refers to beliefs that pain and suffering are challenges sent by God as a test of faith in the process of earning salvation. Such suffering is not to be mitigated, as palliative care strives to do, but rather endured with dignity (Crawley et al., 2000).

Hispanic American Perspectives

Hispanic Americans, with 37 million counted in the 2000 census, compared to 36.2 million African Americans, are now the largest minority and the fastest-growing segment of the American population (Clemetson, 2003). It is a heterogeneous group, comprised of multiple, often divergent, subcultures originating in Mexico, Cuba, Puerto Rico, and Central and South America. Talamantes, Gomez, and Braun (2000) provide insight regarding spiritual influences common among members of this group. Hispanic Americans tend to rely strongly on spiritual values to cope with illness and death. Life is valued as a temporary gift, with death as its natural conclusion and afterlife as its reward. God is a source of strength during suffering and illness for both the sick and their caregivers. For some, good and evil spirits influence well-being, and the spirit of the deceased may linger near the body for days after death. Cultural traditions ensure that the dead remain honored and esteemed through numerous faith-based rituals. Family, rather than individual, decision making is the norm. Because of cultural inclinations to be oriented to the present rather than to the future, Hispanic Americans are often reluctant to engage in discussions regarding advance care planning. Those who believe in God's power to work miracles may be hesitant to withhold or withdraw life-sustaining treatment. In one study (Blackhall et al., 1999), for example, 78 percent of Mexican Americans opposed removal of life support for this reason, but interview data indicated that this position was based on a belief that physicians, who are highly respected and trusted in this culture, would not initiate life support if recovery were not possible.

Asian/Pacific Islander Perspectives

Americans of Asian/Pacific Islander heritage trace their origins to more than thirty countries, which represent numerous subcultures. Many cultural traditions and beliefs regarding the end of life are rooted in Eastern religions, including Confucian, Taoist, Buddhist, Hindu, Muslim, and Sikh faiths. Although it is impossible to generalize, several themes common to many Asian cultures include reverence for elders and ancestors, familial duty to provide care for elderly or sick people, family-based rather than autonomous decision making, a reticence to discuss death or disclose the prognosis to the patient, stoicism in the face of suffering, and tendencies to eschew advance directives while favoring life support (Yeo and Hikoyeda, 2000). Several examples from research findings illustrate these points. Chinese followers of Buddhist, Taoist, and Confucian traditions are similar to African Americans in believing that there is a natural time for death; this view contributes to reluctance to engage in advance planning (Eleazer et al., 1996). Buddhists and persons with a high degree of religiosity have been found to favor life support, whereas many Korean Americans would not personally want life support but would expect family members to make decisions to prolong their lives as long as possible, by whatever means, in keeping with the duty of "filial piety" (Blackhall et al., 1999).

Organizational Cultures

One other important but often overlooked cultural influence deserves mention. Most people in this country spend their final days in health care institutions. The organizational cultures and environments of these facilities can serve to respect or diminish the dying person's dignity and integrity, depending on how institutional values, beliefs, and priorities are operationalized (Nolan and Mock, 2004). Work by Teno and colleagues (2004) suggests that much remains to be done within hospitals and nursing homes to correct numerous perceived deficiencies in the quality of end-of-life care. For example, it is necessary to alleviate family concerns about insufficient respect for the patient during the terminal phase of illness—a condition that robs the person of dignity and increases the risk for spiritual distress.

Methodological Issues

Study design and instrumentation are especially challenging in end-of-life research that focuses on religious and spiritual issues. Prominent issues and opportunities for future improvement are considered here.

Research Design Considerations

Specific studies of religiosity and spirituality at the end of life are limited in number in comparison to other relevant dimensions. Much of this work has been qualitative in design. This method is often chosen as a starting point when little is known about a particular topic. Its value is considerable and lies in eliciting descriptions and explaining phenomena from the perspectives of the participants rather the researcher, helping investigators to prioritize topics for future study, generating testable hypotheses, and providing culturally appropriate language for use in instrument development (Tennstedt, 2002; Stefanek et al., 2005). Qualitative studies of terminally ill cancer patients consistently attest to the importance of religion and spirituality in coping with their illness (Stefanek et al., 2005).

Methodological lessons learned from more extensive research concerning the link between religion and health inform similar research at the end of life (see McCullough et al., 2000; Powell, Shahabi, and Thoresen, 2003). Recent analyses provide evidence of common design weaknesses that future researchers would do well to avoid. Deficiencies, such as the absence or poor operationalizing of conceptual definitions, the lack of specific hypotheses, inappropriate research design that fails to match the research question, inadequate sample sizes, convenience sampling, the use of only single-item measures of religiosity or spirituality, and mistaking correlation for cause, have been criticized (Hill and Pargament, 2003; Miller and Thoresen, 2003; Sloan and Bagiella, 2002). Stefanek and colleagues (2005) urge that when researchers plan studies of religiosity and spirituality in terminal illness, more attention be paid to controlling for possible confounding variables, developing explanatory models that describe the pathways linking key variables, and developing instruments that are comprehensive enough to measure the scope of religiosity/spirituality and sufficiently sensitive to capture changes over time.

Because the end of life represents a relatively new field of inquiry, it is understandable that most quantitative studies to date have employed correlational and cross-sectional designs (Tennstedt, 2002). Yet the need is pressing for prospective longitudinal research to follow issues, such as spiritual concerns and spiritual well-being, that patients themselves rate as important, through the dying process (George, 2002). Logistical problems inherent in longitudinal designs, such as recruitment and retention, are amplified when working with those who are terminally ill and elderly, but investigators have demonstrated that these obstacles can be successfully overcome with careful planning (e.g., Emanuel, Fairclough, and Emanuel, 2000; Murray et al., 2004). There is new evidence that, contrary to common assumptions, participating in structured interviews about death and dying is not usually stressful, and in fact may be helpful, for dying patients and their caregivers (Emanuel, Fairclough, Wolfe, and Emanuel, 2004).

Involvement of terminally ill and elderly persons in research at the end of life is based on the premise that they are able and ready to be so involved. But older and sicker persons may have cognitive, sensory, and/or functional impairments that hinder their ability to provide informed consent and affect the validity, reliability, and usefulness of instruments selected to measure complex constructs such as religiosity and spirituality (Tilden, Tolle, Drach, and Hickman, 2002). Of the roughly 2.4 million people who die each year in the United States, about 80 percent are older adults (Lunney et al., 2003). In a study of Medicare decedents, most succumbed to the frailties of advancing age (47%), terminal cancer (22%), or organ failure (16%) (Lunney, Lynn, and Hogan, 2002). At first glance, one might assume that such circumstances, in contrast to sudden-death situations, provide an opportunity to anticipate and prepare for the inevitable end of life, with religious and spiritual needs possibly figuring prominently in this groundwork. The reality, though, is that numerous factors may limit awareness or acceptance of dying, such as cognitive impairment, unpredictable illness trajectories, continuing pursuit of cure or remission, and poor patient-provider communication (Seale, 1991; Kaufman, 2002). In fact, between 30 and 50 percent of decedents in the above groups are cognitively incapacitated for a significant period of time before death (Emanuel et al., 2000).

When terminally ill patients' conditions prevent them from providing information, current or retrospective proxy reports are sometimes obtained from close relatives or caregivers. The validity of such data is likely to be compromised, however, because recall is influenced by both emotions and perceptions (Addington-Hall and McPherson, 2001). Proxy accounts correspond more closely to patient reports for observable signs than for subjective symptoms, and accuracy of retrospective recall declines in the months following the patient's death (Hinton, 1996; Klinkenberg et al., 2004; McPherson and Addington-Hall, 2003). Because religious and spiritual needs are highly personal and private matters, proxy reports for these factors are likely to be even less reliable. Depending on the study aims, longitudinal designs may help to reduce reliance on proxy reports if sufficiently large samples are recruited initially to account for anticipated attrition due to incapacity.

Convenience sampling has been the norm in most end-of-life research to date. Population-based random sampling, however, which allows for generalizability of findings, may not be feasible in many cases. More realistic alternatives include use of multiple sites and settings, explication of inclusion and exclusion criteria, and specification of participation rates, including reasons for refusal (George, 2002).

Instrumentation

In their discussion of measurement issues affecting research on religiosity and spirituality, Hill and Pargament (2003) note that a considerable number of published studies have included brief measures of one or the other of these variables in large-scale epidemiological or sociological studies that were designed to focus on other issues. These measures have frequently been single or global items, such as religious denomination, religious service attendance, or subjective religiosity. Simple items such as these fail to capture the multidimensional complexity of religiosity and spirituality, which include cognitive, emotional, behavioral, social, and even physiological components.

Sulmasy (2002) described four domains of religiosity and spirituality of special relevance to end-of-life researchers. *Religiosity,* the most widely studied of these domains, includes religious denomination (the least predictive of health) as well as religious behaviors, such as religious service attendance and private religious practices (the best predictors). While little is known about the relationship between religiosity and the end of life, it may not be useful to pursue, and questions concerning it may even cause distress to religious individuals whose illness prevents their active participation. *Religious coping* provides more clinically pertinent information in work with dying patients. *Spiritual well-being,* the opposite of spiritual distress, has excellent potential as either an independent or dependent variable in end-of-life research. When included as a dimension of quality of life, it accounts for much of the variance unexplained by psychological dimensions. The domain of *spiritual needs* is also important to both research and practice, but adequate measures are needed.

When choosing instruments to measure religiosity/spirituality at the end of life, it is essential that researchers, in the absence of standardized definitions or "gold-standard" measures, first articulate clear conceptual meanings of the construct(s) to be studied. They then must select valid, reliable instruments that effectively operationalize these definitions and that are suitable for use with the population being studied.

Instruments designed to measure religiosity and spirituality at the end of life are few in number, and the extent of psychometric testing varies. In their critique of eight well-known, published measures of religiosity and spirituality that have been used in medical studies for at least 10 years, Mytko and Knight (1999) reported that only three demonstrated internal consistency reliability over time, and while all had evidence of construct validity, none had yet clearly established predictive validity. In addition, conceptual overlap between spirituality and other psychological variables, such as optimism and self-esteem, has not yet been adequately addressed.

Comparisons of religiosity/spirituality measures are rare. Tuck, McCain, and Elswick (2001) conducted such an investigation to determine the most reliable measure of spirituality for a longitudinal study of spirituality and psychosocial factors among HIV-positive men. The Existential Well-Being subscale of the Spiritual Well-Being Scale (Paloutzian and Ellison, 1982) yielded the most significant correlations with variables such as quality of life, social support, and coping when compared with the Spiritual Health Inventory (Highfield, 1992), which had more items and fewer significant relationships, and the Spiritual Perspectives Scale (Reed, 1986, 1987), in which all relationships were nonsignificant.

Some quality-of-life instruments contain spiritual or religious subscales, but such instruments are generally not transferable to terminally ill populations; furthermore, quality of life differs conceptually from quality of dying (George, 2002). A possible exception may be the spiritual subscale of the World Health Organization's Quality of Life Assessment (WHOQOL) (WHOQOL Group, 1998). This four-item measure ($\alpha = .85$) reflects meaning in life as well as the influence of personal beliefs on coping with difficulties in life. The unique multicultural, multilingual development process for the WHOQOL may make this subscale appealing to researchers working with culturally and linguistically diverse populations (Power, Bullinger, Harper, and WHOQOL Group, 1999).

The *Toolkit of Instruments to Measure End-of-Life Care* (TIME) (Puchalski, 2001) is a bibliography of instruments for measuring the quality of care for dying patients. This project was funded by the Nathan Cummings Foundation and the Robert Wood Johnson Foundation. The toolkit contains a section on spirituality. It briefly describes 25 measures published between 1967 and 1997 and grouped into four categories (quality of life, attitudes, religiosity, and spirituality). Nine of the most promising are discussed in detail. Of these, four instruments contain especially relevant items that the author suggested could be selected to form a shorter composite to be tested with dying patients. These four measures are the Spiritual Well-Being Scale (Paloutzian and Ellison, 1982), the Death Transcendence Scale (VandeCreek and Nye, 1993), the Herth Hope Scale (Herth, 1992), and the Meaning in Life Scale (Warner and Williams, 1987).

Another potentially valuable reference contains several subscales that have been used in end-of-life studies. The *Multidimensional Measurement of Religiousness/Spirituality for Use in Health Research* (Fetzer Institute, 1999) represents a collaborative effort of a working group of experts supported by the Fetzer Institute and the National Institute on Aging. The volume contains recommended instruments, including their psychometric properties, for 12 key domains of religiosity/spirituality for use in the study of health outcomes. These domains are Daily Spiritual Experiences, Meaning, Values, Beliefs, Forgiveness, Private Religious Practices, Religious/Spiritual Coping, Religious Support, Religious/Spiritual History, Commitment, Organizational Religiousness, and Religious Preference. Of these, the Religious/Spiritual Coping and the Daily Spiritual Experience Scale have been the most widely used and may be the most helpful to end-of-life researchers. Conceptual development and psychometric testing have been reported in detail (Idler et al., 2003).

Relevant Research Findings

Research findings that concern religiosity and spirituality at the end of life are organized according to three contexts: life-threatening illness, being near the end of life, and bereavement.

Religiosity and Spirituality in Life-Threatening Illness

Because research concerning the relationship between religiosity/spirituality and serious illness is relatively recent, it is not surprising that the studies described below are relatively few in number. Their designs were cross-sectional; most employed single settings and convenience samples that varied in size. Patients with cancer, HIV infection, and acute medical illness were the most common populations studied. Conceptual categories included patient meanings, coping with serious illness, maintaining hope, adjustment to illness, relationship to health outcomes, advance planning, and mastery.

Patient Meanings

The meanings that persons with serious illness ascribe to terms such as *religious* or *spiritual* are poorly understood. Two studies have addressed this issue.

The first was a qualitative study of Australians living from three to eight years with hematological malignancies (McGrath, 2004). Patients described spirituality primarily in secular terms as an existential journey that will continue for the remainder of their lives. Their illness forced them to confront issues of mortality and to find meaning and purpose in both their lives and their illness. As a result the patients found opportunities for *spiritual comfort,* including feelings of protection that calmed fears, personal growth, and a share in the responsibility for recovery. But the comfort was balanced by *spiritual pain,* in which positive meanings were challenged as a result of suffering endured from unwanted illness.

The second study used mostly structured interviews to elicit seriously ill patients' views on their own spirituality and religiosity (Woods and Ironson, 1999). Findings were consistent with deductively derived definitions. Those who self-identified as religious were more likely to view God as an external, powerful force *to* whom they were connected through a system of beliefs, rules, and rituals shared with members of a religious community in which the goal is to earn salvation. Those who described themselves as spiritual, in contrast, were more likely to find God within themselves, with a stronger focus on personal beliefs and values and with greater emphasis on connections *with* God, others, and the environment.

Coping with Serious Illness

Results of several studies suggest an association between religious/spiritual beliefs and active cognitive coping styles in the presence of life-threatening illness. This coping approach refers to accepting one's illness and reframing it in a positive and meaningful way. Holland et al. (1999) found that patients with malignant melanoma who had strong religious and spiritual beliefs were more likely to cope with their illness in an active cognitive style, even when differences in age, gender, education, and stage of illness were taken into account. Daugherty et al. (2005) found a similar coping pattern among advanced cancer patients who volunteered for phase 1 clinical trials. Subjects in this study had higher levels of spirituality than nonvolunteers with similarly poor prognoses, and frequently these subjects used a collaborative style of religious problem solving, in which they reported working with (rather than deferring to or ignoring) God in seeking solutions; this style extended to working with their doctors to find an effective treatment. In response to open-ended questions, they discussed being simultaneously realistic about their expectations of experimental treatment and hopeful for positive outcomes. As a result, some could plan their own funerals while also discussing long-term plans for the future.

In two large samples of older, mostly Protestant, hospitalized medical patients in North Carolina, active religious participation and strong intrinsic religious attitudes prevailed, and participants relied on their religious beliefs as the predominant means of coping with their illnesses (Koenig, 1998; Koenig, George, and Titus, 2004). In the later study, religiosity and spirituality were also associated with stronger social support and less depressive symptomatology.

One of the most common religious coping practices is prayer. Although widely assumed to be helpful, there is preliminary evidence that prayer can be associated with spiritual conflicts and even interfere with coping with serious illness, depending on personal meanings attached to it (Taylor, Outlaw, Bernardo, and Roy, 1999).

Maintaining Hope

Several investigations have reported evidence of a relationship between hope and religious/spiritual beliefs/practices among those living with HIV. Heinrich's (2003) study of HIV-positive men at various stages of illness demonstrated that spirituality had a direct, positive effect on hope. In a similar study, HIV-positive women prayed significantly more than did a comparable group of uninfected women, but while prayer was less useful to them as a coping mechanism, more frequent prayer did predict higher levels of optimism (Biggar et al., 1999).

Adjustment to Illness

Spiritual well-being has been shown to be positively related to psychosocial adjustment among women receiving hemodialysis for end-stage renal disease (Tanyi and Werner, 2003), men living with HIV (Tuck et al., 2001), and women with breast cancer (Cotton et al., 1999). In the breast cancer study, though, spiritual well-being contributed minimally to quality of life after controlling for demographic variables and social support. Schnoll, Harlow, and Brower (2000) found that spiritual well-being served as a mediator between demographic variables and psychosocial adjustment in a heterogeneous sample of cancer patients. Their mediational model accounted for 64 percent of the variance in psychosocial adjustment. In a qualitative study, older HIV-positive adults described numerous positive psychosocial benefits derived from religious and spiritual beliefs and practices, including comfort, strength, reduced emotional burden, social and spiritual support, reduced fear, and self-acceptance (Siegel and Schrimshaw, 2002).

Relationship to Health Outcomes

Findings regarding the relationship between religiosity/spirituality and health outcomes are mixed. Koenig (1998) found that religiosity was associated with higher social support, lower depression, and lower illness burden (number and severity of comorbid conditions). Heinrich (2003), however, found no direct effect of spirituality on health, whereas King, Speck, and Thomas (1994) observed that hospitalized patients with strong religious and/or spiritual beliefs had poorer health outcomes. This negative preliminary finding was duplicated in King, Speck, and Thomas's 1999 study in which hospitalized cardiac and gynecological patients with stronger spiritual beliefs, regardless of religiosity, were more than twice as likely to have experienced either no improvement or a decline in health status nine months later. These discrepant findings could be attributable to methodological or sample differences.

Advance Planning

Although religious denomination is generally considered to have little predictive value, investigators who used hypothetical scenarios with a group of hospitalized veterans found that Catholics, compared to other Christians, consistently preferred to forgo life-sustaining treatment (Heeren, Menon, Raskin, and Ruskin, 2001). This difference, however, was statistically significant only for tube feedings. Using a similar strategy with older black and white participants, Cicirelli (1997) found that greater subjective religiosity was one of several variables associated with preferences for continuing life-sustaining treatment regardless of illness severity. One study of hospitalized HIV-positive patients found that those with negative religious attitudes and low religious participation were less likely to engage in advance care planning and more likely to fear death (Kaldjian, Jekel, and Friedland, 1998).

Mastery

One study was found in which spiritual beliefs and attitudes among HIV-positive patients were shown to predict mastery over stress (Gray and Cason, 2002).

Religiosity and Spirituality Near the End of Life

The studies in this section primarily use quantitative methods. While limited in number, several are particularly well designed, with large, randomly selected samples recruited from multiple sites and/or more than one data collection point. Topics include the meaning of a good death, patterns of religiosity/spirituality near the end of life, the place of death, and the desire for a hastened death.

The Meaning of a Good Death

In a study of factors considered important at the end of life, most seriously ill patients included aspects of a religious or spiritual nature—achieving a sense of life completion, being able to help others, coming to peace with God, and praying—as attributes of a good death (Steinhauser et al., 2000a). These characteristics, however, were considered significantly less important by physicians. Coming to peace with God and freedom from pain achieved nearly identical top rankings from both dying patients and a separate group of recently bereaved family members.

Achieving peace with God also emerged as a component of a good death in a qualitative study of men with terminal cancer or end-stage heart disease (Vig and Pearlman, 2004). Conversely, being "not right with God" was identified as an attribute of a bad death (p. 979).

A good death may include spirituality in the absence of a religious component, as evidenced by a case report describing preparations for the end of life by a man with terminal cancer (Block, 2001). This person was able to transcend his experience of suffering as he prepared to take leave of loved ones by finding meaning in his connection with the natural rhythm of the universe.

Patterns of Religiosity/Spirituality Near the End of Life

Data drawn from the Established Populations for Epidemic Logic Studies for the Elderly examined patterns of religious practice and belief in the last year of life (Idler, Kasl, and Hays, 2001). This longitudinal study, conducted between 1982 and 1996, used a stratified weighted sample of elderly people drawn from the New Haven, Connecticut, area. Attendance at church declined in the six months before death in conjunction with deteriorating health and functional levels, but even then occurred about once a month. Subjective religiosity, assessed by how religious the participants considered themselves to be and how much comfort and strength they derived from their faith, which had been high in earlier data collection points, did not decline and even slightly increased as death neared.

Murray et al. (2004) found that spiritual needs of older patients dying from lung cancer or heart failure followed different trajectories that paralleled their illness courses. In this qualitative study conducted in Scotland, patients and their caregivers were interviewed up to five times over the course of a year. For lung cancer patients, spiritual needs peaked at the time of initial diagnosis and then again when they were near death. For the heart failure patients, spiritual needs remained constant throughout their illness and were associated with feelings of isolation, hopelessness, and loss of confidence. Both patients and caregivers had spiritual needs, and while some welcomed the opportunity to discuss them, others considered attempts to discuss them an invasion of personal privacy and not within the purview of health professionals. Those who were reticent to address spiritual concerns struggled alone for often extended periods.

The Place of Death

Between 1980 and 1998, there was a steady decline in hospital deaths (from 54% to 41%), with a concomitant rise in deaths occurring at home or in nursing homes (both 22% in 1998) in the United States (Flory et al., 2004). Considerable racial differences in place of death persist, with whites less likely to die in acute care settings; this pattern cannot be explained by other demographic variables (Iwashyna and Chang, 2002). Little is known about the quality of care at the end of life in general, and religious/spiritual care in particular, in non-hospital settings. The concept of hospice, which encompasses physical, emotional, and spiritual comfort at the end of life and can be provided in a variety of settings, is considered the "gold standard" of care, but only 7 percent of dying elders receive hospice care (Mezey, Dubler, Mitty, and Brody, 2002).

Two studies examined the quality of life, including spirituality, of terminally ill patients enrolled in hospice programs. Among cancer patients admitted to one of five palliative care units, Cohen, Boston, Mount, and Porterfield (2001) noted a significant improvement in existential well-being after one week. Supplemental qualitative interviews provided evidence of increases in spiritual awareness, thoughts about the afterlife, and acceptance, as well as both greater and lesser degrees of hope and religious participation. In Tang, Aaronson, and Forbes's (2004) research, participants were mostly older cancer patients who had been receiving in-home hospice care for almost 29 days at the time of data collection. In this sample, spirituality was positively correlated with quality of life and, along with social support and living-with-caregiver status, was a significant predictor of quality of life.

The Desire for a Hastened Death

A growing number of studies have documented that a transient desire for a hastened death is not uncommon among terminally ill patients. It is typically associated with one or more symptoms of psychological or existential suffering, including depression, hopelessness, not feeling appreciated, or frustration with dependency, but not usually with physical suffering such as pain or declining physical function. Breitbart et al. (2000) found that palliative-care patients with clinical depression were four times more likely than nondepressed patients to wish to die sooner. Several investigators have reported an association between such wishes and low scores on measures of spiritual well-being

(Chibnall, Videen, Duckro, and Miller, 2002; McClain et al., 2003; McClain-Jacobson et al., 2004). These clinical manifestations have been variously termed *death distress* (Chibnall et al., 2002) or *death despair* (McClain et al., 2003) but are also indicative of spiritual distress. Chibnall and colleagues (2002) suggest that spirituality may buffer the death-related anxiety and depression that some people experience as they approach the end of their lives.

Several points regarding wishes for hastened death are clinically important. (1) Such wishes are not stable: vacillating between wishing to die sooner and hoping to survive longer is common. Typical predictors of such waverings have not yet been established (Wolfe et al., 1999; Emanuel et al., 2000; Kelly et al., 2002). (2) Wishes for a hastened death are not synonymous with suicidal ideation, a rare occurrence among the dying (Block, 2001; Kelly et al., 2002). (3) The underlying suffering is treatable if recognized, underscoring the need for ongoing assessment as well as attention to both psychological and spiritual needs among dying patients (Emanuel et al., 2000; Kelly et al., 2002; McClain-Jacobson et al., 2004).

Religiosity and Spirituality in Bereavement

Research concerning religiosity/spirituality and bereavement is limited. Three unrelated studies discussed here illustrate both the opportunity and the need for further work in this area.

Fry (2001) found that spiritual self-efficacy was one of a number of predictors of life satisfaction and self-esteem among older, white, generally healthy Canadian widows, but this did not hold true for widowers. In a separate prospective study of bereaved spouses, children, or close friends, those with strong spiritual beliefs experienced gradual but steady grief resolution over 14 months, those with weaker beliefs continued to grieve for 9 months before experiencing a more rapid resolution of symptoms, and those without spiritual beliefs had unresolved grief at 14 months following the death of a loved one (Walsh et al., 2002). This finding is consistent with earlier work cited by Koenig (2002). Keeley (2004) conducted a qualitative study of survivors' recollections of final conversations with a dying loved one. Most of these discussions included religious or spiritual themes that served to comfort the bereaved and guide them as they faced the future without the deceased.

The Clinical Relevance of Religiosity/Spirituality in End-of-Life Care

This section examines patients' views regarding the role of health care providers in addressing their religious/spiritual needs, issues related to providers' involvement in this area, and the kinds of religious and spiritual care being offered or suggested in clinical practice for those who are terminally ill.

Patients' Perspectives on Clinicians' Involvement in Religious/Spiritual Issues

While patients consistently acknowledge the importance of religion/spirituality as they face serious illness and death, their views regarding the physician's role in addressing these concerns vary a great deal. Their views regarding the involvement of other clinicians is less known. Generalizability of the findings described here is in most cases limited by undefined terms, nonrandom sampling at single sites, untested investigator-developed instruments, and geographic bias.

Assessment

Generally, patients favor physician awareness of their religious/spiritual beliefs and find assessment of these beliefs acceptable under certain circumstances, but not as a routine part of medical practice. In a small Vermont study, 52 percent of participants agreed that physicians had a right to ask about spiritual beliefs, but only 21 percent considered it an obligation (Maughans and Wadland, 1991). A multisite survey of primary care patients in North Carolina, Florida, and Vermont found that two-thirds believed their physicians should be aware of their religious or spiritual beliefs, but only one-third felt that this dimension should be routinely assessed in office visits, and still fewer (10%) would be willing to trade time spent on medical problems for discussion of spiritual issues (MacLean et al., 2003). In contrast, 77 percent of a convenience sample of 200 hospital inpatients in Kentucky and North Carolina wanted their doctors to take their spiritual needs into consideration, and 37 percent would welcome more frequent discussions of their religious beliefs, but 68 percent had never had this opportunity (King and Bushwick, 1994). In an Ohio family practice setting, 83 percent of survey respondents said that it was appropriate for physicians to inquire about spiritual beliefs, primarily under circumstances of serious illness or bereavement, with the main purpose limited to understanding the patient's or family's perspective (McCord et al., 2004). And in a Philadelphia study, 45 percent of pulmonary outpatient study participants reported holding religious beliefs that would affect treatment preferences, and most participants agreed that their physicians should ask about such beliefs in the event of serious illness, but only 15 percent could recall having had such conversations (Ehman et al., 1999).

Intervention

In terms of spiritual care, preferences appear to be mixed, and patients' wishes for direct physician intervention primarily concern prayer. Fully 48 percent of hospitalized participants in King and Bushwick's (1994) southeastern U.S. study wanted their doctors to pray with them. More than two-thirds of a sample representative of the same geographic region indicated a desire for spiritual intervention if they became seriously ill or injured, but only 2 percent preferred to have physicians assume this responsibility (Mansfield et al., 2002). Their own ministers would be their first choice for such assistance, followed by hospital chaplains at a distant second (5%). In another study, the degree of acceptability of physicians' spiritual ministration varied as a function of illness severity, with acceptability of prayer increasing to 50 percent only if patients were near death (MacLean et al., 2003). A 1998 national phone survey using random-digit dialing found that 35 percent of respondents engaged in prayer in response to health concerns, and most of these found prayer to be helpful, but only 11 percent of those who used prayer discussed it with their physicians (McCaffrey et al., 2004). Daaleman and Nease (1994) reported that patients found physician referrals to clergy acceptable (although they were likely to refer themselves if spiritual issues arose) but did not perceive physicians to be qualified to address religious or spiritual concerns. Other patient reports corroborate this perspective: 82.6 percent of oxygen-dependent patients with chronic lung disease in a Seattle study reported that their physicians did not ask about their spiritual beliefs and that those who did were not skilled at such assessment (Curtis et al., 2004).

Clinicians Providing Religious/Spiritual Care

This section addresses what is known about religious/spiritual care in current practice, identifies the barriers and some of the ethical issues that clinicians encounter in providing such care, and considers recent initiatives to enhance clinical competence to meet patients' religious/spiritual needs at the end of life.

Current Practice

Patients without close family or religious community support may rely more heavily on health care providers for help with religious/spiritual tasks that arise at the end of life (Koenig, 2002). And attending to patients' values, including respecting religious beliefs, has been identified by patients, families, and clinicians alike as one of the essential domains of high-quality end-of-life care (Curtis et al., 2001).

For the most part, physicians agree that they should be cognizant of patients' religious/spiritual beliefs, but they are reluctant to discuss matters of faith or participate in prayer except under limited conditions. In a cross-sectional survey of primary care physicians practicing primarily in North Carolina, 84.5 percent agreed that they should be aware of patients' beliefs, but they were most likely to engage in discussions about these beliefs or offer a silent prayer only when death approached, and at the patient's request (Monroe et al., 2003). In the same study, family physicians, whose training placed more emphasis on psychosocial and spiritual factors, were more likely to take a spiritual history than were internists, but these two groups were otherwise similar in their approach to faith issues.

Nurses, who espouse a holistic philosophical orientation to practice, consider spiritual needs of patients an integral part of their practice domain. They are responsible for assessing religious/spiritual needs, facilitating and supporting patient and family religious/spiritual practices, and making referrals to chaplains or clergy as patients wish. When caring for patients at the end of life, they are often instrumental in helping them to achieve existential comfort and peace. Hospice nurses in particular are noted for their attention to spiritual needs, one of the hallmarks of this mode of care.

When asked who was accountable for addressing spiritual/existential distress among their patients, 37.5 percent of oncologists and 47.5 percent of oncology nurses claimed primary responsibility (Kristeller, Zumbrun, and Schilling, 1999). Although more than 85 percent of both groups identified chaplains as the ideal group to intervene, such referrals were infrequent, especially among physicians. Both physicians and nurses assigned spiritual distress a mid- to low-level priority in relation to other patient problems; the majority nevertheless believed that their help, when provided, was at least somewhat effective. Several studies have reported minimal documentation of spiritual histories or interventions in medical records of dying patients, lending further credence to perceptions of the relatively low priority of spiritual assessment and intervention in terminal care (Fins, Guest, and Acres, 2000; King and Wells, 2003).

Barriers to Religious/Spiritual Care

A qualitative study examined factors cited by physicians as barriers to psychosocial-spiritual care of the dying (Chibnall et al., 2004). Cultural barriers began during training with the professional socialization process in medicine in which psychosocial-spiritual aspects of the person were marginalized, gradually desensitizing young physicians to them. Organizational barriers included escalating bureaucratic regulations, excessive paperwork, and mounting workloads, which resulted in serious time constraints. Clinically, physicians felt insufficiently skilled to undertake the complex communications involved in addressing these issues. Monroe et al. (2003) suggested, based on their data, that difficulties identifying patients who wish to talk about spiritual issues and worries about projecting personal beliefs onto patients may be the most significant barriers.

Nurses experience many of the same roadblocks as physicians, including inadequate educational preparation, time, staffing, and privacy to provide spiritual care (Tanyi, 2002). Skill levels are likely to vary widely as well, given the broad range of specialties and educational backgrounds within the nursing profession. When Taylor, Highfield, and Amenta (1999) compared the perspectives and practices of one group of hospice nurses with those of a group of oncology nurses, hospice nurses had higher religiosity and spirituality scores, offered spiritual care more frequently and with greater confidence and comfort in their abilities, had more positive attitudes about spiritual caregiving, reported better training to provide such care, and enjoyed stronger organizational support for it.

Although widely assumed, the adequacy of the preparation of pastoral care staff and religious congregations to minister to the spiritual needs of patients and families at the end of life is not well documented (Field and Cassel, 1997). Crawley et al. (2000) cautioned that clergy members, who play a pivotal role in the care of the dying within the African American community, may not be sufficiently informed about palliative care and hospice and are thus not in a position to encourage their use among those in their congregation who could benefit from such services. Findings from a qualitative study involving Christian religious representatives in multicultural Honolulu suggest that faith-based communities have the potential to play an expanded role in helping their members with the end-of-life issues (Braun and Zir, 2001). These roles include preparing members spiritually and practically for death, facilitating reconciliation and forgiveness, clarifying ethical and moral principles for decision making, administering rituals, and providing outreach to sick, dying, and bereaved members.

Finally, clinicians who lack religious/spiritual beliefs, who are struggling with their own needs or conflicts, or who ascribe to a belief system differing from that of the patient may experience greater challenges in addressing religious or spiritual needs (Koenig, 2002; McSherry and Cash, 2003).

Ethical Issues

Clinician involvement with religious/spiritual issues at the end of life raises several important ethical issues. Sloan, Bagiella, and Powell (1999) argued that, while physicians who support patients' religious beliefs during times of crisis are acting respectfully, they are not religious experts. Patients' religious perspectives are important to take into account, but prescription of religious interventions for health problems is inappropriate for two reasons. First, because these researchers judge the link between religious activity and health outcomes to be weak at best, they believe there is insufficient scientific evidence to justify it. Second, they believe that clinician involvement in this area may be harmful if it engenders guilt in religious patients who interpret illness as moral failure. An additional concern is that using religion instrumentally to achieve health trivializes religion, which has intrinsic worth regardless of its effects on health (Sloan et al., 2000).

Post, Puchalski, and Larson (2000) addressed ethical concerns regarding spiritual needs assessment, professional boundaries, and patient requests for physician prayer. While many physicians are reluctant to assess spiritual needs, Post and colleagues encourage the use of brief initial screenings, which can be done quickly and respectfully. These assessments are intended to identify patients' needs and perspectives related to their care, and they provide opportunities for referral to chaplains or other spiritual counselors that are frequently missed for patients experiencing spiritual distress. Patients may in some cases blur the boundaries between physician and pastoral caregiver, but Post and colleagues contend that physicians must maintain clear distinctions. This applies particularly to patient requests for physicians to pray with them. Whenever possible, they advise that such prayer be led by clergy to avoid misunderstanding or perceived coercion. Physicians should lead prayer only if a religious leader is unavailable, if the patient initiates the request, and if the physician can do so comfortably. Otherwise, respectful listening while the patient prays is an acceptable option.

Conflicts between medical recommendations and patients' religious beliefs are not unusual in clinical practice. Physicians report managing such differences through accommodation of patients' or families' views with openness and flexibility, and through persuasion when warranted if religious convictions risk harm or suffering (Curlin et al., 2005). Brett and Jersild (2003) proposed that, when patients or families justify their treatment requests with religious beliefs, physicians may offer alternative religious interpretations in attempting to persuade a change, preferably in collaboration with clergy. Lo and others (2002) would likely disagree with this approach, given their recommendations in similar circumstances to explore and respect the patient's or family's views and recognize the limits of their own expertise by avoiding theological debates; these authors also suggest that clinicians not compromise their integrity by acting contrary to their own spiritual or religious beliefs (such as by feigning agreement) during such interactions.

Initiatives to Enhance Clinical Competence

Achieving and maintaining competence in end-of-life care is an essential goal for all professional caregivers. It requires widespread educational and organizational reform within the health care system. Until recently, medical and nursing education have given little attention to end-of-life care, including religious/spiritual needs of dying patients and their loved ones. In response to numerous initiatives (Sullivan et al., 2004), this situation appears to be changing quickly. For example, the number of accredited medical schools in this country that include courses on spirituality in medicine in the curriculum rose from 17 to 84 between 1994 and 1998 (Fortin and Barnett, 2004). To effect change through nursing education, the Robert Wood Johnson Foundation in 2000 funded the End-of-Life National Education Consortium (Sherman et al., 2002). Membership represents numerous professional organizations. The consortium uses a "train the trainer" approach to teach quality end-of-life care to nurse educators, who then implement curriculum change that incorporates this new knowledge.

Several prominent examples illustrate attempts to enhance seasoned health care providers' competence in providing end-of-life care. In 2000 the *Journal of the American Medical Association* instituted a bimonthly series of articles entitled "Perspectives on Care at the Close of Life" (McPhee et al., 2000) to guide professional caregivers in the management of difficult but important issues that arise at the end of life, including those concerning religion and spirituality. The *American Journal of Nursing* launched a similar monthly series in 2002 (Ferrell and Coyle, 2002). Members of both professions have also undertaken efforts to encourage authors and editors to incorporate palliative care principles and practices into the content of leading textbooks (Carron, Lynn, and Keaney, 1999; Ferrell, Virani, Grant, and Juarez, 2000). Valuable references for both clinicians and the lay public are also increasingly available (e.g., Lynn and Harrold, 1999; Lynn, Schuster, and Kabcenell, 2000).

Religious/Spiritual Care at the End of Life

Religious/Spiritual Assessment

The inclusion of questions about religious/spiritual beliefs and values in medical histories remains controversial among many care providers. Such assessment, however, is becoming part of expected standards of practice. In its evaluations of the quality of care provided by health care facilities, for instance, the Joint Commission on the Accreditation of HealthCare Organizations (2001) now includes expectations that patients' spiritual orientation will be promptly assessed and that facilities will provide adequate pastoral care resources to meet patients' needs.

The main reason for asking patients nearing the end of their lives about religious/spiritual issues is because of these issues' impact on overall well-being (Sulmasy, 2002). Information gained in a spiritual history provides valuable insight regarding whether, and to what extent, the person relies on a belief system to cope with crises, to guide medical treatment decision making, and as a source of personal or social support; evidence of religious struggle or spiritual distress may also be uncovered that may be amenable to counseling (Koenig, 2004). When a clinician takes a spiritual history, it is critical that it be done within the context of an accepting relationship, with the patient willing, and with the clinician remaining open and nonjudgmental, not proselytizing or challenging patients' beliefs (Kaut, 2002; Koenig, 2004).

Several useful tools have been created to assist clinicians in conducting spiritual histories near the end of life. The *FICA*, developed by Puchalski, assesses *F*aith, beliefs, meanings in life; *I*mportance and influence of faith in caring for self; *C*ommunity membership or support (religious/spiritual); and how the patient wants the clinician to *A*ddress any needs (Lynn, Schuster, and Kabcenell, 2000). The *HOPE* questions (Anandarajah and Hight, 2001) assess sources of *H*ope, strength, comfort, meaning, peace, love, and connection; *O*rganized religion and its role in the patient's life; *P*ersonal spirituality and practices; and *E*ffects on medical care and end-of-life decisions. Kub et al. (2003) recommend inquiring about the importance of religion in the patient's life and frequency of attendance at religious services before illness in addition to the standard demographic question regarding religious denomination. Sulmasy's (2002) personal preference is to ask just one question ("What role does spirituality or religion play in your life?"), allowing subsequent discussion to flow from the patient's initial response.

Spiritual Interventions

Appropriate strategies to enhance spirituality or prevent or treat spiritual distress at the end of life relate primarily to the existential rather than to the religious. Health care providers rarely have the qualifications to provide religious counseling. They do, however, have the obligation to learn and appreciate the role of religion in the patient's life, to facilitate the patient's ability to engage in comforting religious coping and worship practices, to help the patient to maintain connections with a supportive religious community, and to recognize signs of religious/spiritual distress, offering referral to religious clergy with the patient's consent.

In order to intervene effectively with spiritual needs of an existential nature, clinicians need to be comfortable with discussing spiritual concerns, demonstrate empathy, and possess excellent listening and communication skills (Rousseau, 2000). When patients are experiencing spiritual suffering, these skills will help the clinician to refrain from trying to "fix" the problem with quick reassurances when the most therapeutic strategies may be listening and being present as the patient shares thoughts and feelings (Kaut, 2002; Lo et al., 2002).

Preparation for dying involves, for many, the process of accomplishing tasks such as clarifying the meaning, purpose, and value of their lives; redefining hopes and goals; and leaving a legacy (Koenig, 2002). Various strategies have been reported to facilitate the accomplishment of these tasks. Which are most effective, for whom, when, and in what amount are worthy topics for future research.

Interventions often used with elderly people, such as life review and reminiscence therapy, can be helpful for loved ones who listen as well as for the people who share their life stories. Breitbart, Gibson, Poppito, and Berg (2004) reported helping patients to find meaning and purpose through meaning-centered group therapy that includes reading, didactics, personal reflections, and guided discussions. Revising hopes and goals is often a gradual process, accomplished as the person becomes ready to accept the possibility of death. Back, Arnold, and Quill (2003) offer guidance through case examples on helping seriously ill patients to hope for the best yet prepare for the worst while they are still well enough to do so. Life projects, such as videotapes, audiotapes, letter-writing, journal-writing, or participating in a "dignity psychotherapy" protocol may help people find comfort in leaving behind a legacy that will survive beyond their passing (Chochinov, 2002). Chandler (1999) described the spiritual comfort and peace that the dying may derive through the arts as well as through complementary therapies. Music and art can calm anxiety and fear by providing a peaceful environment. Some patients derive psycho-spiritual benefit from interventions such as meditation, guided imagery, massage, and aromatherapy, which can alleviate suffering by comforting both body and soul.

Recommendations to Advance the Development of Knowledge

A number of priorities for knowledge development can ultimately lead to improvements in the religious and spiritual care of dying people and their loved ones. Those most salient to this discussion concern the pressing needs for improved conceptual clarity and more rigorous research design.

The Need for Improved Conceptual Clarity

While consensus regarding the meanings of religiosity and spirituality is gradually developing among scholars, much work remains to be done. Conceptual definitions of these terms need to be compatible with the belief systems of the group(s) being studied. When the intent is to produce findings generalizable to large populations, definitions must be broad enough to encompass the diversity of prevalent cultural, ethnic, and denominational meanings. This implies moving beyond primarily Christian and Euro-American viewpoints to incorporate perspectives of those who ascribe to nondominant values and belief systems.

The process of conceptual clarification should include reaching consensus on the key dimensions of religiosity and spirituality. This step is important for several reasons. Clearly delineated components of these complex constructs will (1) make it easier for researchers to specify and operationalize conceptual definitions; (2) provide direction for instrument development and refinement; (3) allow for the range of beliefs influenced by culture, ethnicity, and organized belief systems to be more easily measured; (4) provide for consistency that will permit comparisons across studies; and (5) facilitate cumulative knowledge.

Meanings are by nature dynamic and will undoubtedly continue to change over time. But this should not preclude efforts to reduce ambiguity. Conceptual clarification of religiosity and spirituality can be enhanced by using a multidisciplinary approach, with scholars from wide variety of backgrounds working together to reach agreement. While this seems to be occurring naturally over time, more concerted efforts, through such avenues as expert consensus conferences or Delphi studies, could help to hasten achievement of this goal.

The Need for Enhanced Methodological Rigor

As previously noted, the study of religiosity and spirituality at the end of life is an emerging field. It has been characterized by numerous exploratory studies that are typically either qualitative or descriptive in design, with one data collection point. Most of the studies are conducted with relatively small samples of terminally ill patients who have specific diseases (usually cancer or advanced HIV infection) and who were recruited from single sites. While much has been learned from these studies, their inherent limitations have often prevented their findings from being generalized beyond the immediate study population.

George (2002) made a strong case for the need for longitudinal designs to move the science beyond correlations to determinations of causal relationships among variables associated with religiosity and spirituality. As these relationships are elucidated, intervention studies are likely to follow.

Although there is a continuing need for, and value in, qualitative and descriptive studies that are well-designed and well-executed, future research should place greater emphasis on generating and/or testing explanatory models that link variables known to be associated with religiosity and spirituality at the end of life. Such work will require more sophisticated data analytic techniques than have been commonly used in this field to date. To improve generalizability of results, researchers will need to give careful consideration to several factors in the design stage, including use of power analysis to determine adequate sample size, recruitment of participants who are representative of the population being studied, and use of collaborative teams of coinvestigators from multiple, diverse sites.

Work of this caliber will require talent, backed by funding, to execute more sophisticated research designs. To expand the cadre of qualified researchers, it will be essential to invest in postdoctoral training for young or midcareer investigators to acquire the expertise necessary to build programs of research devoted to the study of religiosity and spirituality at the end of life. Ensuring that federal and private funding sources recognize the importance of this agenda to the American public will also be necessary so that adequate funds will be available to implement such research and translate clinically relevant findings promptly into practice for the benefit of dying patients and their loved ones.

Conclusion

This chapter reviewed the current status of knowledge development on religiosity and spirituality at the end of life. Contemporary conceptual challenges include definitional inconsistencies, a body of existing knowledge that is largely atheoretical, and cultural diversity that limits shared meanings and values—all of which can be effectively addressed as the science grows. Methodological challenges reflect both the relative newness of this field of inquiry and the often-fragile health conditions of those whose lives are drawing to a close. Researchers will need to employ more rigorous research designs that allow for generalizable results, rely on psychometrically sound instruments with greater consistency, and conduct more longitudinal studies of religiosity and spirituality across illness and aging trajectories. Recent research on religiosity and spirituality in life-threatening illness, at the close of life, and during bereavement was also examined. These studies, despite their limitations, have yielded intriguing results that should stimulate further work in these and related areas to move the science forward.

Despite the challenges that investigators face, the opportunities are both considerable and exciting. Time, talent, and funding will be required to achieve conceptual clarity, methodological rigor, and clinically relevant findings. All of us, ultimately, stand to be the beneficiaries of such investments.

Acknowledgments

The author gratefully acknowledges the support and assistance of Rachel A. Pruchno, Ph.D., and Edward P. Lemay Jr., M.S., in the development of this chapter. This work was supported by a grant from the National Institute of Nursing Research to Dr. Pruchno (RO1 NR 05237).

REFERENCES

Addington-Hall, J., and McPherson, C. 2001. After-death interviews with surrogate/bereaved family members: Some issues of validity. *Journal of Pain and Symptom Management* 22:784–90.

Ainlay, S. C., and Smith, D. R. 1984. Aging and religious participation. *Journal of Gerontology* 39:357–63.

Anandarajah, G., and Hight, E. 2001. Spirituality and medical practice: Using the HOPE questions as a practical tool for spiritual assessment. *American Family Physician* 63:81–88.

Atchley, R. C. 2005. On including religious and spiritual faith and practice in gerontological research. *Journal of Gerontology: Social Sciences* 60B:52.

Back, A. L., Arnold, R. M., and Quill, T. E. 2003. Hope for the best and prepare for the worst. *Annals of Internal Medicine* 138:439–44.

Biggar, H., Forehand, R., Devine, D., Brody, G., Armistead, L., Morse, E., et al. 1999. Women who are HIV infected: The role of religious activity in psychosocial adjustment. *AIDS Care* 11:195–99.

Blackhall, L. J., Frank, G., Murphy, S. T., Michel, V., Palmer, J. M., and Azen, S. P. 1999. Ethnicity and attitudes towards life-sustaining technology. *Social Science and Medicine* 48:1779–89.

Block, S. D. 2001. Psychological considerations, growth, and transcendence at the end of life: The art of the possible. *Journal of the American Medical Association* 285:2898–2905.

Braun, K. L., and Zir, A. 2001. Roles for the church in improving end-of-life care: Perceptions of Christian clergy and laity. *Death Studies* 25:685–704.

Breitbart, W., Gibson, C., Poppito, S. B., and Berg, A. 2004. Psychotherapeutic interventions at the end of life: A focus on meaning and spirituality. *Canadian Journal of Psychiatry* 49:366–72.

Breitbart, W., Rosenfeld, B., Pessin, H., Kaim, M., Funesti-Esch, J., Galietta, M., et al. 2000. Depression, hopelessness, and desire for hastened death in terminally ill patients with cancer. *Journal of the American Medical Association* 284:2907–11.

Brett, A. S., and Jersild, P. 2003. "Inappropriate" treatment near the end of life: Conflict between convictions and clinical judgment. *Archives of Internal Medicine* 163:1645–49.

Carron, A. T., Lynn, J., and Keaney, P. 1999. End of life care in medical textbooks. *Annals of Internal Medicine* 130:82–86.

Chandler, E. 1999. Spirituality. *Hospice Journal* 14:63–74.

Chibnall, J. T., Bennett, M. L., Videen, S. D., Duckro, P. N., and Miller, D. K. 2004. Identifying barriers to psychosocial-spiritual care at the end of life: A physician group study. *American Journal of Hospice and Palliative Medicine* 21:419–26.

Chibnall, J. T., Videen, S. D., Duckro, P. N., and Miller, D. K. 2002. Psychosocial-spiritual correlates of death distress in patients with life-threatening medical conditions. *Palliative Medicine* 16:331–38.

Chochinov, H. M. 2002. Dignity-conserving care: A new model for palliative care. *Journal of the American Medical Association* 287:2253–60.

Cicirelli, V. G. 1997. Relationship of psychosocial and background variables to older adults/end-of-life decisions. *Psychology and Aging* 12:72–83.

Clarfield, A. M., Gordon, M., Marwell, H., and Alihhai, S. M. H. 2003. Ethical issues in end-of-life geriatric care: The approach of three monotheistic religions—Judaism, Catholicism, and Islam. *Journal of the American Geriatrics Society* 51:1149–54.

Clemetson, L. 2003. Hispanics now largest minority, census shows. *New York Times,* January 22. Retrieved from www.nytimes.com.

Cohen, S. R., Boston, P., Mount, B. M., and Porterfield, P. 2001. Changes in quality of life following admission to palliative care units. *Palliative Medicine* 15:363–71.

Copp, G. 1998. A review of current theories of death and dying. *Journal of Advanced Nursing* 28:382–90.

Corr, C. A. 1992. A task-based approach to coping with dying. *Omega* 24:81–94.

Cotton, S. P., Levine, E. G., Fitzpatrick, C. M., Dold, K. H., and Targ, E. 1999. Exploring the relationships among spiritual well-being, quality of life, and psychological adjustment in women with breast cancer. *Psycho-Oncology* 8:429–38.

Crawley, L., Payne, R., Bolden, J., Payne, T., Washington, P., and Williams, S. 2000. Palliative and end-of-life care in the African American community. *Journal of the American Medical Association* 284:2518–21.

Curlin, F. A., Roach, C. J., Gorawara-Bhat, R., Lantos, J. D., and Chin, M. H. 2005. When patients choose faith over medicine: Physician perspectives on religiously related conflicts in the medical encounter. *Archives of Internal Medicine* 165:88–91.

Curtis, J. R., Engelberg, R. A., Nielsen, E. L., Au, D. H., and Patrick, D. L. 2004. Patient-provider communication about end-of-life care for patients with severe COPD. *European Respiratory Journal* 24:200–205.

Curtis, J. R., Wenrich, M. D., Carline, J. D., Shannon, S. E., Ambrozy, D. M., and Ramsey, P. G. 2001. Understanding physicians' skill at providing end-of-life care: Perspectives of patients, families, and health care workers. *Journal of General Internal Medicine* 16:41–49.

Daaleman, T. P., Cobb, A. K., and Frey, B. B. 2001. Spirituality and well-being: An exploratory study of the patient perspective. *Social Science and Medicine* 53:1502–11.

Daaleman, T. P., and Nease, D. E. 1994. Patient attitudes regarding physician inquiry into spiritual and religious issues. *Journal of Family Practice* 39:564–68.

Daaleman, T. P., and VandeCreek, L. 2000. Placing religion and spirituality in end-of-life care. *Journal of the American Medical Association* 284:2514–17.

Daugherty, C. K., Fitchett, G., Murphy, P. E., Peterman, A. H., Banik, D. M., Hlubocky,

F., et al. 2005. Trusting God and medicine: Spirituality in advanced cancer patients: Volunteering for clinical trials of experimental agents. *Psycho-Oncology* 14:135–45.

Ehman, J. W., Ott, B. B., Short, T. H., Ciampa, R. C., and Hansen-Flaschen, J. 1999. Do patients want physicians to inquire about their spiritual or religious beliefs if they become gravely ill? *Archives of Internal Medicine* 159:1803–6.

Eleazer, G. P., Hornung, C. A., Egbert, C. B., Egbert, J. R., Eng, C., Hedgepeth, J., et al. 1996. The relationship between ethnicity and advance directives in a frail older population. *Journal of the American Geriatrics Society* 44:938–43.

Emanuel, E. J., Fairclough, D. L., and Emanuel, L. L. 2000. Attitudes and desires related to euthanasia and physician-assisted suicide among terminally ill patients and their caregivers. *Journal of the American Medical Association* 284:2460–68.

Emanuel, E. J., Fairclough, D. L., Wolfe, P., and Emanuel, L. L. 2004. Talking with terminally ill patients and their caregivers about death, dying, and bereavement: Is it stressful? Is it helpful? *Archives of Internal Medicine* 104:1999–2004.

Ferrell, B. R., and Coyle, N. 2002. An overview of palliative nursing care. *American Journal of Nursing* 102(5):26–31.

Ferrell, B., Virani, R., Grant, M., and Juarez, G. 2000. Analysis of palliative care content in nursing textbooks. *Journal of Palliative Care* 16:39–47.

Fetzer Institute. 1999/2003. *Multidimensional Measurement of Religiousness/Spirituality for Use in Health Research*. Retrieved from www.fetzer.org/Programs.aspx?PageID= Programs&NavID=3&ProgramID=93.

Field, M. J., and Cassel, C. K., eds. 1997. *Approaching Death: Improving Care at the End of Life*. Washington, DC: National Academy Press.

Fins, J. J., Guest, R. S., and Acres, C. A. 2000. Gaining insight into the care of hospitalized dying patients: An interpretive narrative analysis. *Journal of Pain and Symptom Management* 20:399–407.

Flory, J., Young-Xu, Y., Gurol, I., Levinsky, N., Ash, A., and Emanuel, E. 2004. Place of death: U.S. trends since 1980. *Health Affairs* 21:194–200.

Fortin, A. H., and Barnett, K. G. 2004. Medical school curricula in spirituality and medicine. *Journal of the American Medical Association* 291:2883.

Fry, P. S. 2001. Predictors of health-related quality of life perspectives, self-esteem, and life satisfaction of older adults following spousal loss: An 18-month follow-up study of widows and widowers. *Gerontologist* 41:787–98.

Gallup Poll. 2004. Religion. May 2–4. Retrieved from www.pollingreport.com/religion .htm.

George, L. K. 2002. Research design in end-of-life research: State of science. *Gerontologist* 42 (Special Issue III): 86–98.

Gray, J., and Cason, C. L. 2002. Mastery over stress among women with HIV/AIDS. *Journal of the Association of Nurses in AIDS Care* 13:43–57.

Hall, B. A. 1997. Spirituality in terminal illness: An alternative view of theory. *Journal of Holistic Nursing* 15:82–96.

Hall, B. A. 1998. Patterns of spirituality in persons with advanced HIV disease. *Research in Nursing and Health* 21:143–53.

Heeren, O., Menon, A. S., Raskin, A., and Ruskin, P. 2001. Religion and end of life treatment preferences among geriatric patients. *International Journal of Geriatric Psychiatry* 16:203–8.

Heinrich, C. R. 2003. Enhancing the perceived health of HIV seropositive men. *Western Journal of Nursing Research* 25:367–82.

Hermann, C. P. 2001. Spiritual needs of dying patients: A qualitative study. *Oncology Nursing Forum* 28:67–72.

Herth, K. 1992. Abbreviated instrument to measure hope: Development and psychometric properties. *Journal of Advanced Nursing* 17:1251–59.

Highfield, M. F. 1992. Spiritual health of oncology patients. *Cancer Nursing* 15:1–8.

Hill, P. C., and Pargament, K. I. 2003. Advances in the conceptualization and measurement of religion and spirituality. *American Psychologist* 58:64–74.

Hinton, J. 1996. How reliable are relatives' retrospective reports of terminal illness? Patients' and relatives' accounts compared. *Social Science and Medicine* 43:1229–36.

Holland, J. C., Passik, S., Kash, K. M., Russak, S. M., Gronert, M. K., and Sison, A., et al. 1999. The role of religious and spiritual beliefs in coping with malignant melanoma. *Psycho-Oncology* 8:14–26.

Hopp, F. P., and Duffy, S. A. 2000. Racial variations in end-of-life care. *Journal of the American Geriatric Society* 48:658–63.

Idler, E. L., Kasl, S. V., and Hays, J. C. 2001. Patterns of religious practice and belief in the last year of life. *Journal of Gerontology: Social Sciences* 56B:S326–34.

Idler, E. L., Musick, M. A., Ellison, C. G., George, L. K., Krause, N., Ory, M. G., et al. 2003. Measuring multiple dimensions of religion and spirituality for health research: Conceptual background and findings from the 1998 General Social Survey. *Research on Aging* 25:327–65.

Iwashyna, T. J., and Chang, V. W. 2002. Racial and ethnic differences in place of death: United States, 1993. *Journal of the American Geriatrics Society* 50:1113–17.

Joint Commission on Accreditation of Healthcare Organizations. 2001. Spiritual assessment. *Behavioral Health Care,* July 31. Retrieved from www.jcaho.org/.

Kagawa-Singer, M., and Blackhall, L. J. 2001. Negotiating cross-cultural issues at the end of life: "You got to go where he lives." *Journal of the American Medical Association* 286:2993–3001.

Kaldjian, L. C., Jekel, J. F., and Friedland, G. 1998. End-of-life decisions in HIV-positive patients: The role of spiritual beliefs. *AIDS* 12:103–7.

Kaufman, S. R. 2002. A commentary: Hospital experience and meaning at the end of life. *Gerontologist* 42 (Special Issue III): 34–39.

Kaut, K. P. 2002. Religion, spirituality, and existentialism near the end of life. *American Behavioral Scientist* 46:220–34.

Keeley, M. P. 2004. Final conversations: Survivors' memorable messages concerning religious faith and spirituality. *Health Communication* 16:87–104.

Kelly, B., Burnett, P., Pelusi, D., Badger, S., Verghese, F., and Robertson, M. 2002. Terminally ill cancer patients' wish to hasten death. *Palliative Medicine* 16:339–45.

King, D. E., and Bushwick, B. 1994. Beliefs and attitudes of hospital inpatients about faith healing and prayer. *Journal of Family Practice* 39:349–52.

King, M., Speck, P., and Thomas, A. 1994. Spiritual and religious beliefs in acute illnesses: Is this a feasible area for study? *Social Science and Medicine* 38:631–36.

King, M., Speck, P., and Thomas, A. 1999. The effect of spiritual beliefs on outcome from illness. *Social Science and Medicine* 48:1291–98.

King, D. E., and Wells, B. J. 2003. End-of-life issues and spiritual histories. *Southern Medical Journal* 96:391–93.

Klinkenberg, M., Willems, D. L., Onwuteaka-Philipsen, B. D., Deeg, D. J. H., and van der Wal, G. 2004. Preferences in end-of-life care of older persons: After-death interviews with proxy respondents. *Social Science and Medicine* 59:2467–77.

Koenig, H. G. 1998. Religious attitudes and practices of hospitalized medically ill older adults. *International Journal of Geriatric Psychiatry* 13:213–24.

Koenig, H. G. 2002. A commentary: The role of religion and spirituality at the end of life. *Gerontologist* 42 (Special Issue 3): 20–23.

Koenig, H. G. 2004. Taking a spiritual history. *Journal of the American Medical Association* 291:2881.

Koenig, H. G., George, L. K., and Titus, P. 2004. Religion, spirituality, and health in medically ill hospitalized older adults. *Journal of the American Geriatrics Society* 52:554–62.

Koenig, H. G., Moberg, D. O., and Kvale, J. N. 1988. Religious activities and attitudes of older adults in a geriatric assessment clinic. *Journal of the American Geriatric Society* 36:362–74.

Kristeller, J. L., Zumbrun, C. S., and Schilling, R. F. 1999. "I would if I could": How oncologists and oncology nurses address spiritual distress in cancer patients. *Psycho-Oncology* 8:451–58.

Kub, J. E., Nolan, M. T., Hughes, M. T., Terry, P. B., Sulmasy, D. P., Astrow, A., et al. 2003. Religious importance and practices of patients with a life-threatening illness: Implications for screening protocols. *Applied Nursing Research* 16:196–200.

Kübler-Ross, E. 1969. *On Death and Dying.* New York: Macmillan.

Lo, B., Ruston, D., Kates, L. W., Arnold, R. M., Cohen, C. B., Faber-Langendoen, K., et al. 2002. Discussing religious and spiritual issues at the end of life: A practical guide for physicians. *Journal of the American Medical Association* 287:749–54.

Lunney, J. R., Foley, K. M., Smith, T. J., and Gelband, H., eds. 2003. *Describing Death in America: What We Need to Know.* Washington, DC: National Academy Press.

Lunney, J. R., Lynn, J., and Hogan, C. 2002. Profiles of older Medicare decedents. *Journal of the American Geriatrics Society* 50:1108–12.

Lynn, J., and Harrold, J. 1999. *Handbook for Mortals: Guidance for People Facing Serious Illness.* New York: Oxford University Press.

Lynn, J., Schuster, J. L., and Kabcenell, A. 2000. *Improving Care for the End of Life: A Sourcebook for Health Care Managers and Clinicians.* New York: Oxford University Press.

MacLean, C. D., Susi, B., Phifer, N., Schultz, L., Bynum, D., Franco, M., et al. 2003. Patient preference for physician discussion and practice of spirituality: Results from a multicenter patient survey. *Journal of General Internal Medicine* 18:38–43.

Mansfield, C. J., Mitchell, J., and King, D. E. 2002. The doctor as God's mechanic: Beliefs in the southeastern United States. *Social Science and Medicine* 54:399–409.

Maugans, T. A., and Wadland, W. C. 1991. Religion and family medicine: A survey of physicians and patients. *Journal of Family Practice* 32:210–13.

Mazanec, P., and Tyler, M. K. 2003. Cultural considerations in end-of-life care. *American Journal of Nursing* 103(3):50–58.

McAuley, W. J., Pecchioni, L., and Grant, J. A. 2000. Personal accounts of the role of God in health and illness among older rural African American and white residents. *Journal of Cross-Cultural Gerontology* 15:13–35.

McCaffrey, A. M., Eisenberg, D. M., Legdza, A. T. R., Davis, R. B., and Phillips, R. S. 2004.

Prayer for health concerns: Results of a national survey on prevalence and patterns of use. *Archives of Internal Medicine* 164:858–62.

McClain, C. S., Rosenfeld, B., and Breitbart, W. 2003. Effect of spiritual well-being on end-of-life despair in terminally ill cancer patients. *Lancet* 361:1603–7.

McClain-Jacobson, C., Rosenfeld, B., Kosinski, A., Pessin, H., Cimino, J. E., and Breitbart, W. 2004. Belief in an afterlife: Spiritual well-being and end-of-life despair in patients with advanced cancer. *General Hospital Psychiatry* 26:484–86.

McCord, G., Gilchrist, V. J., Grossman, S. D., King, B. D., McCormick, K. F., Oprandi, A. M., et al. 2004. Discussing spirituality with patients: A rational and ethical approach. *Annals of Family Medicine* 2:356–61.

McCullough, M. E., Hoyt, W. E., Larson, D. B., Koenig, H. G., and Thoresen, C. 2000. Religious involvement and mortality: A meta-analytic review. *Health Psychology* 19:211–22.

McGrath, P. 2004. Reflection on serious illness as spiritual journey by survivors of haematological malignancies. *European Journal of Cancer Care* 13:227–37.

McPhee, S. J., Rabow, M. W., Pantilat, S. Z., Markowitz, A. J., and Winker, M. A. 2000. Finding our way: Perspectives on care at the end of life. *Journal of the American Medical Association* 284:2512.

McPherson, C. J., and Addington-Hall, J. M. 2003. Judging the quality of care at the end of life: Can proxies provide reliable information? *Social Science and Medicine* 56:95–109.

McSherry, W., and Cash, K. 2004. The language of spirituality: An emerging taxonomy. *International Journal of Nursing Studies* 41:151–61.

Mezey, M., Dubler, N. N., Mitty, E., and Brody, A. A. 2002. What impact do setting and transitions have on the quality of life at the end of life and the quality of the dying process? *Gerontologist* 42:54–67.

Miller, W. R., and Thoresen, C. E. 2003. Spirituality, religion, and health: An emerging research field. *American Psychologist* 58:24–34.

Monroe, M. H., Bynum, D., Susi, B., Phifer, N., Schultz, L., Franco, M., et al. 2003. Primary care physician preferences regarding spiritual behavior in medical practice. *Archives of Internal Medicine* 163:2751–56.

Mouton, C. P. 2000. Cultural and religious issues for African Americans. In K. L. Braun, J. H. Pietsch, and P. L. Blanchette, eds., *Cultural Issues in End-of-life Decision Making,* pp. 71–82. Thousand Oaks, CA: Sage.

Murray, S. A., Kendall, M., Boyd, K., Worth, A., and Benton, T. F. 2004. Exploring the spiritual needs of people dying of lung cancer or heart failure: A prospective qualitative interview study of patients and their careers. *Palliative Medicine* 18:39–45.

Mytko, J. J., and Knight, S. J. 1999. Mind, body, and spirit: Towards the integration of religiosity and spirituality in cancer quality of life research. *Psycho-Oncology* 8:439–50.

Nolan, M. T., and Mock, V. 2004. A conceptual framework for end-of-life care: A reconsideration of factors influencing the integrity of the human person. *Journal of Professional Nursing* 20:351–60.

Paloutzian, R. F., and Ellison, C. W. 1982. Loneliness, spiritual well-being, and quality of life. In L. A. Peplau and D. Perlman, eds. *Loneliness: A Sourcebook for Current Therapy,* pp. 224–37. New York: Wiley.

Post, S. G., Puchalski, C. M., and Larson, D. B. 2000. Physician and patient spirituality: Professional boundaries, competence, and ethics. *Annals of Internal Medicine* 132: 578–83.

Powell, L. H., Shahabi, L., and Thoresen, C. E. 2003. Religion and spirituality: Linkages to physical health. *American Psychologist* 58:36–52.

Power, M., Bullinger, M., Harper, A., and WHOQOL Group. 1999. The World Health Organization WHOQOL-100: Tests of the universality of quality of life in 15 culture groups worldwide. *Health Psychology* 18:495–505.

Puchalski, C. 2001. *TIME: Toolkit of Instruments to Measure End-of-Life Care: Spirituality.* Retrieved from www.chcr.brown.edu/pcoc/Spirit.htm.

Reed, P. G. 1986. Religiousness among terminally ill and healthy adults. *Research in Nursing and Health* 9:35–41.

Reed, P. G. 1987. Spirituality and well-being in terminally ill hospitalized adults. *Research in Nursing and Health* 10:335–44.

Rousseau, P. 2000. Spirituality and the dying patient. *Journal of Clinical Oncology* 18:2000–2002.

Schnoll, R. A., Harlow, L. L., and Brower, L. 2000. Spirituality, demographic and disease factors, and adjustment to cancer. *Cancer Practice* 8:298–304.

Seale, C. 1991. Communication and awareness about death: A study of a random sample of dying people. *Social Science and Medicine* 32:943–52.

Sherman, D. W., Matzo, M. L., Rogers, S., McLaughlin, M., and Virani, R. 2002. Achieving quality care at the end of life: A focus of the End-of-Life Nursing Education Consortium (ELNEC) curriculum. *Journal of Professional Nursing* 18:255–62.

Siegel, K., and Schrimshaw, E. W. 2002. The perceived benefits of religion and spirituality among older adults living with HIV/AIDS. *Journal for the Scientific Study of Religion* 41:91–102.

Sloan, R., and Bagiella, E. 2002. Claims about religious involvement and health outcomes. *Annals of Behavioral Medicine* 24:14–21.

Sloan, R. P., Bagiella, E., and Powell, T. 1999. Religion, spirituality, and medicine. *Lancet* 353:664–67.

Sloan, R. P., Bagiella, E., VandeCreek, L., Hover, M., Casalone, C., Hirsch, T. J., et al. 2000. Should physicians prescribe religious activities? *New England Journal of Medicine* 342:1913–16.

Stefanek, M., McDonald, P. G., and Hess, S. A. 2005. Religion, spirituality, and cancer: Current status and methodological challenges. *Psycho-Oncology* 14:450–63.

Steinhauser, K. E., Christakis, N. A., Clipp, E. C., McNeilly, M., McIntyre, L., and Tulsky, J. A. 2000a. Factors considered important at the end of life by patients, family, physicians, and other caregivers. *Journal of the American Medical Association* 284: 2476–82.

Steinhauser, K. E., Clipp, E. C., McNeilly, M., Christakis, N. A., McIntyre, L. M., and Tulsky, J. A. 2000b. In search of a good death: Observations of patients, families, and providers. *Annals of Internal Medicine* 132:825–32.

Sullivan, A. M., Warren, A. G., Lakoma, M. D., Liaw, K. R., Hwang, D., and Block, S. D. 2004. End-of-life care in the curriculum: A national study of medical education deans. *Academic Medicine* 79:760–68.

Sulmasy, D. P. 2002. A biopsychosocial-spiritual model for the care of patients at the end of life. *Gerontologist* 42 (special issue 3): 24–33.

Talamantes, M. A., Gomez, C., and Braun, K. L. 2000. Advance directives and end-of-life care: The Hispanic perspective. In K. L. Braun, J. H. Pietsch, and P. L. Blanchette, eds., *Cultural Issues in End-of-life Decision Making*, pp. 83–100. Thousand Oaks, CA: Sage.

Tang, W. R., Aaronson, L. S., and Forbes, S. A. 2004. Quality of life in hospice patients with terminal illness. *Western Journal of Nursing Research* 26:113–28.

Tanyi, R. 2002. Towards clarification of the meaning of spirituality. *Journal of Advanced Nursing* 39:500–509.

Tanyi, R. A., and Werner, J. S. 2003. Adjustment, spirituality, and health in women on hemodialysis. *Clinical Nursing Research* 12:229–45.

Taylor, E. J., Highfield, M. F., and Amenta, M. 1999. Predictors of oncology and hospice nurses' spiritual care: Perspectives and practice. *Applied Nursing Research* 12:30–37.

Taylor, E. J., Outlaw, F. H., Bernardo, T. R., and Roy, A. 1999. Spiritual conflicts associated with praying about cancer. *Psycho-Oncology* 8:386–94.

Tennstedt, S. L. 2002. Commentary on "Research design in end-of-life research: State of science." *Gerontologist* 42 (special issue 3): 99–103.

Teno, J. M., Clarridge, B. R., Casey, V., Welch, L. C., Wetle, T., Shield, R., et al. 2004. Family perspectives on end-of-life care at the last place of care. *Journal of the American Medical Association* 291:88–93.

Tilden, V. P., Tolle, S., Drach, L., and Hickman, S. 2002. Measurement of quality of care and quality of life at the end of life. *Gerontologist* 42 (special issue 3): 71–80.

Tuck, I., McCain, N. L., and Elswick, R. K. 2001. Spirituality and psychosocial factors in persons living with HIV. *Journal of Advanced Nursing* 33:776–83.

VandeCreek, L., and Nye, C. 1993. Testing the death transcendence scale. *Journal for the Scientific Study of Religion* 32:279–83.

Vig, E. K., and Pearlman, R. A. 2004. Good and bad dying from the perspective of terminally ill men. *Archives of Internal Medicine* 164:977–81.

Walsh, K., King, M., Jones, L., Tookman, A., and Blizard, R. 2002. Spiritual beliefs may affect outcome of bereavement: Prospective study. *British Medical Journal* 324:1551–54.

Warner S. C., and Williams, J. I. 1987. The meaning in life scale: Determining the validity and reliability of a measure. *Journal of Chronic Diseases* 40:503–12.

Waters, C. M. 2001. Understanding and supporting African Americans' perspectives of end-of-life care planning and decision making. *Qualitative Health Research* 11:385–98.

Werth, J. L., Blevins, D., Toussaint, K. L., and Durham, M. R. 2002. The influence of cultural diversity on end-of-life care and decisions. *American Behavioral Scientist* 46:204–19.

WHOQOL Group. 1998. The World Health Organization Quality of Life Assessment: Development and general psychometric properties. *Social Science and Medicine* 46:1569–85.

Wolfe, J., Fairclough, D. L., Clarridge, B. R., Daniels, E. R., and Emanuel, E. J. 1999. Stability of attitudes regarding physician-assisted suicide and euthanasia among oncology patients, physicians, and the general public. *Journal of Clinical Oncology* 17:1274–79.

Woods, T. E., and Ironson, G. H. 1999. Religion and spirituality in the face of illness:

How cancer, cardiac, and HIV patients describe their spirituality/religiosity. *Journal of Health Psychology* 4:393–412.

Yeo, G., and Hikoyeda, N. 2000. Cultural issues in end-of-life decision making among Asian and Pacific Islanders in the United States. In K. L. Braun, J. H. Pietsch, and P. L. Blanchette, eds., *Cultural Issues in End-of-life Decision Making*, pp. 101–25. Thousand Oaks, CA: Sage.

Part II / The Future
of Family Responsibility

CHAPTER FIVE

The Family and the Future

Challenges, Prospects, and Resilience

Norella M. Putney, Ph.D., Vern L. Bengtson, Ph.D., and Melanie A. Wakeman, Ph.D.

Demographic and economic transformations in the past few decades have disrupted patterns of work and family that most people had taken for granted for more than a century. With globalization, the workplace as a stable institution is eroding, and individuals and families are presented with greater uncertainties and risks as companies continually restructure and outsource in search of greater flexibility and profits. Not even persons with higher education and professional status are immune to the dislocations produced by globalization. Accompanying these changes has been the blurring of the boundaries between work and family, so that the uncertainties of the workplace have spilled over into family life. What constitutes men's and women's work and men's and women's family roles has become more ambiguous, and time pressures have increased.

As a consequence of population aging and globalization, families are changing in both form and meaning. Longer lives and fewer children, high divorce rates and the increase in single parent families, the movement of mothers into the labor force and greater economic insecurity—all have profoundly affected the direction and experience of individual lives. Relations between parents, children, grandparents, and grandchildren seem different than they used to be, the feelings of attachment less certain.

But does all this mean that the family is in decline? We will argue that a defining feature of the family has been, and continues to be, its ability to adapt to changing socioeconomic, political, and cultural conditions. We suggest that in uncertain times, the nurturance and support provided by family may be more important than ever for individual well-being. We will also assert that family diversity and fluidity are now "normal" and that families are adapting by expanding beyond the nuclear family structure to involve a variety of kin and nonkin relationships. While the late modern family condition, particularly as represented by the individualized life course, presents potentially threatening levels of insecurity, it also opens up the possibility of more egalitarian and democratic forms of intimacy. To the extent that nuclear families are challenged in their ability to provide the socialization, nurturance, and support needed by family members, kin across several generations and in a variety of family structures will increasingly be called upon to provide these essential family functions. In late modern society, relations across generations and kinship types are becoming increasingly important to individuals and families.

In this chapter we discuss the challenges and stresses as well as the prospects we see for American families in the near future. We first focus on the larger societal forces and conditions that will constrain and challenge families: population aging, the globalization phenomenon and the expansion of individualization and risk, changes in social welfare regimes, the economic challenges faced by middle-class families, and changes in the institutionalized life course and their implications for the patterning of the work life and family expectations. Next, we examine three microlevel outcomes of these larger social changes that will continue to challenge family members. These include marital instability and its consequences, the demands of balancing work and family, and the growing challenge of providing care to elderly family members.

We then focus on the opportunities for families in the next decade. At the macrosocial level, we consider the emergence of the "latent kin matrix" and the modified extended family form as signs of family resilience, offering expanded potentials for emotional and social support. We then consider four microsocial prospects for family members in late modern society. The story is one of adaptability. First, we discuss the surprising strength of intergenerational family bonds and suggest that families are adapting to changing conditions by expanding support across generations. We find that grandparents may represent an increasingly important source of family strength and resilience. Second, we present research showing that compared to intact families a generation ago, today's two-parent intact families seem to be especially successful in fulfilling their family responsibilities. Third, we call attention to a phenomenon that is occurring more frequently today because of changing economic conditions: prolonged parenting. This occurs when adult children delay departure from the family nest while they obtain additional education, or when they return home because they have problems. Our research suggests this pattern is adaptive and will contribute to stronger family bonds in the future. Fourth, we consider changing cultural norms and whether familism has increased in the past few decades. We point to research suggesting that in the past decade, younger cohorts, including baby boomers, have become more collectivist in their value orientations and in the importance they give to families. Finally, we present some projections for families in the future. It is our belief that despite unprecedented changes over the past four decades, the family will remain strong and central in people's lives.

Social Change and the Family: Demographic, Socioeconomic, and Political Contexts

To assess the challenges and stresses facing contemporary families, it is important that we consider their larger demographic, socioeconomic, and political contexts. We discuss several macrostructural trends that will affect families in the twenty-first century. These include population aging, globalization, neoliberalism, and changes in the typical life course.

Population Aging

Arguably, the major macrolevel change affecting families in the next several decades will be population aging. Population aging is more than a demographic phenomenon; it affects the social, political, economic, and cultural conditions of life for the entire society. The worldwide decline in fertility coupled with dramatic increases in average life expectancy will mean greater numbers and proportions of elders in all nations, especially persons 85 or older. Around the world, there is much concern about the consequences of population aging for national economies and governments. What is less obvious, but equally important, is that population aging will profoundly affect families. Population aging as well as later marriage and childbearing is altering family structures and reducing the number of younger family members available to care for aging parents and grandparents. As a result, population aging will strain the existing health care and support resources of all nations and families. For families and states in the twenty-first century, the question is, Who will support and care for elderly people?

Actually, population aging represents a human success story. Societies now have the luxury of aging. But the steady, sustained growth in life expectancy also poses many challenges. We point to three changes during the past fifty years that are associated with population aging and the challenges they pose for nations and families: the dramatic extension of life, changes in the age structures of nations, and changes in family structures and relationships.

Extension of the Life Course

Over the past six decades, there has been a remarkable increase in life expectancy, especially in industrialized societies. In the United States the average life expectancy increased from 46 years in 1900 to 77 years in 2002 (Population Reference Bureau, 2003). Improved health and longevity and lower fertility have generated growing numbers and proportions of older population throughout most of the world. Europe has the highest proportion of population age 65 or older (ranging from 18% to 20%). By 2030, most western European nations will have an elderly population (65 or older) of 24 to 26 percent, and 7 percent are projected to be age 80 or older (U.S. Bureau of the Census, 2002a). However, Japan, with the highest life expectancy in the world (78 years for men and 85 years for women), is projected to be the oldest country for the next several decades (Population Reference Bureau, 2003). It is estimated that by 2030, 29 percent of the Japanese population will be age 65 or older. By these standards, the United States is comparatively young. Currently those 65 or older make up just 13 percent of the population; the percentage will increase to 21 by 2030 as baby boomers move into retirement (U.S. Bureau of the Census, 2002a).

Changes in the Age Structures of Nations

Lower fertility and increased longevity are altering the age structures of all nations. In the span of just one century, age pyramids have become rectangularized in most industrialized societies. Age structures—representing age cohorts of different sizes relative to one another as they move through historical time—have profound implications for the economic, political, and social well-being of a nation and its people. The shape of an age structure tells a great deal about dependency relationships between individuals and families, their government, and the economic and social resources that may be available to meet the needs of elderly people. Shifts in population age structures generally result in changing service demands and economic needs. With an increasingly older age structure comes change in the relative numbers of people who can support public health and pension programs for elderly people.

Changes in Family Structures and Relationships

There have also been widespread changes in family structures and relationships over the past six decades. Some of these are the consequences of the expanded life course, others the result of trends affecting family structures, notably higher divorce rates and increases in childbearing by single women. This means that the age structure of most American families has changed from a pyramid to what might be described as a "beanpole"—that is, a family structure with a long, thin shape, having more family generations alive but fewer members in each generation (Bengtson, Rosenthal, and Burton, 1990). Today there are many more three- and four-generation families than in the past. These changes in demographic distribution by age within families are remarkable and have important implications for family functions and relationships. In particular, the decrease in mortality rates over the past century is increasing the availability of extended intergenerational kin—grandparents and great-grandparents—who can care for family members in need and serve as resources for children as they grow up (Bengtson, 2001).

Wachter (1997) estimated the future availability of kin for family members. He found that while low fertility rates in the late twentieth century will lead to a shortage of kin for those reaching retirement around 2030, the effects of divorce, remarriage, and family blending are expanding the numbers and types of step-kin, thus "endowing the elderly of the future with kin networks that are at once problematic, rich, and varied" (Wachter, 1997, p. 1181). The implications are that step-kin are increasing the kin supply across generations while also becoming potential sources of nurture and support for family members in need and that this phenomenon may compensate in part for lower fertility rates (Amato and Booth, 1997).

Globalization and Late Modern Society

Globalization, the growing power of transnational corporations, and increasing fluidity as well as uncertainty—all define the current postindustrial period, or what some refer to as "late modernity" (Giddens, 1991; Heinz, 2003; Phillipson, 2003b). In the United States, the last quarter of the twentieth century was marked by increasing economic turbulence: waves of company restructuring and job loss, followed by the shifting of manufacturing and professional jobs to lower-wage developing countries. This process was made possible by the rapid advance of information and communication technology. Globalization represents the triumph of capitalism and the technological revolution. As part of the globalization phenomenon, multinational corporations and financial institutions are able to move capital- and labor-intensive productive activities around the globe, seeking the most favorable economic conditions, blurring national boundaries, and compressing time and space. Its major actors are transnational corporations and financial institutions and the political and professional elites associated with them (Sklair, 2002).

Underlying these changes has been the expansion of "individualism," regarded by many as the master trend of our times (Bellah, Madsen, Sullivan, and Tipton, 1985; Binstock, 1999). Under globalization and its reorganization of work, the implicit employment contract, with its provisions for a lifetime career and economic security, has moved toward increasing individualization and privatization, transferring substantially more "risk" to individuals and families (O'Rand, 2003). Long-term work careers and stable employment are less certain, and unemployment is rising because of more volatile and deregulated labor markets (Heinz, 2001). Jobs have become increasingly insecure. These trends have accelerated in the past few years, and the "outsourcing of American jobs" has emerged as a major political issue.

These larger economic changes and the trends toward increasing individualism that they embody are implicated in higher divorce rates and changing family structures, weakened kinship norms, the stresses related to juggling work and family roles, and pervasive ambivalence and uncertainty. At the same time, there are more choices (in work and life style) and more opportunities. These changes reflect tendencies of the late modern period and how they have permeated family life and intimate relations. Some social theorists believe these developments have prompted a heightened degree of instability in social relations. Individuals are faced with distinctive pressures in managing everyday life, and day-to-day interactions entail a greater degree of openness as well as uncertainty (Giddens, 1991). How will families respond to these twenty-first-century challenges? Will families continue to be important, or will the obligations across generations and kinship structures become less relevant?

Neoliberalism and the Retrenchment of Social Welfare Programs

In the context of expanding capitalism and the growing importance of global markets, globalization tends to weaken the role of governments in providing for its most vulnerable citizens (Estes, 2003; Phillipson, 2003a). Transnationals are exerting increasing influence on social policy agendas, pressuring for the expansion of market forces in the provision of social services and the reduction of public welfare programs. This is particularly evident with regard to retirement programs and provisions for families. Phillipson (2003a) argues that the growing power of global finance and private transnational entities raises fundamental questions about a society's collective obligations and the rights of its citizens to health and support in old age.

In the United States, there are increasing pressures to transfer more and more of the risks associated with aging—the threat of poverty, the need for long-term care, and the likelihood of severe illness—to individuals and their families (in particular, women caregivers and elderly people). O'Rand (2003) argues that as individuals and their families have become increasingly responsible for health, retirement provisions, and dependency needs, risk now characterizes the life course in late modern societies. "The idea of life course risk was founded on social insurance formulations, which sought institutionalized solutions to individual risks" (O'Rand, 2003, p. 694). O'Rand notes this has now reversed. Under the sway of market forces, individualized solutions are being sought for institutional risks, and individuals are increasingly "on their own." The issue of risk is now central to policy debates over aging, income security, and health care.

This shift amounts to the unraveling of the social safety net. Individuals are being required to assume new risk-taking roles and responsibilities in terms of their health and financial security. While individual autonomy and choice increase in the process, privatization brings with it increasing disparities and new high-risk groups (O'Rand, 2003). As a consequence of these trends, income inequality has increased in the United States (Korpi and Palme, 1998). O'Rand points to an increasing education gap in pension coverage (it is less available to those with a high school education or less) as well as new "gender gaps" in pension coverage. Another risk is the decline in employer-paid health insurance coverage for workers and their families. In the current environment, lower-class workers are no longer able to obtain pension coverage or private sources of insurance for health and income loss.

Yet contrary trends may be emerging—a potential shift away from a politics of liberalism to a global politics of social concern. Laissez-faire economic liberalism and its wrenching structural adjustments appear to have prompted a concern on the part of some international organizations (the World Bank, IMF, and U.N. agencies) with the negative social consequences of globalization (Phillipson, 2003b). Some U.S. politicians are beginning to challenge free trade policies to protect U.S. jobs. Others suggest that the growing antiglobalization movements (such as those demonstrating against the World Trade Organization), using the arguments of class polarization and ecological unsustainability, will work to replace capitalist globalization with a globalization of economic and social human rights (Sklair, 2002).

Consequences: Challenges to Families

At the beginning of the twenty-first century, evidence is mounting of the growing economic insecurity of middle-class U.S. families. As part of a Harvard University study of changing bankruptcy patterns in the United States, Warren and Tayagi (2003) found that two-income, two-parent middle-class families in 2001 were less well off financially than single-income, two-parent middle-class families were in 1970. Findings indicate that the high costs of housing, health care, education, and child care have left contemporary middle-class, two-income families with much greater financial commitments and less discretionary income than their 1970 single-income family counterparts. Savings rates have declined from 11 percent to almost zero, and today's two-income families are at much higher risk for financial distress through job loss, unexpected medical expense, or divorce. The study documents that over the past generation, the number of middle-class U.S. families who have found themselves in serious financial trouble has increased dramatically, regardless of prevailing economic conditions. The authors project that if current trends continue, more than 5 million families with children will file for bankruptcy by 2010. That means that almost one of every seven families with children will have declared itself broke, "losers in the great American economic game" (Warren and Tayagi, 2003, p. 6). These economic dilemmas will present families with new challenges in the coming decade.

The Changing Life Course: Linking Social Contexts and Individual Lives

The Life-Course Perspective

The life course is both a social phenomenon and a widely used theoretical perspective in the study of families and aging. The life course of individuals is conceptualized as a sequence of age-graded roles and transitions that are embedded in social institutions and history. Applying a life-course perspective, family researchers can assess the importance of larger social and historical contexts, such as wars, economic recessions, political movements, or cultural changes, for the health and well-being of individuals and families across the life span. It is through the use of age distinctions and birth cohorts that the transitions of the adult life can be marked and families can be linked to historical contexts (Elder and Johnson, 2001).

The *institutional* structuring of lives is at the core of life-course analysis (Mortimer and Shanahan, 2003). Institutional contexts—the family, schools, work and labor markets, church, government—define both the normative pathways of social roles, including key transitions, and the psychological, behavioral, and health-related trajectories of persons as they move through them. Within pluralistic contemporary societies, life-course trajectories and transitions display considerable variability. At the same time, continuity remains a predominant feature of individual psychological and behavioral trajectories.

Deinstitutionalization of the Life Course

Education, entering the work force, marriage, becoming a parent, the completion of child rearing, and retirement—these involve key transitions in the adult life course, but their timing has shifted during the last century. Governed by age norms, the timing of these transitions had become increasingly sequenced and uniform through the first half of the twentieth century. Specific age norms rather than the less structured or idiosyncratic needs of families came to regulate transition timing and duration (Hareven, 1996). Phases of the life course became more differentiated; its patterning became institutionalized (Kohli, 1986). This was particularly evident in the 1950s. One consequence, for example, was that by midcentury the "empty nest" phase emerged for parents at midlife because age norms now specified a narrower time frame for child-bearing, schooling, and exit from home (Hareven, 1996). An uninterrupted working career, beginning in young adulthood and lasting through midlife, was expected and realized (for white men, at least), culminating in a specific age for retirement. In the past three decades, however, the strict timing patterns of life-course transitions have loosened and become more flexible—representing a deinstitutionalization, or destandardization, of the life course (Heinz, 2003). Some social theorists suggest that it occurred because economic turbulence and globalization rendered the normal life course and its institutionalized pathways less certain. In late modern society, labor markets are increasingly fluid and contingent. At the same time, individuals are allowed greater freedom to shape their own life course (Beck, 1992; Giddens, 1991; Heinz, 2003; Phillipson, 2003b).

Implications for Families

In late modernity, a "contingent work life course" presents new challenges for building a work career with any continuity or security (Heinz, 2003). One consequence is that family life and its rhythms are less certain. The timing of individual life-course transitions has been affected, as reflected in the increasingly later ages of marriage and childbearing. Delayed completion of education as well as delayed and interrupted retirement are more common (Heinz, 2003). Have these historical shifts in work and family life been detrimental for family cohesiveness?

Within families over time, there are countervailing forces of change and continuity. On the one hand, it may be said that in a rapidly changing world, grandparents, parents, and children share less culture and historical experience and that family solidarity is thereby challenged. On the other hand, increased longevity means that multigenerational family members will live longer "shared lives," with more opportunity for shared activities and mutual support and assistance, thereby promoting solidarity and continuity. Phillipson (2003b) proposes that the current process of "detraditionalization," a characteristic of late modernity, is most likely a "reworking" rather than an abandonment of the family practices of trust and reciprocity. He suggests that these principles underpinning family relations continue to exert considerable force.

Stresses on Family Members

What are the microlevel consequences of the dramatic demographic and economic transformations and increasing "risks" in late modern society? We suggest three issues that will continue to stress families and individuals in the next decade: marital instability and its consequences, the difficulty of balancing work and family, and the increasing need to care for elderly family members in the face of reduced public resources.

Marital Instability and Its Consequences

Census statistics reveal just how much family structures in the United States have changed over the past quarter century. Changing patterns of family formation and dissolution, childbearing, and other types of kinship arrangements have altered family configurations and dramatically increased the diversity of family forms. In 2000, 53 percent of the adult population were married, compared to 72 percent in 1970; 11 percent were separated or divorced in 2000, up from 4.5 percent in 1970 (U.S. Bureau of the Census, 2001). The 2000 census demonstrates the continued shift from two-parent to one-parent families. The proportion of all households consisting of married couples with their own children (which can include stepchildren) declined from 40 percent in 1970 to 24 percent in 2000 (Casper and Bianchi, 2002), while those consisting of one parent with children increased from 11 percent in 1970 to 16 percent in 2000. Approximately half of the first marriages of the baby boom cohort will end in divorce (a rate that may be lower for more recent cohorts), and about 60 percent of second marriages end in divorce (Emery, 1999). Cohabitation has increased dramatically since the 1950s; however, unmarried couples make up just 6 percent of U.S. households at any one time (Casper and Bianchi, 2002).

Marriage Patterns. In the United States, more than 90 percent of every female birth cohort since the mid-1800s has eventually married (Cherlin, 1999), although the timing of marriage has varied significantly across cohorts. The median age of marriage for women increased from 20 years in 1956 to 25 years in 2001, and for men from 23 to 27 years over the same period (Bianchi and Casper, 2001). During the post–World War II years, marriages were more universal and people married earlier than in any other period in the twentieth century. However, since the early 1970s, there has been a dramatic decline in marriage rates in the United States (Goldstein and Kenney, 2001). Also having declined are remarriages, and they are more likely to end in divorce than first marriages.

It is unclear whether the decline in marriage rates reflects an increasing proportion of women who will remain single their entire lives, or merely a postponement of marriage to older ages. A related question is whether greater economic independence has made women more likely to remain single, or whether the effect has primarily meant a later age at first marriage. A century ago, remaining single was more common among the more highly educated, probably because these women were more likely to pursue careers—until lately seen as incompatible with marriage. Goldstein and Kenney (2001) found evidence that a new pattern is emerging in which marriage will be more common for women with college degrees than for those without. That is, women's economic independence is becoming associated with higher rates of marriage rather than lower rates of marriage. For older cohorts of women, the opposite was true (Elder, 1999). Some researchers suggest that marriage has become less important in the United States (Cherlin, 1999; Spain and Bianchi, 1996). However, using forecast models, Goldstein and Kenney (2001) conclude that marriage in the United States remains a strong social institution and that it will not be overtaken by cohabitation as a long-term substitute for marriage, as has been observed in the Scandinavian countries.

In recent years, as divorce has become easier to obtain and less stigmatized, and because women have far greater occupational opportunities and fewer children, married couples who are unhappy are much less likely to stay married (Wolfinger, 1998). Factors which have been found to predict divorce include an early age of marriage, the duration of the marriage, and women's increased labor force participation, which provides them with some degree of economic independence and makes them less dependent on the marriage for their financial well-being.

Changes in Fertility. In the past decade, birthrates have plunged to below replacement level in most industrialized nations and in several rapidly developing nations (notably South Korea and China). Several western European nations, as well as Japan, are now losing population (Bengtson and Putney, 2000). The U.S. birth rate in 2002 (13.9 per 1,000 women between ages 15–44) dropped 1 percent from 2001 to its lowest level since 1909. The total fertility rate in 2002 was at 1.9, slightly less than replacement level. This decline is attributed to women bearing fewer children, the continuing decline in teen births (down 28% since 1990), and the steadily growing senior population (Centers for Disease Control and Prevention, 2003). Spain and Bianchi (1996) characterize the recent decline in childbearing seen among baby boom and Generation X women as representing a practical response to the economic and time constraints of contemporary family life. In recent years, a disconnect has appeared between marriage and parenthood: in 2002 more than one-third of all U.S. births occurred outside of marriage (Centers for Disease Control and Prevention).

Changes in Family Structures and the Implications for Family Well-Being. Increases in divorce and remarriage and in childbearing outside of marriage are forcing reconsideration of how families and kinship relations are defined. In fact, the definition of *family* has become ambiguous (Stacey, 1991). No longer is there a single culturally dominant family pattern, but rather a multiplicity of family and household arrangements whose forms change frequently in response to changing personal and occupational circumstances. For poor and minority families in particular, young women have come to rely less on marriage and husbands and more on other kinship ties for support—mothers who help them in raising their children, grandparents, siblings, other relatives, and fictive kin. In general, African Americans are more likely than whites to reside in extended family households with other kin nearby and to report having "fictive kin" (Chatters and Jayakody, 1995). Latinos are also more likely to reside in multigenerational households than whites (Himes, Hogan, and Eggebeen, 1996).

Changes in family configurations brought about by divorce, single parenthood, and remarriage have important implications for individual and family well-being. Duncan and Morgan (1985) found that the economic environment faced by most people is not stable but volatile and that much of the volatility can be explained by frequent changes in marital status and hence family composition. They found such family composition changes to be far more important for the family's economic status than were changes in the labor force participation and wage rates of the adults in the household or any of the initial characteristics of the adults, such as educational attainment or attitudes. In particular, divorce had devastating effects on the economic status of women and children, whereas marriage or remarriage had almost equally beneficial effects.

Divorce affects fathers in a different way. Research findings suggest that father–adult child bonds are more conditional than mother–adult child bonds and may be especially vulnerable when there is a divorce, which can lower the divorced father's reserves of family support when he becomes elderly (Lawton, Silverstein, and Bengtson, 1994). This corresponds to other research findings concerning the negative effects of divorce, the parent's divorce as well as the child's, on the quality of the adult child–parent relationships (Kaufman and Uhlenberg, 1998; Marks, 1995; Uhlenberg, 1993). In a longitudinal study of cross-generational family influences and achievement orientations, Bengtson, Biblarz, and Roberts (2002), found that divorced fathers have become increasingly disadvantaged in terms of their emotional bonds with their children when compared to mothers, whether the mothers are divorced or not. In fact, parental divorce has reduced to almost nonexistent the ability of baby boomer fathers to *influence* their Generation X children's aspirations, self-esteem, and values.

Trends in Family Income. Primarily as a result of the 2001 economic recession, poverty rates in the United States rose almost a full percent in a two-year period (from 11.3% in 2000 to 12.1% in 2002), and real median household income declined over the same period (U.S. Bureau of the Census, 2002b, 2003). The poverty rate increased across a broad range of population groups, including all families, non-Hispanic whites, and people 18 to 64 years old. In 2002, 17 percent of all children lived in families with incomes below the poverty level. In mother-only households, 38 percent of children lived in families with incomes below the poverty level (for children in father-only households, 19% lived in poverty) (U.S. Bureau of the Census, 2003). There is a growing disparity in income in the United States, exacerbated by the 2000–2001 recession and "jobless" recovery. Some suggest the disparity reflects the conservative politics in the United States in recent years, the growing domination of global market ideology, and the greater shifting of risk to individuals and families (Parrott, Mills, and Bengtson, 2000).

A surprising trend over the past few years also points to these disparities in family resources: the *increase* in the number of stay-at-home mothers in the later half of the 1990s. The 2000 census showed a significant decline since 1998 in the labor force participation rate of mothers with infants (from 59% to 55%), the first decline since the government began reporting these statistics. These mothers were characterized as married, mostly white, over age 30, and having a college education. While this trend is likely due to the economic expansion and stock market gains in the latter half of the 1990s, it also suggests that "stay-at-home mothering" may be regaining its popularity, even if only available to those who can afford it (Bachu and O'Connell, 2001).

Balancing Work and Family Life

The difficulty of balancing work with family life has emerged as a pressing problem for families in late modern America, and this is particularly true for women. Moen (1992) argues that the dilemma created by the conflicting demands of family work and wage work is not new; it is an issue that has been paramount for women since the beginning of the twentieth century. Other researchers suggest its priority only emerged when mothers of young children began to flood into the labor market beginning in the 1970s (coincident with the rapid increase in divorce) and the crisis of child care and time constraints intensified (Hochschild, 1989, 1997). Also, contemporary women are more likely to be heads of household than were women of the 1950s. Consequently, by the 1990s mothers were carrying heavier and more diverse burdens than many of their mothers or grandmothers had known (Blackwelder, 1997).

This balancing act has been difficult for women, given the traditional primacy of family and child care in their lives. Gerson (1985) suggests it is particularly difficult for younger cohorts of women because of the contradictory signals given by parents, employers, and educational and political institutions and because gender norms are no longer clear-cut. In one longitudinal study of baby boom women who graduated from college in 1967, the proportion reporting that they felt family-career conflict increased from 25 percent in 1967 to 50 percent in 1981 (Tangri and Jenkins, 1993). The authors found that these women felt a real sense of difficulty in reconciling high performance standards in both areas with the limitations imposed by finite time and energy. Gerson (1985) suggests that whereas these changes in educational and occupational opportunities created many new options for women over the past four decades, when coupled with persistent gender inequality, they have also created new and intensified personal dilemmas and social conflicts.

Time Pressures. A key issue emerging from the ongoing debates concerning work-family balance has to do with time: the time that employment requires as well as the timing of occupational demands in relation to those of family, in particular the "daily juggling" done by working mothers and fathers and the resulting stress (Parcel and Cornfield, 2000). How much time parents spend at work and at home is a recent research focus (Hochschild, 1997). In her study of two-income middle- and upper-middle-class families at a large manufacturing firm, Hochschild suggested that mothers in particular are finding the balancing of work and home so stressful that many now see work as a haven. However, in an empirical test of Hochschild's findings (using data from the General Social Survey), Kiecolt (2003) found no evidence that working mothers in two-parent households preferred work over home. In fact, she found the opposite. Between 1973 and 1994, women shifted away from finding work more satisfying toward finding home a haven. No changes were found among men.

The unequal amount of time that mothers and fathers spend on housework is another source of stress in families (Coltrane, 2000). Hochschild (1989) found that on average, women work in and out of the home 15 hours a week more than men work, or an extra month of 24 days a year. Men's share of domestic work has improved only slightly in more recent years, partly because women spend less time doing domestic work. And despite the trend toward greater acceptance of egalitarian gender roles, both husbands and wives believe it is women who should have responsibility for family relationships and care (Aronson, 1992).

Changing Strategies for Balancing Work and Family. For a century or more, women have used various strategies for balancing the claims of work and family, including not marrying, delaying childbearing, and having fewer children. More than 25 percent of American women born in the first decade of the twentieth century never bore children (Rosenberg, 1992). Another strategy was to work part-time. A third was to time child-rearing and market work sequentially. As recently as 1980, most married mothers followed a sequential pattern of labor force participation, leaving the labor force during their prime child-rearing years, and reentering the labor force when their children grew older (Moen, 1992; Spain and Bianchi, 1996). Baby boom women were more likely to enact their work and family roles simultaneously and more likely to remain in the labor force during their prime child-rearing years.

By the 1990s, the difficulty of balancing work and family in dual-income families had given rise to new strategies. In a qualitative study, Becker and Moen (1999) investigated the contemporary work-family adaptive strategies of middle-class dual-earning couples. They define "adaptive strategies" as the processes family members engage in to (re)construct and modify their roles, resources, and relationships. What they found was that most couples were *not* pursuing two high-powered careers, but typically engaged in strategies that reduced and restructured their commitments to paid work over the life course and thereby buffered the family from work encroachments. Three "scaling back" strategies were identified: placing limits (disproportionately done by the wife); having a one-career and one-job (usually the woman's) marriage; and trading off. For women, placing limits was most typically associated with having young children at home. However, unlike men, women engaged in placing limits on paid employment across all ages and life-course stages, even when there were no children in the home.

Maternal Employment and Practices. The employment of mothers of young children has emerged as a contentious issue in the last two decades. Some researchers suggest it is precisely this issue that brought the work-family balance problem to public, and scholarly, awareness (Perry-Jenkins, Repetti, and Crouter, 2000). A common hypothesis is that changing gender roles and increased maternal employment have been detrimental to children's well-being. The assumption is that the time a mother spends in the labor force is inversely related to the time she spends with her children (Coleman, 1988). However, psychological studies have found little evidence that mothers in dual-earner households interact with their children less frequently than mothers who stay at home with their children (Turner and Troll, 1994; Parcel and Menaghan, 1994).

Researchers have found that the effect of maternal employment on young children varies by the mother's education and occupational status (Kalmijn, 1994; Moen, 1992). Women's working experiences can be an asset to the learning environment at home. Because of changing roles for women, mothers have become increasingly important role models for occupational achievement for their children, especially their daughters. Ironically, it is the mothers in non-professional full-time jobs, which usually provide less flexibility to meet family needs, who may feel greater pressures at work and thus more work-family imbalance and distress.

The persistence of gendered roles and time allocations puts more demands on employed women than on employed men across the life course (Kiecolt, 2003). Women remain disadvantaged in the accumulation of work-related returns because they tend to spend more time on domestic and caring work than do men (Heinz, 2003). In a study of U.S. dual-earner couples and their pathways through work and marriage, Han and Moen (2001) verified the persistence of unequal comparative advantages and life chances between men and women at the nexus of work and home. They found that working women had more marital instability than did working men, and the wives' employment sequences were highly contingent on their husbands' careers.

Who Will Care for Elderly People?

As family structures and functions change, will contemporary families be able to meet the needs of their elderly members? One of the major functions of multigenerational families is the provision of care and support to dependent members—in childhood, youth, and old age. In the United States, for example, almost 80 percent of informal caregiving is provided by family members (Bengtson, 2001). Longer lives and the changes in family structure that ensue have important implications for family functions and relationships, because they affect the availability of potential caregivers and the chances of receiving family support. Longer lives have meant a dramatic increase in the number of midlife adults who have surviving parents. An increasing proportion of those parents will survive to very old ages, although not without serious impairments. At the same time, declines in fertility have meant that fewer potential caregivers are available for the growing numbers of elderly people.

The increased longevity of grandparents, great-grandparents, and other family members represents a resource of kin available for help and support that can be, and frequently is, activated in times of need (Silverstein, Parrott, and Bengtson, 1995). However, as the aged increase both in numbers and in proportions, and in the context of finite state and family resources, important social and political questions arise about how the elderly population will be cared for—and by whom.

Two decades ago, Elaine Brody called attention to an impending crisis—that "having a dependent elderly parent was becoming a normative experience for many individuals and families *and exceeding the capacities of some of them*" (Brody, 1985, p. 20, italics added). Brody pointed to two converging demographic and socioeconomic trends and their likely effects on family caregiving: the accelerated rate of increase in the very old population—those most likely to need care; and the rapid entry of middle-aged women—the traditional providers of parent care—into the workforce, affecting their availability for parent care and constituting a major claim on their time and energy. This middle generation of women with multiple and potentially conflicting roles has been referred to as the "sandwich generation." Subsequent investigations of the sandwich generation phenomenon have focused on three issues: the need to use representative samples (Brody used a small convenience sample), the nature and prevalence of multiple role occupancies and their demographic potential for "overlapping," and the consequences of having multiple roles for well-being. Enacting multiple roles can have negative effects because of stress and burden (Goode, 1960), or it can have positive effects by providing benefits, such as gratification or feelings of self-efficacy or buffering the stress from other roles (Thoits, 1986), or it can have varied effects, depending on context (Moen, Robison, and Dempster-McClain, 1995).

Findings indicate that in general the psychological health effects of occupying concurrent roles are small, suggesting that multiple role occupancy per se may not consistently affect the perceived well-being of parental caregivers. It is unclear whether the "myth" of the sandwich generation will have more validity for the upcoming cohorts of adult children who will bring very different work and family life experiences and expectations to their midlife roles.

Who Will Be the Primary Caregiver? The person within the family who is given the primary caregiving role varies from one society to another. Cultural values play an important part in the hierarchy of caregiver selection. For example, in East Asian societies, under the norm of filial piety and as embodied in law, adult children, especially eldest sons, have responsibility for elderly parents, physically as well as financially (although it is typically a son's wife who provides the daily care to her in-laws, whether coresiding or not) (Youn, Knight, Jeong, and Benton, 1999). In Germany, the spouse is the first source of care, and the second-choice scenario is for the elderly person to try to manage without help. Informal care provided by adult children, other relatives, or friends is the third choice, followed by professional care. In the United States, the spouse is the first choice; secondarily an adult child, typically a daughter, becomes the primary caregiver. Responsibility next passes to a daughter-in-law (Gatz, Bengtson, and Blum, 1991). Cultural beliefs and rules of caregiver selection, the existence of state support for elder care, and the availability of kin are of course confounded. These facts complicate the issues facing policymakers as populations age.

Changing Values concerning Family Care. Norms of filial piety figure prominently in the way Asian families and nations care for their elderly population. Sung (2000) describes filial piety as characterized by close interdependent ties, responsibility and sacrifice, harmony, and viewing individuals in relation to the family. Filial familism contrasts with Western individualism and its emphasis on independence, self-reliance, and self-fulfillment. However, researchers have begun to observe that because of industrialization and urbanization, the significance of filial piety among Asians has been weakened—its power to compel exchange and support between parents and their children is now greatly diminished (Yoon, Eun, and Park, 2000). For example, in South Korea extensive migration now makes it more difficult for children to be filially pious through coresidence. As a result, parents have reduced their expectation of being able to rely on their children for support. Recent surveys show that South Korean elderly people prefer to live separately from adult children and not to burden them with their needs. Intergenerational relationships are becoming more affection-based, and younger generations tend to exchange support based more on feelings of reciprocity (Sung, 2000). These changes suggest an emergent trend in the expression of filial piety, a move from authority-dependency relationships to egalitarian and reciprocal patterns of mutual support between generations, more similar to patterns in Western nations. Today, Korean society presents a mixture of Western and traditional Korean cultures where norms of familism and individualism coexist, and attitudes among the young toward family care of elderly people are changing.

The Paradox of Elder Care. Providing care for elderly family members is a growing concern in nations of both East and West. Yet in all societies, the primary responsibility for providing care and support to elderly people remains with families. For Western states, population aging means that a growing number of elderly people will be dependent on the tax support of decreasing numbers of working adults, both in terms of their main income source, public pensions, and in terms of government-sponsored health care. In the past decade, however, most Western nations have come under considerable economic and political pressure to reduce their social welfare programs. Longer lives, smaller family sizes, and perhaps fewer potential caregivers are creating a need for wider sources of support for elderly people. The paradox in Western nations is that, as a consequence of increasing budgetary pressures and policy changes, the role of the family as caregivers is being reemphasized, but this is occurring as families are less able to care for their elderly members (Parrott, Mills, and Bengtson, 2000).

In recently industrialized East Asian nations, it is now widely believed that population aging will overwhelm the family's continued ability to meet the dependency needs of its elders unless there is support from the wider society (Yoon, Eun, and Park, 2000). Yet Eastern states have been reluctant to move away from exclusive reliance on the family for care of elderly people. Expanding the state's role in caring for elderly people will not come easily to traditional Eastern societies because it conflicts with deeply held cultural beliefs about the family's duty to its elders. Moreover, filial piety seems to strongly discourage the family from accepting care services from nonfamily members. In Eastern societies, the particular form of support for elderly people will be guided as much by the principle of filial piety as by the imperatives of demography or the rules of the market.

Macrostructural Changes and Prospects: Family Resilience

How are families responding to the changing economic environment, to the threatened downsizing of government-sponsored health and old age programs, and to the increasing risks of late modern society? Have the dramatic social changes of the past four decades weakened family bonds such that the family is less able to provide nurturance and support? In this section we consider how families in the United States are adapting to the growing diversity of family forms, such as those resulting from divorce and remarriage, gay and lesbian families, a growing array of "ex" kin who remain in the family network, and fictive kin.

The Latent Kin Matrix

Family structures and functions are dynamic in that relationships are characterized by latent support that has the potential, when needed, to become enacted over time. This dynamic aspect of family life is defined by Riley and Riley (1993) as the *latent-kin matrix*, a family network that remains dormant, or in reserve, until a need arises to activate its support potential. Some scholars suggest that the greater diversity of family structures that results from divorce and remarriage can form the basis for this type of family network (Riley and Riley, 1993; Silverstein and Bengtson, 1997). These contemporary family structures and support arrangements place greater emphasis on the voluntary relationships between kin and ex-kin or fictive kin.

What needs to be investigated is how and under what conditions these latent family intergenerational networks become activated, how one charts the complex ebb and flow of intergenerational support over time, and how cultural, political, and economic environments condition the likelihood that latent support will be transformed into enacted support. The decoupling of these dimensions by itself signifies the late modern notion that the family is a complex and evolving social institution whose members continually negotiate with each other to achieve both day-to-day and enduring intergenerational arrangements.

How useful is the concept of the "latent kin matrix?" In a study of intergenerational relations typologies, Silverstein and Bengtson (1997) demonstrate that while there is significant diversity among American families across the dimensions of solidarity, most types do possess the latent solidarity resources needed to evoke intergenerational support and assistance in times of need. This study found that "latent kin" attachments are an important characteristic of intergenerational relations, a fact overlooked by the "family values" contingent in their pronouncements of family decline (Silverstein and Bengtson, 1997).

The Modified Extended Family

More than a half century ago, Parsons (1944) concluded that the nuclear family form, with its breadwinner father and stay-at-home mother, was the most functional for an industrial society. He theorized that although the extended family would remain important for older family members, its functions were no longer central or vital. But history has shown that Parsons was incorrect in his conclusion. In the past few decades, which have seen rapid social and economic change, this traditional nuclear family form has become less prominent. Instead, research on intergenerational relations indicates that the extended family may be stronger now than ever before (Bengtson, Biblarz, and Roberts, 2002). This development is based on two factors. First, people are now living far longer than they did in the past, so there are far greater opportunities for multigenerational families to form. Second, 35 years of data collected from members of three- and four-generation families demonstrate that family feelings of kinship solidarity, affection, and exchange of services have remained constantly high despite the vast social changes that have taken place.

The form of the extended family in a postindustrial society is different from that of the past. The *modified extended family* is characterized by moderate to infrequent face-to-face contact and relatively large distances between family members, but also high rates of communication and strong norms of filial obligation. The contemporary modified extended family no longer requires a common household or close proximity of nuclear subunits, because services, through technology and advanced communications, can be exchanged over geographic distance (Litwak, Silverstein, Bengtson, and Hirst, 2003). At the same time, the basic reason for kinship dispersal—that is, occupational demands—pertains less to retirees. Further, under the current conditions of occupational uncertainty, the need for young adults to move away from kin for occupational advancement may be less compelling. Also, because of the need for additional education, financial support, or delays in family formation, adult children remain in the family home far longer than they did four decades ago. This trend is evident in all Western nations (Goldscheider, 1997).

In contemporary times, it is important to understand how the meaning of family, as well as its functions, has been expanded. In addition to family members, friends, neighbors, work friends, and other types of primary groups provide a network of support for individuals. Without taking these groups into account, it might seem that traditional extended family functions have been completely lost and taken over by large formal organizations (Litwak et al., 2003). In late modern society, the extended family has taken on a new form; it has retained some key functions but has also gone into partnership with large formal organizations and a host of new primary groups. While the structures of primary groups and formal organizations are completely different, they nonetheless depend upon each other for achieving common goals. These different structures provide for distinct ways of motivating members: bureaucracies motivate through economic market incentives, emphasizing civil but impersonal relationships, and the family motivates by internalized commitments of duty and/or affection to the relationship as an end in itself. Family functions have not been lost. The extended family (although no longer living in near proximity), the nuclear family household, and other types of primary groups remain supportive of each other. Some services require a large family unit, such as extending help with cash flow problems, helping during periods of emotional crisis (e.g., conflicts between spouses), and helping during health crises. Current studies show that these services are retained by the modified extended family and supplied to the nuclear family structure (Attias-Donfut and Wolff, 2000; Bengtson, 2001; Spilerman, 2000).

Microsocial Consequences of Change: Family Members' Adaptability

At the macrosocial level, trends relating to the family as an institution are important to understand because they can reveal the contexts and forces that circumscribe family responses to challenge. At the microsocial level, however, it is important to focus on what the trends mean for individuals and how they may or may not adapt to changes in their lives as members of families.

The Surprising Strength of Intergenerational Family Bonds

What have been the consequences of changing societal and family age structures and the creation of "more years of shared lives" across generations? In contrast to those who say families and kinship relationships have weakened in the past several decades, research demonstrates that intergenerational family bonds remain strong over time. With data from the Longitudinal Study of Generations, we have charted the course of intergenerational solidarity dimensions over three decades (from 1971 to 2003) of unprecedented social change. Results show consistently high levels of emotional closeness between grandparents and parents, parents and youth, and grandparents and grandchildren over the time period. What these results suggest is that despite the challenges and stresses emanating from the shift to postindustrial conditions, families have found ways to adapt and thrive.

Expanding Support across Generations

Longitudinal research on the functioning of multigenerational families affirms that families are adapting by expanding support across generations—beyond the nuclear family to enlist support from grandparents, grandchildren—and laterally through the modified extended family. There is increasing interdependence and exchange across several generations of family members, and this expansion has protected and enhanced the well-being of new generations of children. Bengtson, Biblarz, and Roberts (2002) examined how well contemporary families are fulfilling their responsibilities to prepare youth for the future. When parental influences on youths' aspirations, self-esteem, and values—measures of the family's success in the socialization of its children—were examined, these authors found that parents' ability to influence their children had not declined over recent generations. Intergenerational transmission processes were still working effectively to shape achievement orientations of youth. The effects of parental divorce on younger generations were not that significant. The evidence showed that three core dimensions of children's identity—aspirations, self-esteem, and values—were not strongly affected by the rise in divorce rates over the three decades. Further, the experience of parental divorce did not erode the self-confidence of Generation X youth. Both Generation X youth who experienced parental divorce and those from traditional families had high and roughly equivalent levels of self-esteem.

It may be that the apparent resiliency of Generation X children who have experienced recent changes in family structure and roles can be accounted for by the adaptive and compensatory processes that their families have drawn on, particularly in times of need. These processes may often involve expanding the family to bring additional parentlike figures and family members into the lives of children, such as grandparents or extended and fictive kin relations. The influence of extended and fictive kin is particularly evident in African American families.

The Increasing Importance of Grandparents

Grandparents may represent an increasingly important source of family strength and resilience. Grandparents are considerably more financially secure than they were just 25 years ago, with a higher standard of living and economic well-being (Treas, 1995). Also, grandparents today are healthier and have many more active years ahead of them after retirement. Grandparents, as they age, can expect fewer years of chronic illnesses and limiting disabilities (Hayward and Heron, 1999). Emotional closeness and support from grandparents could potentially mitigate divorce-related family problems and custodial-parent role-overload that can negatively affect the well-being of both adult children and grandchildren (Silverstein, Giarrusso, and Bengtson, 1998). Greater grandparent involvement with grandchildren could compensate for the temporary declines in mother's attention and time with her children following divorce. In this situation, children would continue to receive the adult-family-member time investment so essential to their development.

The number of grandchildren in the care of grandparents has risen dramatically over the last two decades. Grandparents were the leading child-care providers for preschoolers who were in some type of child-care arrangement in 1997 (U.S. Bureau of the Census, 2002c). By 2000, more than 4.5 million grandchildren were coresiding with head-of-household grandparents, representing more than 1 in 18 children under age 18 in the United States. This represents a 30 percent increase over 1990 in the number of grandchildren in grandparent-headed households (AARP, 2002). In a nationally representative sample, using the grandparent as the reference, as many as 30 percent of black grandmothers, 19 percent of Hispanic grandmothers, and 12 percent of white grandmothers have been surrogate parents for a grandchild at some point in their lives (Szinovacz, 1998). Often grandparents become surrogate parents when the middle generation is disabled or otherwise unable to fulfill parental obligations—the so-called skipped generation. Grandparents' care of grand-children does put increased pressure on some older Americans' physical and financial resources. Yet many grandparents find the experience rewarding (Silverstein, Giarrusso, and Bengtson, 1998). These trends may make grandparent-grandchildren involvement more important than ever before.

Today's Successful Families

In *How Families Still Matter*, Bengtson, Biblarz, and Roberts (2002) found that the aspirations, self-esteem, and values of the Generation Xers from intact families were significantly more positive than those of comparable two-parent families in the previous generation. This result suggests that today's non-divorced, two-parent families are more successful than their counterparts a generation ago. Most surprising is the discovery of strengths in a family type that is typically used as a reference category but not as often explored in its own right: the two-biological-parent family of the 1990s.

In several respects, these two-parent intact families seem to be more effective in the socialization of their children than yesterday's two-parent intact families. It is likely that these families are a select group. Less happily married or dysfunctional parents of Generation X children would have already divorced (unlike similarly predisposed marital partners of earlier generations who would have found divorce much more difficult to accomplish). Nevertheless, it is important to uncover how today's two-parent intact families have been successful in navigating the late modern social structure—balancing work and home, negotiating the division of labor, and finding self-fulfillment while at the same time maintaining a high level of commitment and investment in their children.

The uniquely high levels of humanistic and collectivistic values among Generation X children from two-parent intact families in our study may be related to a greater egalitarianism between still married mothers and fathers in the baby boom generation. Increases in women's educational attainment over the past three decades has meant that marriages in which women are better educated than their husbands have become more likely (Qian, 1998). Women's greater education and economic power within marriage may mean that they participate in household decision making about child rearing, consumption, and other life choices not only in their roles as wives and mothers but as educational equals and breadwinners. This change within marriages may have served children well.

Prolonged Parenting

Prolonged parenthood—when children remain home longer than expected, or don't leave, or return, not because of their parents' needs but because of their own economic needs—can be a challenge for families. But it also represents new possibilities for families, demonstrating how families adapt. The completion of child rearing is a key transition point in the adult life course, but its timing has shifted during the past century (Goldscheider and Goldscheider, 1994; Hareven, 1996). By the middle of the twentieth century, the pattern of leaving home at increasingly younger ages resulted in the emergence of the "empty nest" phase for parents at midlife (Hareven, 1996). In the past few decades, however, the relaxation of these timing norms as well as unfavorable employment prospects have delayed young adults' departure from the family home—and parenting has been extended (Putney and Bengtson, 2001). This new phenomenon has been called "the cluttered nest." As featured in *Newsweek* (Tyne, 2002), "adultolescence" may represent a new phase in the family life cycle.

What does this all mean for intergenerational relationships in the future? Is prolonged parenting disruptive or disappointing for midlife parents—or beneficial and satisfying? While it is still normative for young adults to leave their parents' home and establish independent residences before marriage (Goldscheider, 1997; Ward and Spitze, 1996), recent cohorts have delayed leaving and are increasingly returning to the family home during periods of economic hardship or marital problems. It is estimated that about 40 percent of recent cohorts of young adults have returned home after some period away. Those who leave to marry continue to be less likely to return. Those who leave to seek independence—including those who leave for cohabiting relationships—are more likely to return than was the case for previous cohorts. The never married are the most likely to move back into the parental home (Goldscheider, 1997).

Research shows that it is the characteristics and needs of adult children that account for coresidence with middle-aged and older parents (White and Rogers, 1997). In contemporary economic conditions, adult children benefit from coresidence with parents into their mid-20s, particularly in terms of educational attainment (White and Lacy, 1997). As a result of the trend of delayed nest-leaving, young adults receive a significant amount of parental support from midlife parents, both tangible and emotional, over a longer period of time. It is a stream of assistance that does not shift in the other direction until quite late in parents' lives, when the parents finally become net recipients of intergenerational transfers (Bengtson and Harootyan, 1994; Eggebeen and Hogan, 1990; Rossi and Rossi, 1990).

Less is known about the quality of their relationship and how it is affected by the coresidence experience. Do the economic and instrumental benefits of coresidence come at the expense of feelings of closeness and affection between parents and adult children? The findings are varied, depending on the context, the age of the adult child, and whether the adult child left and returned home or never left. In a study of parents of coresiding adult children, Aquilino and Supple (1991) found generally high parent satisfaction and positive parent-child interactions, but also some strains. These are often associated with frustrated expectations about the timing of leaving home and independence, particularly among adult children. Coresidence is more likely to intensify parent-child relations and the potential for conflict over money, household tasks, values, and lifestyles (Ward and Spitze, 1992).

There are ethnic differences in attitudes toward intergenerational coresidence. Among the major ethnic groups in the United States, Hispanics and non-Hispanic Catholics are most supportive of coresidence (Goldscheider and Lawton, 1998), while white, nonfundamentalist Protestants are the least supportive. Attitudes among blacks toward coresidence are more ambiguous in that their family structure has become more rather than less extended over the last several decades (Ruggles, 1996). For blacks, preferences are confounded with other determinants of coresidence such as inadequate resources and need for assistance.

There is some indication among younger cohorts that the norms prescribing an independent household as a sign of successfully transitioning to adulthood may be weakening (Alwin, 1996). It may be that delayed departure from the parental home or returning after attempting to establish an independent residence, as is now occurring, is adaptive and will positively affect intergenerational relations in the future by increasing interpersonal contacts and investments in parent-child relationships now.

Changing Cultural Norms: Will the Importance of Family Increase?

Has familism—the belief that family and family relationships are of central importance—declined across generations? To what degree has individualism overwhelmed the values of familism? Researchers have documented the weakening of norms governing interpersonal and family behaviors in American society. From the mid-1960s through the 1980s, there were remarkable changes in attitudes and behaviors related to gender roles, marriage and divorce, cohabitation, and childbearing outside of marriage (Alwin, 1996; Brewster and Padavic, 2000; Hareven, 1996; Ruggles, 1996; Scott, Alwin, and Braun, 1996; Thornton, 1989). One consequence is that marriages, in particular, are increasingly based on individual choice and sensitivities rather than on norms of obligation (Cherlin, 1999; Giddens, 1991; Hareven, 1996).

Giddens (1991) theorizes that the nature of social relationships—especially marital relationships—has changed in the late modern period. Giddens refers to the emergence of the "pure relationship" in which the cultural norms prescribing role behaviors and obligations have fallen away, and intimate relationships rest almost entirely on emotional sensitivity and trust. But Giddens offers a caveat. Kin relationships, especially those between parent and child, are exceptions. Even if kin relations appear quite weak, there are obligations that relatives have toward one another that are specified by the bonds of kinship. Such norms of obligation underlie traditional understandings of familism. Being familistic can provide a social and emotional mooring, a sense of personal security that rests within one's group.

The increasing prevalence of parent–adult child coresidency suggests that a shift back to more familistic values may be occurring, at least among younger cohorts. Using national data, Alwin (1996) examined attitudes toward coresidence between 1973 to 1991 and found a gradual shift toward greater approval of coresidence among more recently born cohorts (born after 1940). The older cohorts were significantly less favorable toward parent–adult child coresidence. Also, younger cohorts had higher levels of contact with kin than older cohorts, and contact with kin was positively associated with endorsement of subjective norms of coresidence.

Parent–adult child coresidence has also increased in European nations. Age at marriage has been pushed back, due in part to unfavorable economic conditions, but also because marriage is less appealing to young adults (Cherlin, 1999; Rossi, 1997). Scabini and Cigoli (1997) found that in several western European countries, adult children's relationships with parents are generally positive, making coresidence more likely and attractive. They note that today's young adults, raised in more egalitarian homes, have more positive relations with their midlife parents than young adults did even 30 years ago and less reason to leave home. Hence, among younger cohorts, understandings of egalitarianism and familism may have changed such that younger cohorts now see these values as complementary and positive.

There are other indications of a cultural shift toward more familistic values. Bengtson, Biblarz, and Roberts (2002) found that Generation X young adults are turning toward a more collectivist value orientation compared to their parents when they were young adults. A study of baby boom women found that they had become significantly more familistic in their values between young adulthood and midlife, and this contributed to their psychological well-being (Putney and Bengtson, 2003). In a recent study of changing attitudes of different generations toward work life balance, Radcliffe's Public Policy Center (2000) found that most Americans have become more family-focused. Younger workers, particularly young men, indicated they consider family issues of primary importance and are willing to forgo money or prestige for more time with their families.

Social commentators writing about the plight of Generation Xers have found that today's youth are less supportive of the liberal political values held by their parents. They are returning to religion, have family-orientated aspirations, and are actively searching for a moral compass to guide their lives (Halstead, 1999). Parental divorce may be playing a role. Bengtson, Biblarz, and Roberts (2002) found that Generation X daughters whose parents divorced were more humanistic and less materialistic than Generation X daughters whose parents did not divorce. Perhaps some compensatory process in the context of traditional gender roles is at work, with daughters placing greater importance on the expressive values of caring and commitment to others—a consequence of their experience of family disruption.

Projections and Prophecies

What challenges and new prospects will families face in the next decade? Here are a few predictions, each representing an important research agenda for the next decade.

- We expect that the nuclear family will remain a prominent form, but far less isolated than in the past. It will rely increasingly on intergenerational family bonds for emotional and social support. We suggest that close multigenerational ties are adaptive and much needed in a fast-changing world.

- As we broaden our understanding of what a family is—a diverse, multigenerational family form whose relations are both ascribed and created—we will see an institution that is both resilient and functional. There are many strengths evolving from these family arrangements—including, perhaps, shared parenting, authoritative parenting practices (not necessarily just by parents, but also by additional parent-like figures), egalitarian household arrangements, and more collectivistic and humanistic value orientations. In a late modern society marked by diversity, fluidity, and choice, the multigenerational family retains its cohesiveness and solidarity. The family will remain the fundamental site of trust and mutual support.

- The individual life course will continue its trend toward destandardization and deinstitutionalization. As noted by Heinz (2003), delayed completion of education and delayed and interrupted retirement are growing in prevalence, along with longer-term patterns of delayed marriage and fertility and increased job mobility. O'Rand (2003, p. 695) projects that "we can expect the life course to be longer and, for many, healthier, temporally more complex in its education, work and family transition sequences—and increasingly unequal in its fortunes."

- Population aging will pose a major challenge for families and nations over the next half century. At the societal level, aging may become a source of intergenerational conflict, or at least strain. The question of who will bear the burden of caring for elderly people—whether it is the family or the state—may increasingly evoke generational tension. Because generational conflict involves more than economic considerations, it could develop into a heated political issue that becomes international in scope.

- But it is also possible that the huge growth in the older population over the next four decades, along with the increasing saliency of the caregiving experience, may lead to a resurgence of more humanistic and familistic values and a greater commitment to others. Some scholars suggest that as the baby boom generation ages and caregiving becomes increasingly salient, we are likely to see the emergence of "an ethics of care" (Polivka, 2000, p. 248).

Conclusion

We can look forward to the continuing influence and enduring importance of families. The family is still fulfilling its basic functions, but in a world very different from that of the 1950s. Family forms are far more diverse. We suggest that under conditions of globalization, the deinstitutionalized life course, and economic uncertainty, this diversity of forms is adaptive. Less bound by their biological moorings, late modern family relations and commitments now assume a more voluntaristic and "intentional" quality, more similar to the "created" kinship ties found among minority groups, friendship circles, or same-sex partners. In contemporary marriages where the gendered division of labor is less pronounced or less prescribed by gender norms (which prevailed in the postwar years), men and women are less economically and emotionally dependent upon one another. Thus there are opportunities for greater intimacy, but also more uncertainty. In this more fluid, deinstitutionalized late modern era, marital and family relationships may require more constant nurturance and tending.

In late modern society, there are pressures and the opportunities to shift more familial responsibility to the extended family. Our research suggests families are moving beyond the confines of the traditional nuclear family to the broader support and emotional resources of multigenerational family relationships. This trend can be seen in the growing incidence of grandparents raising grandchildren, where the middle generation's marriages dissolve, or where there are other difficulties (such as drug addiction) that interfere with the younger adult's ability to parent.

Given the new economic reality of late modern society, midlife parents still have their young adult children at home. Today's youth will be in college far longer than their parents were, extending the time when they will be economically dependent on the resources of their parents. Research finds that, perhaps unlike earlier periods in our history, many midlife parents are quite satisfied with these arrangements. The extended period of intergenerational exchange and support tends to strengthen the bonds of solidarity as well.

In our consideration of family stresses and prospects at the beginning of the twenty-first century, we return to an age-old question posed by philosophers and writers, and now social scientists—what Mannheim (1952) called "the problem of generations"—the ongoing tension between continuity and change, affirmation and innovation, and their reconciliation in the human social order over time. This paradox of continuity and change has relevance for our study of families and their well-being at this time in history. At the macrosocial level, we recognize the force of demography—the age structure of a given society, its distinct social metabolism that inheres in changing rates of births, deaths, and migration. The socioeconomic conditions of a society, its structures of organization and opportunity, its culture and its history, all set the boundaries of individual choice and action and family functioning. At the intersection of the macro and the micro, the life-course perspective calls us to inquire about how human development, historical location, and individual choice interact to affect generational differences and continuities. And at the microsocial level, our focus is on the processes by which generations, within families, pass on the knowledge and values, the material and psychological resources, that its members need to live successfully in society.

It is within the family that the paradox of continuity and change, the problem of balancing individuality and allegiance, is most immediate. It is a fluid, unending process and sometimes contentious. At times we think that surely a "break" from the past has occurred: families aren't what they used to be; families are in trouble. Yet if we look closely, we can see threads of continuity across generations, patterns of family resilience, and individual adaptation. Recognizing the serendipity of human events and the choices that individuals make in determining their life path, we continue to look to the family as the context for negotiating these questions of individuality and integration, continuity and change, in late modern society.

Acknowledgments

This research was supported by National Institute on Aging Grants R01-AG07977 and T32-AG00037.

REFERENCES

AARP. 2002. *Census 2000 Number and Percentage Change since 1990: Children under 18 Living in Grandparent-Headed Households.* Washington, DC: AARP Grandparent Information Center. Retrieved from www.aarp.org/confacts/grandparents/grand-facts.html (site discontinued; last accessed March 15, 2004).

Alwin, D. F. 1996. Coresidence beliefs in American society—1973–1991. *Journal of Marriage and the Family* 58:393–403.

Amato, P., and Booth, A. 1997. *A Generation at Risk: Growing Up in an Era of Family Upheaval.* Cambridge, MA: Harvard University Press.

Aquilino, W. S., and Supple, K. R. 1991. Parent-child relations and parent's satisfaction with living arrangements when adult children live at home. *Journal of Marriage and the Family* 53:13–27.

Aronson, J. 1992. Women's sense of responsibility for the care of old people: "But who else is going to do it?" *Gender and Society* 6:8–29.

Attias-Donfut, C., and Wolff, F.-C. 2000. Complementarity between private and public transfers. In S. Arber and C. Attias-Donfut, eds., *The Myth of Generational Conflict: The Family and State in Aging Societies,* pp. 47–68. London: Routledge.

Bachu, A. and O'Connell, M. 2001. *Fertility of American Women, June 2000.* Current Population Reports. Washington, DC: U.S. Bureau of the Census.

Beck, U. 1992. *Risk Society: Towards a New Modernity.* London: Sage.

Becker, P. E., and Moen, P. 1999. Scaling back: Dual-earner couples' work-family strategies. *Journal of Marriage and Family* 62:995–1007.

Bellah, R. N., Madsen, R., Sullivan, W. M., and Tipton, S. M. 1985. *Habits of the Heart: Individualism and Commitment in American Life.* Berkeley: University of California Press.

Bengtson, V. L. 2001. Beyond the nuclear family: The increasing importance of multigenerational relationships in American society. The 1998 Burgess Award Lecture. *Journal of Marriage and Family* 63:1–16.

Bengtson, V. L., Biblarz, T. J., and Roberts, R. E. L. 2002. *How Families Still Matter: A Longitudinal Study of Youth in Two Generations.* New York: Cambridge University Press.

Bengtson, V. L., and Harootyan, R. A. 1994. *Intergenerational Linkages: Hidden Connections in American Society.* New York: Springer Publishing Co.

Bengtson, V. L., and Putney, N. M. 2000. Who will care for the elderly? Consequences of population aging East and West. In K-D. Kim, V. L. Bengtson, G. D. Meyers, and K-S. Eun, eds., *Aging in East and West: Families, States, and the Elderly,* pp. 263–85. New York: Springer Publishing Co.

Bengtson, V., Rosenthal, C., and Burton, L. 1990. Families and aging: Diversity and heterogeneity. In R. H. Binstock and L. K. George, eds., *Handbook of Aging and the Social Sciences,* 3rd ed., pp. 263–87. San Diego: Academic Press.

Bianchi, S. M., and Casper, L. M. 2001. *American Families Resilient after Fifty Years of Change.* Washington, DC: Population Reference Bureau.

Binstock, R. H. 1999. Challenges to United States policies on aging in the new millennium. *Hallym International Journal of Aging* 1:4–13.

Blackwelder, J. 1997. *Now Hiring: The Feminization of Work in the United States, 1900–1995.* College Station: Texas A&M University Press.

Brewster, K. L., and Padavic, I. 2000. Changes in gender-ideology, 1997–1996: The contributions of intracohort change and population turnover. *Journal of Marriage and the Family* 62:477–88.

Brody, E. M. 1985. Parent care as normative family stress. *Gerontologist* 25:19–29.

Casper, L. M., and Bianchi, S. M. 2002. *Continuity and Change in the American Family.* Thousand Oaks, CA: Sage.

Centers for Disease Control and Prevention. 2003. News release: U.S. birth rate reaches record low. June. In *Births: Preliminary Data for 2002.* National Vital Statistics Report 51(11). Retrieved from www.cdc.gov/nchs/releases/03/news/lowbirth.htm (site discontinued; last accessed March 15, 2004).

Chatters, L. M., and Jayakody, R. 1995. Commentary: Intergenerational support within African-American families: Concepts and methods. In V. L. Bengtson, K. W. Schaie, and L. M. Burton, eds., *Adult Intergenerational Relations: Effects of Social Change,* pp. 97–118. New York: Springer Publishing Co.

Cherlin, A. J. 1999. *Public and Private Families: An Introduction.* 2nd ed. New York: McGraw-Hill.

Coleman, J. S. 1988. Social capital in the creation of human capital. *American Journal of Sociology* 94 (suppl.): S95–120.

Coltrane, S. 2000. Research on household labor: Modeling and measuring the social embeddedness of routine family work. *Journal of Marriage and the Family* 62:1209–33.

Duncan, G. J., and Morgan, J. N. 1985. The panel study of income dynamics. In G. H. Elder Jr., ed., *Life Course Dynamics: Trajectories and Transitions, 1968–1980,* pp. 50–71. Ithaca, NY: Cornell University Press.

Eggebeen, D. J., and Hogan, D. P. 1990. Giving between generations in American families. *Human Nature* 1:211–32.

Elder, G. H., Jr. 1999. *Children of the Great Depression: Social Change in Life Experience.* 25th anniversary ed. Boulder, CO: Westview Press.

Elder, G. H., Jr., and Johnson, M. K. 2001. The life course and aging: Challenges, lessons, and new directions. In R. A. Settersten Jr., ed., *Invitation to the Life Course: Toward New Understandings of Later Life,* pp. 49–81. Amityville, NY: Baywood.

Emery, R. E. 1999. *Marriage, Divorce, and Children's Adjustment.* 2nd ed. Thousand Oaks, CA: Sage.

Estes, C. L. 2003. Theoretical perspectives on old age policy: A critique and a proposal. In S. Biggs, A. Lowenstein, and J. Hendricks, eds., *The Need for Theory: Critical Approaches to Social Gerontology.* Amityville, NY: Baywood.

Gatz, M., Bengtson, V. L., and Blum, M. J. 1991. Caregiving families. In J. E. Birren and K. W. Schaie, eds., *Handbook of the Psychology of Aging,* 3rd ed., pp. 405–26. San Diego: Academic Press.

Gerson, K. 1985. *Hard Choices: How Women Decide about Work, Career, and Motherhood.* Berkeley: University of California Press.

Giddens, A. 1991. *Modernity and Self-identity: Self and Society in the Late Modern Age.* Stanford, CA: Stanford University Press.

Goldscheider, F. 1997. Recent changes in U.S. young adult living arrangements in comparative perspective. *Journal of Family Issues* 18:708–24.

Goldscheider, F. K., and Goldscheider, C. 1994. Leaving and returning home in twentieth-century America. *Population Bulletin* 48:2–33.

Goldscheider, F. K., and Lawton, L. 1998. Family experiences and the erosion of support for intergenerational coresidence. *Journal of Marriage and the Family* 60:924–38.

Goldstein, J. R., and Kenney, C. T. 2001. Marriage delayed or marriage forgone? New cohort forecast of first marriage for U.S. women. *American Sociological Review* 66:506–19.

Goode, W. J. 1960. A theory of role strain. *American Sociological Review* 25:483–96.

Halstead, T. 1999. A politics for Generation X. *Atlantic Monthly,* August, pp. 33–42.

Han, S-K., and Moen, P. 2001. Coupled careers: Pathways through work and marriage in the United States. In H. P. Blossfeld and S. Drobnic, eds., *Careers of Couples in Contemporary Societies: From Male Breadwinner to Dual Earner Families,* pp. 201–31. New York: Oxford University Press.

Hareven, T. K. 1996. Historical perspectives on the family and aging. In R. Blieszner and V. H. Bedford, eds., *Aging and the Family: Theory and Research,* pp. 13–31. Westport, CT: Praeger.

Hayward, M. D., and Heron, M. 1999. Racial inequality in active life among adult Americans. *Demography* 36:77–91.

Heinz, W. R. 2001. Work and the life course: A cosmopolitan-local perspective. In V. M. Marshall, W. R. Heinz, H. Kruger, and A. Verma, eds., *Restructuring Work and the Life Course,* pp. 3–22. Toronto: University of Toronto Press.

Heinz, W. R. 2003. From work trajectories to negotiated careers: The contingent work life course. In J. T. Mortimer and M. J. Shanahan, eds., *Handbook of the Life Course,* pp. 185–204. New York: Kluwer Academic/Plenum.

Himes, C. L., Hogan, D. P., and Eggebeen, D. J. 1996. Living arrangements of minority elders. *Journal of Gerontology: Social Sciences* 51B:S42–48.

Hochschild, A. R. 1989. *The Second Shift: Working Parents and the Revolution at Home.* New York: Viking.

Hochschild, A. R. 1997. *The Time Bind: When Work Becomes Home and Home Becomes Work.* New York: Metropolitan Books.

Kalmijn, M. 1994. Mother's occupational status and children's schooling. *American Sociological Review* 59:257–75.

Kaufman, G., and Uhlenberg, P. 1998. Effects of life course transitions on the quality of relationships between adult children and their parents. *Journal of Marriage and the Family* 60:924–38.

Kiecolt, K. J. 2003. Satisfaction with work and family life: No evidence of a cultural reversal. *Journal of Marriage and the Family* 56:23–35.

Kohli, M. 1986. The world we forgot: A historical review of the life course. In V. W. Marshall, ed., *Later Life: The Social Psychology of Aging,* pp. 271–303. Beverly Hills, CA: Sage.

Korpi, W., and Palme, J. 1998. The paradox of redistribution and strategies of equality: Welfare state institutions, inequality, and poverty in the western countries. *American Sociological Review* 63:661–87.

Lawton, L., Silverstein, M., and Bengtson, V. L. 1994. Affection, social contact and geographic distance between adult children and their parents. *Journal of Marriage and the Family* 56:57–68.

Litwak, E., Silverstein, M., Bengtson, V. L., and Hirst, Y. W. 2003. Theories about families, organizations, and social supports. In V. L. Bengtson and A. Lowenstein, eds., *Global Aging and Challenges to Families,* pp. 54–74. New York: Aldine de Gruyter.

Mannheim, K. 1952. The problems of generations. In D. Kecskemeti, ed., *Essays on the Sociology of Knowledge,* pp. 276–322. London: Routledge & Kegan Paul. Original work published 1922.

Marks, N. 1995. Midlife marital status differences in social support relationships with adult children and psychological well-being. *Journal of Family Issues* 16:5–28.

Moen, P. 1992. *Women's Two Roles: A Contemporary Dilemma.* New York: Auburn House.

Moen, P., Robison, J., and Dempster-McClain, D. 1995. Caregiving and women's well-being: A life course approach. *Journal of Health and Social Behavior* 36:259–73.

Mortimer, J. T., and Shanahan, M. J. 2003. Preface to *Handbook of the Life Course.* New York: Kluwer Academic/Plenum.

O'Rand, A. 2003. The future of the life course: Late modernity and life course risks. In J. T. Mortimer and M. J. Shanahan, eds., *Handbook of the Life Course,* pp. 693–701. New York: Kluwer Academic/Plenum.

Parcel, T. L., and Cornfield, D. R., eds. 2000. *Work and Family: Research Informing Policy.* Thousand Oaks, CA: Sage.

Parcel, T. L., and Menaghan, E. G. 1994. *Parents' Jobs and Children's Lives.* New York: Aldine de Gruyter.

Parrott, T. M., Mills, T. L., and Bengtson, V. L. 2000. The United States: Population demographics, changes in the family, and social policy challenges. In K-D. Kim, V. L. Bengtson, G. D. Meyers, and K-S. Eun, eds., *Aging in East and West: Families, States, and the Elderly,* pp. 191 224. New York: Springer Publishing Co.

Parsons, T. 1944. The social structure of the family. In R. N. Anshen, ed., *The Family: Its Function and Destiny,* pp. 173–201. New York: Harper.

Perry-Jenkins, M., Repetti, R. L., and Crouter, A. C. 2000. Work and family in the 1990s. *Journal of Marriage and the Family* 62:981–98.

Phillipson, C. 2003a. From family groups to personal communities: Social capital and social change in the family life of older adults. In V. L. Bengtson and A. Lowenstein, eds., *Global Aging and Challenges to Families,* pp. 54–74. New York: Aldine de Gruyter.

Phillipson, C. 2003b. Globalization and the reconstruction of old age: New challenges for critical gerontology. In S. Biggs, A. Lowenstein, and J. Hendricks, eds., *The Need for Theory: Critical Approaches to Social Gerontology,* pp. 163–79. Amityville, NY: Baywood.

Polivka, L. 2000. Whither goest the baby boom? Politics and values in an aging society. *Gerontologist* 40:246–51.

Population Reference Bureau. 2003. *2003 World Population Data Sheet.* Washington, DC: Population Reference Bureau. Retrieved from www.prb.org/pdf/WorldPopulation DS03_Eng.pdf (site discontinued; last accessed March 15, 2004).

Putney, M. N., and Bengtson, V. L. 2001. Families and intergenerational relations at midlife. In M. E. Lachman, ed., *Handbook of Midlife Development,* pp. 528–70. New York: Wiley.

Putney, M. N., and Bengtson, V. L. 2003. Baby boom women at midlife: Familism and self-esteem. Paper presented at the annual meeting of the Gerontological Society of America, San Francisco.

Qian, Z. C. 1998. Changes in assortive mating: The impact of age and education, 1970–1990. *Demography* 35:279–92.

Radcliffe Public Policy Center. 2000. *Life's Work: Generational Attitudes toward Work and Life Integration.* Cambridge, MA: Radcliffe Institute for Advanced Study.

Riley, M. W., and Riley, J. W. 1993. Connections: Kin and cohort. In V. L. Bengtson and W. A. Achenbaum, eds., *The Changing Contract across Generations,* pp. 169–89. New York: Aldine de Gruyter.

Rosenberg, R. 1992. *Divided Lives: American Women in the Twentieth Century.* New York: Hill and Wang.

Rossi, A. S., and Rossi, P. H. 1990. *Of Human Bonding: Parent-Child Relations across the Life Course.* New York: Aldine de Gruyter.

Rossi, G. 1997. The nestlings: Why young adults stay at home longer. The Italian case. *Journal of Family Issues* 18:627–44.

Ruggles, S. 1996. Living arrangements of the elderly in America: 1880–1980. In T. K. Hareven, ed., *Aging and Generational Relations over the Life Course: A Historical and Cross-Cultural Perspective,* pp. 254–71. New York: Walter de Gruyter.

Scabini, E., and Cigoli, V. 1997. Young adult families: An evolutionary slowdown or a breakdown in the generational transition? *Journal of Family Issues* 18:608–26.

Scott, J., Alwin, D. F., and Braun, M. 1996. Generational changes in gender-role attitudes: Britain in a cross-national perspective. *Sociology* 30:471–92.

Silverstein, M., and Bengtson, V. L. 1997. Intergenerational solidarity and the structure of adult child–parent relationships in American families. *American Journal of Sociology* 103:429–60.

Silverstein, M., Giarrusso, R., and Bengtson, V. L. 1998. Intergenerational solidarity and the grandparent role. In M. Szinovacz, ed., *Handbook on Grandparenthood,* pp. 144–58. Westport, CT: Greenwood Press.

Silverstein, M., Parrott, T. M., and Bengtson, V. L. 1995. Factors that predispose middle-aged sons and daughters to provide social support to older parents. *Journal of Marriage and the Family* 57:465–75.

Sklair, L. 2002. *Globalization: Capitalism and Its Alternatives.* New York: Oxford University Press.

Spain, D., and Bianchi, S. M. 1996. *Balancing Act: Motherhood, Marriage, and Employment among American Women.* New York: Russell Sage Foundation.

Spilerman, S. 2000. A wealth and stratification process. *Annual Reviews of Sociology* 16:497–524.

Stacey, J. 1991. *Brave New Families: Stories of Domestic Upheaval in Late Twentieth Century America.* New York: Basic Books.

Sung, K-T. 2000. An Asian perspective on aging east and west: Filial piety and changing families. In K-D. Kim, V. L. Bengtson, G. D. Meyers, and K-S. Eun, eds., *Aging in East and West: Families, States, and the Elderly,* pp. 41–56. New York: Springer Publishing Co.

Szinovacz, M. E. 1998. Grandparents today. A demographic profile. *Gerontologist* 38:37–52.

Tangri, S. S., and Jenkins, S. R. 1993. The University of Michigan class of 1967. In K. D. Hulbert and D. T. Schuster, eds., *Women's Lives through Time: Educated American Women in the Twentieth Century,* pp. 259–81. San Francisco: Jossey-Bass.

Thoits, P. A. 1986. Multiple identities: Examining gender and marital status differences in distress. *American Sociological Review* 51:259–72.

Thornton, A. 1989. Changing attitudes toward family issues in the United States. *Journal of Marriage and the Family* 51:873–93.

Treas, J. 1995. Commentary: Beanpole or beanstalk? Comments on "The demography of Changing Intergenerational Relations." In V. L. Bengtson, K. W. Schaie, and L. M. Burton, eds., *Adult Intergenerational Relations: Effects of Social Change,* pp. 26–29. New York: Springer Publishing Co.

Turner, B. F., and Troll, L. E., eds. 1994. *Women Growing Older: Psychological Perspectives.* Thousand Oaks, CA: Sage.

Tyne, P. 2002. Back with mom and dad: Enter the adultolescents. *Newsweek,* March 25, pp. 38–40.

Uhlenberg, P. 1993. Demographic change and kin relationships in later life. In G. L. Maddox and M. P. Lawton, eds., *Annual Review of Gerontology and Geriatrics,* 13:219–38. New York: Springer Publishing Co.

U.S. Bureau of the Census. 2001. America's families and living arrangements, 2000. In *Current Population Reports,* P20–537. Retrieved from www.census.gov/population/www/socdemo/hh-fam/p20–537_00.html (site discontinued; last accessed March 15, 2004).

U.S. Bureau of the Census. 2002a. *International Data Base.* Washington, DC: U.S. Government Printing Office.

U.S. Bureau of the Census. 2002b. *Poverty Rate Rises, Household Income Declines.* CB02-124. Retrieved from www.census.gov/Press-Release/www/releases/archives/income_wealth/000390.html (last accessed October 31, 2006).

U.S. Bureau of the Census. 2002c. *Who's Minding the Kids? Grandparents Leading Child-Care Providers.* CB02-102. Retrieved from http://148.129.75.3/Press-Release/www/2002/cb02–102.html (site discontinued; last accessed March 15, 2004).

U.S. Bureau of the Census. 2003. Poverty, income see slight changes; child poverty rate unchanged. CB03-153. Retrieved from www.census.gov/Press-Release/www/2003/cb03–153.html.

Wachter, K. W. 1997. Kinship resources for the elderly. *Philosophical transactions of the Royal Society of London* 352:1811–17.

Ward, R. A., and Spitze, G. 1992. Consequences of parent–adult child coresidence: A review and research agenda. *Journal of Family Issues* 13:553–72.

Ward, R. A., and Spitze, G. 1996. Will the children ever leave? Parent-child coresidence history and plans. *Journal of Family Issues* 17:514–39.

Warren, E., and Tayagi, A. W. 2003. *The Two-Income Trap: Why Middle-Class Mothers and Fathers Are Going Broke.* New York: Basic Books.

White, L., and Lacy, N. 1997. The effects of age at home leaving and pathways from home on educational attainment. *Journal of Marriage and the Family* 59:982–95.

White, L. K., and Rogers, S. J. 1997. Strong support but uneasy relationships: Coresidence and adult children's relationships with their parents. *Journal of Marriage and the Family* 59:62–76.

Wolfinger, N. H. 1998. The effects of parental divorce on adult tobacco and alcohol consumption. *Journal of Health and Social Behavior* 39:254–69.

Yoon, H., Eun, K-S., and Park, K-S. 2000. Korea: Demographic trends, sociocultural contexts, and public policy. In K-D. Kim, V. L. Bengtson, G. D. Meyers, and K-S. Eun, eds., *Aging in East and West: Families, States, and the Elderly,* pp. 121–37. New York: Springer Publishing Co.

Youn, G., Knight, G., Jeong, H.-S., and Benton, D. 1999. Differences in familism values and caregiving outcomes among Korean, Korean American, and white American dementia caregivers. *Psychology and Aging* 14:355–64.

CHAPTER SIX

Long-Term Care, Feminism, and an Ethics of Solidarity

Martha B. Holstein, Ph.D.

> Any real society is a caregiving and a care receiving society and we must therefore discover ways of coping with these facts of human neediness and dependency that are compatible with the self-respect of the recipients and do not exploit the caregiver. —NUSSBAUM, 2002
>
> Existing systems of allocating the benefits and burdens of caring for the chronically ill and disabled are unfair.
> —HIRSCHFIELD AND WIKLER, 2003–4

In the early 1960s, during debates about the proposed Medicare legislation, assistance with nonmedical, custodial care was off the table. A commonly held notion even today—that people would take advantage of the public provision of services such as bed making and meal preparation—is rooted in privilege and often serves as the unwarranted justification for limiting public benefits. In fact, families have not abandoned their elders; nor have older people eagerly sought services. In the words of an 85-year-old woman in Oregon, Illinois, "It is hard enough to need help; it is even harder to ask for it" (Holstein and Mitzen, 2004). Caregivers ask not for replacement care but for a "supplement and respite from what they continually provide" (Hooyman and Gonyea, 1999, p. 163).

The consequences of this situation—that long-term care resides primarily in the private or family realm and that consequently its financing is treated differently than financing acute care—raises ethically important questions that touch upon the lives of older people who need help with the tasks of daily living and those who provide this help—most often family members, in particular women, and poorly paid home care aides, also predominantly women.

These individuals are bound together by ties of vulnerability, response to vulnerability, commitment, and concern. They are also fundamentally unequal compared to those who neither need nor give care. This truth signals exploitation of a caregiver's labor, which renders it a problem of justice despite the satisfactions caregiving might bring.

Moving against the contemporary political grain that emphasizes personal responsibility, I will argue that greater collective responsibility for caregiving is essential if we accept a central feature of social justice—that each person has dignity and worth that institutional structures should not violate or exploit (Nussbaum, 2001). Placing the burden of care on women in ways that can result in economic, social, and other physical and mental harms represents such violation and exploitation. Ethical difficulties are compounded because this system can lead to inadequate care while it differentially affects people on the basis of their income when they are the most vulnerable. To mitigate or eliminate these harms requires new ways to think about caring for people of any age who are dependent upon others to make it through the day. Individuals who give care need care to protect their own physical and mental well-being. They also need care to allow them to exercise their rights and obligations as citizens—opportunities to contribute to their communities in meaningful ways, not least by participating actively in defining needs and shaping policy agendas, especially agendas relevant to long-term care. Defining needs, as political theorist Nancy Fraser (1989) reminded us some years ago, is a political rather than an objective or neutral act. Who better to define the needs of the cared-for and the caregiver than people in those roles? But as long as caregiving is on the periphery of public life, "those involved in caring relationships will be perceived as ' other' and their rights as citizens will be attenuated" (Lloyd, 2004, p. 248). As a result of their relative isolation, their anomalous state, and the vagaries of the political process, caregivers rarely participate in public life.

Philosophical reflections about long-term care, until quite recently, have not called attention to these problems. Over the past 20 years or so, this work has focused instead on extending ethical individualism, or the ability to make choices about one's life; autonomy, whether by design or not, became the ethical trump card. While I do not wish to return to the "bad" old days of acting as if the older people had little or nothing to say about how they were to live, I am not convinced that autonomy as now understood ought to carry the weight assigned to it when relationships resulting from dependency constitute the difference between making it and not making it for many older people. An ethics that assigns a central role to the older person and her or his autonomous choices without attending to the context and the relationships that exist in that context is too paltry, too reductionist to account for frailty and the inequalities that caregiving and care receiving create. By obscuring the family, such ethical individualism isolates the elder and negates the interdependencies that exist. In the name of autonomous choice, social justice concerns can easily be effaced. As further evidence of how reductionist approaches to ethics often obscure larger problems, we need only note that the Medicaid system pits needy women and children against elders who need long-term care.

Long-term-care legislation in Illinois—the Older Adult Services Act—signed by the governor in August 2004 focuses almost exclusively on the needs and desires of the older person; families are grouped with professional providers to be activated when the older person needs them. There is no word about their individual capacities to meet these expectations or even their own needs and desires. While the imperative to rebalance care in favor of the community instead of institutions is critically important, achieving this end ought not be won on the backs of "informal" caregivers. This possibility is reminiscent of the increase in such care that followed in the wake of diagnosis-related groups (DRGs) in the 1980s. The emphasis on community care, while serving the anti-institutionalization preference of most older people, can have significant social costs if caregivers are only tangentially considered in the rhetoric of client-centered care and the client rather than the family system is seen as the unit of care. The problem will be exacerbated with long-term care because the patient rarely recovers lost functions and therefore does not cease needing care.

To critique the assumption that families, most often women, are always available and to contest ethical individualism, we need an ethics of solidarity. The older person who has multiple frailties could not be without the many hands that sustain him or her. These hands are both extensions of the person receiving care and an integral part of another human being to whom we also owe respect and concern. As important as the recent efforts to fund caregiver support programs are, they involve no structural change but are targeted at mitigating the stress of individual caregivers. Stress relief is essential, but it is not enough. Caregiver support programs cannot overcome the inequitable burdens and hence the inequality that public policy and gender relations create.

In what follows, I briefly describe the consequences of both implicit and explicit decision making about long-term care. I have selected certain consequences as particularly noteworthy if a more just system is the goal. These consequences give theoretical arguments their factual foundation and their emotional force without which, I suggest, no action will come. Philosopher Elizabeth Wolgast (1987) observed some years ago that we act not in response to eloquent theories of justice but rather in response to a sense of injustice. "Justice," as legal theorist Martha Finemen (1999, p. 14) observes, "is not found in abstract pronouncements." Gendered caregiving, however loving, should provoke strong feelings and stimulate a vigorous debate about justice. While ideal systems of justice, based on universal principles, offer the grounding for a moderate welfare state, even rich theories such as Rawls's (1999) monumental *Theory of Justice* cannot adequately account for either dependency or gender relations (Kittay, 1999). Such theories assume a rough equality of citizens who cooperate because such cooperation serves everyone (Nussbaum, 2001). But this formulation ignores the asymmetrical relations caused by dependency. Neither givers nor receivers of care are able to freely decide about their own lives and act on those decisions in unencumbered ways.

In developing my argument, I rely largely on feminist political and legal theorists who have been, for the past decade or more, concerned with developing a way to think philosophically and politically about dependency. Long-term care raises political questions about how any society should equitably allocate public resources, but it also compels us to ask about and respond to other moral questions related to justice (beyond allocational decisions), human connectedness, responses to vulnerability, solidarity, and mutuality. When we expand our vision to include these moral qualities, we must also revisit the presumption that we are free to choose whether or not to give care. What, philosopher Naomi Scheman (1983) asks, would happen to those among us who cannot care for themselves if we had a single-minded focus on self-actualization and autonomy rather than, let us say, equality or nourishing relationships? Commitments to care have no place in such a moral system. As long as women, but not men, for example, are blamed if they turn their backs on vulnerability no matter how good the reasons they offer, autonomy will inevitably clash with other important moral values. (For an extended discussion of this point, see Holstein, 1999).

In bringing this chapter to a close, I will offer some recommendations of policy choices we might make both in the short and in the long term. The German system provides one example of a social insurance model of long-term care that, while not ideal, takes seriously many of the concerns that this chapter addresses, in particular the commitment to social solidarity.

Sources of Ethical Problems

Because the ethical problems we now see in long-term care are rooted in culture, in attitudes such as that of the 1960s legislator quoted above and in the incremental and disjointed way long-term-care policy has evolved (Cole and Holstein, 1994), solutions to these problems are also complex. Long-term-care policy is a patchwork of add-ons to other pieces of social and health legislation and is grounded in historical notions of the family, the gendered division of labor, the long-held belief that family matters are entirely private, and the production and reproduction of caring activities by generations of women so continually that indeed they became "better" at it than their male counterparts. To solve the problem involves each of these components.

I want to focus here on the more immediate reasons that long-term care relies on the family and the residual welfare state and then trace some of the equally immediate consequences. Public policy makes "informal" care a necessity. Because Medicare, for example, will pay for acute care services and home health care only when they involve rehabilitation, but will not pay for the care that a patient with Alzheimer's disease needs to stay out of a nursing home, families provide the bulk of care to their older members. When there are no families or when more help is needed than families can provide, the affluent pay privately for additional help and the poor rely on the residual, albeit increasingly costly, welfare system. Many in the middle can do neither until such time that they "spend down" and become eligible for Medicaid.

Medicaid, while vitally needed, is no panacea. Recipients often perceive this means-tested program as "welfare" and hence stigmatizing. As a result, they often resist applying and choose to do without the help it might make available. The need to reveal personal details of their lives to qualify, and fear for the well-being of a spouse, makes it even more unattractive. State Medicaid recovery policies, which ask that states recover costs to Medicaid from whatever assets are left at a client's death, adds to their reluctance to apply. Further, Medicaid is so structured that its use to cover the costs of long-term care for older people pits them against younger women and children for whom the program was initially designed.

Women and Caregiving

Women are the primary recipients of long-term care as well as the primary caregivers. This is true for both paid and unpaid care. Most older people who have long-term-care needs—about 65 percent—rely solely on family members for care; another 30 percent supplement this care with paid caregivers. While many men do a yeoman's job of caring for their wives and elderly parents, women provide 60–75 percent of "informal" care and spend 50 percent more time on caregiving activities than do men (Family Caregiver Alliance, 2001). Even when men provide care, they tend to do the instrumental tasks that can be scheduled—paying bills or mowing the lawn—and not the personal-care services like bathing or dressing. In the biblical book of Ruth, a chorus of women affirm that Ruth is for Naomi better than seven sons, a refrain still spoken: "I am alone; I don't have a daughter. I have sons. They are not going to take care of me" (Calumet City, IL; Holstein and Mitzen, 2004).

As Kittay (1999), Goodin (1985), and others have pointed out, the obligation to give care arises out of a response to vulnerability. Women, as a result of ideology, cultural expectations, power relationships within families, and their social experiences, seem to act on—and perhaps experience—this obligation more powerfully than men (Brewer, 2001; Bubeck, 2002). Practically, because women tend to earn less than men, economic rationality (i.e., the maximization of household income) makes it logical for women rather than men to reduce their working hours or quit work entirely. Yet, interestingly, even when the argument from economic rationality fails (e.g., when men are unemployed and women are working), women do more caregiving than men (Bubeck, 2002). We are unlikely to see a change anytime soon (Holstein, 1999; Hooyman and Gonyea, 1999, 1995). A further irony is that in many states, adding hours of family care leads to reduced public benefits. Yet family care is a significant factor in keeping older people out of the nursing homes they dread. Lacking family caregivers, 50 percent of older people with long-term-care needs are in nursing homes; only 7 percent who have a family member to care for them are in institutions (Administration on Aging, 2000).

Women's caregiving, translated into dollars, would amount to more than $195 billion a year (Arno, Levine, and Memmot, 1999). Public costs were around $257 billion in 2000 (Montgomery and Holzhausen, 2003–4). Family caregiving also has enormous social costs. It is estimated that partial absenteeism of workers because of caregiving responsibilities, turnover, and more general absenteeism costs business more than $600 million annually (National Alliance for Caregiving, 2004). In the next 25 years, estimates suggest that one in three workers will be providing some type of long-term care (Gordon, 2001).

Because caring labor is not employment at will and because it constitutes a large part of adult identity (West, 2002), it is inevitable that its consequences are both immediate and long-term. Women who work and also provide care generally face lost wages, part-time work, early retirement, and reduced benefits from Social Security and pensions. Further, women who return to work after caregiving are likely to be employed in a job with few or no benefits, earn lower wages, and receive lower retirement benefits than people who do not provide care. Caregiving is costly more directly—for example, buying medical equipment, installing assistive devices, purchasing drugs, and hiring help can sometimes mean financial hardship (FCA, 2001). These consequences are set against a background of collapsing pensions, climbing medical costs, and the erosion of job security. They further exacerbate the already existing inequality in late life when women are more likely than men to be poor.

There are also personal costs. Depression and anxiety are familiar accompaniments of caregiving (FCA, 2001). Other health effects—such as not filling one's own prescriptions or failing to take advantage of preventive care—are also common. To be fair, however, many women also report satisfaction with caregiving, particularly as caregiving contributes to their sense of purpose in life (Marks, Lambert, and Choi, 2002). Yet, such reliance on the private, family system also makes many care receivers uneasy; few of us wish to burden those we love, although the fear of being a burden is itself gendered.

Many of these consequences flow from the atypical situation of caregivers in a society that presumes most people can take care of themselves and views choice as the essential feature of moral agency. Caregivers are not autonomous agents; caring responsibilities may "impose themselves" in ways that may render the caregiver's "life plans unrealizeable" (Bubeck, 2002, p. 169). But as long as it is assumed that caregiving activities are freely chosen, even among those who give care, the problems of justice and the disregard of other moral values will not be faced. Philosopher Margaret Urban Walker (1998, p. 181) reminds us that "some prejudices are so culturally normative" (i.e., that women make better caregivers) "that they are hardly experienced as problematic, which means that even those who are at the losing end of the prejudices do not deliberate about them." Further, even if women wished to deliberate about them, their absence from the table where decisions about long-term care are made effectively silences them. And, more generally because the "voices of middle- and lower-income groups," who are the most likely to face serious caregiver-related problems, "are largely missing from the public conversation" (Verba, Schlozman, and Brady, quoted in Harrington, 1999, p. 179), the ability to perceive the problems created by the current system is further limited. This omission is important because the first step in moral responsiveness is perceiving that problems exist.

Women give care because it is needed and because they feel responsible and often derive great satisfaction from doing so. That's the prevailing cultural norm. Contrary to the myth of choice, our lives are filled with unchosen obligations (Baier, 1985) even when lovingly given. If some are to live, some must care. To give care is not a free and unfettered choice. To distribute the responsibilities for caregiving differently is partly an individual problem, but in large measure it is also a social one. Until large campaign contributors or legislators change the sheets of an incontinent relative or put a meal on the table, they will have difficulty empathizing with either people who are unable to do such tasks or those who rely on a family member to do them. If decision makers do not change the diapers of the old or prepare a meal or take them on slow walks around the block, they will not see and therefore will not try to deal with the instrumental and personal costs of this commitment.

Feminist philosopher Diana Meyers (1997, p. 197) gets at the radical potential of seeing differently. The importance of moral perception seems indisputable, for how one sees other people, their relations, and one's relations to them has a profound impact on choice and action. Defective moral perception throws moral deliberation and thus moral judgment off course. Moreover, it camouflages social ills and thwarts critical moral reflection.

Partial views inadvertently shape our policy choices and at the same time blind us to the effects of such limited perceptions. Seeing through the lens of gender can lead to alternative perceptions of social reality and value creation while redefining need and hence the manner in which society addresses these issues. Modifying perceptions, often as a result of personal experience, can play an important role in bringing personal problems to public attention. As we learned in the case of Nancy Reagan and her advocacy for embryonic stem cell research, the personal becomes the political when a person in power learns firsthand about the import of a particular disease or condition. As more women become legislators or policy leaders and know what that slow walk around the block feels like, perhaps change will come. In Illinois, as just one example, the Conference of Women Legislators (COWL) has made long-term care a priority area of work. If the current system assumes women's caregiving, "women must have a significant voice in determining how that care is accomplished" (Hooyman and Gonyea, 1999, p. 164).

In addition to family caregivers, the women who are paid low wages to give care to someone else's mother suffer—from their inability to care well for their own families, since their low wages and lack of benefits usually drive them to work at two or more jobs. They are further disadvantaged should they need care themselves, for they have such limited resources. The corrosive effects of not feeling recognized for the work that they do or encountering demanding or unappreciative clients or inadequate supervision mean that many of these caregivers leave as soon as another low-wage job comes along. Caregiver morale is often low, and annual turnover in some parts of the country exceeds 100 percent. These facts affect the quality of care and contribute to the inadequate supply of well-trained caregivers. They also have morally significant consequences because competence and the building and maintaining of trusting relationships are essential moral qualities in any good caregiving relationship (Tronto, 1993; Holstein, 2001).

Caregiving and Class

Our system of providing care to dependents is also closely related to class. Though not wholly divorced from the fact of gender, class creates another cache of ethical problems. Middle-class people—and I mean the traditional working middle class, not those earning upwards of $200,000 a year who are often labeled middle-class—and the working poor are often overwhelmed by the burden of paying for long-term care. "If you are on Medicaid or a millionaire who can afford to pay for LTC, you're okay but most of us in the middle, we get stuck with it. . . . We shouldn't have to hire lawyers to get through the system," said one person in this category (Skokie, IL; Holstein and Mitzen, 2004). Another said, "I'd rather die; I don't want to spend this money. Just let me go" (Moline, IL; Holstein and Mitzen, 2004). For this group, the first source of payment is one's own income or assets, generally followed by Medicaid. While some people transfer their assets before disability to avoid spend-down and to leave a legacy, in itself a morally questionable practice, others simply worry or spend down their lifetime accumulation of assets in order to become eligible for Medicaid. Some older people have even divorced their spouses as a way to qualify for Medicaid without spending down assets. And some buy long-term-care insurance; in that case, some states that participate in the Partnership in Care program permit policyholders who use up their benefits to roll over to Medicaid while protecting their assets. This provision, however, has been changed for people who bought Partnership policies after 1993; their assets are protected while they are alive, but the state can recover assets upon their death (Meiners, McKay, and Mahoney, 2002). Lower-income people, too rich for Medicaid and too poor to pay the premiums on long-term-care insurance, have no way, at this time, to protect their assets. Long-term-care insurance gives individuals greater choice and potentially reduces costs to the state, both morally worthy ends, but it also raises moral questions: namely, it further segments the population who need long-term care and bestows further advantages on the more affluent and the healthier who do not have the medical conditions that may lead to the denial of a policy.

Additionally, as only one among many ironies, while estate taxes are disappearing for most of the population, so that affluent people can pass on the results of their labor (and the hidden public subsidies that supported their accumulation of wealth) to their heirs, people who go onto Medicaid—which is visible as a direct subsidy—know that the state can recover whatever assets remain at their death. For some people, otherwise eligible for Medicaid, that fact keeps them from applying for assistance. Their home may be all that they have to leave to a relative who has taken care of them for months and even years. For the state, in contrast, Medicaid enrollment allows it to maximize the federal match and so bring more money to the always financially strapped program. This ethical balancing act has not received adequate exploration. Such an exploration would examine the issue of individual and community justice. What serves the community often does not serve the individual. With Medicaid it is much more immediately clear than with the estate tax, but both set individual and community into conflict. In the case of the estate tax, legacy is viewed as a good—the central argument for elimination of the estate tax. This isn't surprising. In a society that touts the individual, he or she usually prevails over community—unless one happens to be poor and on Medicaid.

The situation will not be improving. Massive cuts in Medicaid spending are already threatened; the need for long-term-care services will continue to grow no matter how much we exercise and drink green tea. Simultaneously, the language of private responsibility for health and well-being, which includes the purchase of long-term-care insurance, is becoming an ever more dominant motif in public discussions about long-term care.

What, then, are the ethical implications of this sketch of problems rooted in class? With few exceptions, people clearly in the middle or among the working poor have far fewer choices than others. While this fact is true at every other stage of life too, being able to obtain good long-term care when one is old and vulnerable is quite different from making a choice between a Honda and a Lexus. Not only is care often compromised; important ethical values are also elided. With a checklist of tasks to be done and limited time to do them, paid care workers in the home or in the institution are rarely able to attend to identity-preserving activities like talking, or simple touching, or making sure the resident can live in habitual ways, an often ignored component of autonomy (Agich, 2003). Choice remains important, especially as an individual's life space narrows, but choice does not constitute the whole or even the major portion of moral obligations to older, vulnerable individuals. Yet, this minimalist requirement—choice—is what we accept as the standard moral norm for services to the aging.

Equally importantly, elders face additional moral hazards when they are forced to rely strongly on families for care. They often experience a feeling that they are a burden; they may find that it is virtually impossible to leave anything behind—including their home—as a legacy to those who cared for them; and they risk receiving inadequate care either in the home or in an institution. Burden is often the expressed reason for wanting assistance in dying, and legacy is something most treasure. A thoughtful reconsideration of what kind of people we are, accompanied by a refocusing on the relational aspects of the self, might be one path to reconsidering a moral foundation for caregiving practices.

Competition for Resources

Assuming that many working-class poor and middle-class individuals ultimately go on Medicaid, another problem emerges. Relegating long-term care to the residual welfare state means that these individuals directly compete with poor women and children for Medicaid resources. Unless states substantially increase their share of Medicaid funding, there will be an inevitable squeezing in one place or another, and something must give. As we know today, the bulge is occurring at the state level. Medicaid and discretionary services for the poor are among the budget items that state governments tinker with when the squeeze to balance the budget is on. Although this squeeze affects Medicaid services for elderly people, it is often women and children who face the worst consequences. It is unfortunately easier to reduce programs for poor women and children, so easily demonized as less deserving than elderly people, than to imagine 90 people in wheelchairs evicted from a nursing home because Medicaid funding was reduced. A program meant, then, to care for the very poor thus helps to support both poor elders and formerly middle-class elders who have qualified for Medicaid. A systematic examination of the moral questions around such devices as asset transfer is beyond the scope of this chapter, but I suggest that the primary fault lies within a system that demands impoverishment before public dollars become available. How does one decide what allocations are just when we have equally needy populations? Can it ever be made fair, with fairness meaning equal treatment of people with comparable needs? Or will groups always need to contend against one another, with those who have the best image and advocates winning?

Caregiving and Collective Responsibility

Bringing together these observations suggests the outlines of an argument for a new way to think about caring for the dependent among us. My central focus is on solidarity and the need for a stereoscopic vision that sees the person needing care and the person giving it simultaneously. I will argue that care is a collective responsibility of society, as is defense or keeping our cities clean. Let me offer some claims that highlight the discussion above and suggest the conditions that make collective responsibility essential.

- Dependency at some stage in every human life is universal and inevitable; it is a fundamental part of the human condition (Fineman, 1999).
- Care is necessary labor because there will always be people who need care (Bubeck, 2002).
- Caring for people who are dependent is society-preserving; caregivers provide the often-invisible hands that make everything else work; they are the foundation on which the American myth of independence, autonomy, and individualism rests; caregivers give an invisible subsidy to all of us (Fineman, 1999).

- Caregivers experience a "a derivative dependency," because their time, energy, and resources are tied up in caregiving; they must therefore rely on others to provide for their material needs.
- Ideological presuppositions and tradition mean that women assume the responsibilities of care because they are expected to; they have few acceptable reasons for not giving care (Holstein, 1998).
- This caregiving is taken for granted, with minimal attention paid to its gendered nature and the implications of that nature (Fineman, 2002, p. 222).
- The iconic image of marriage and family is no longer the lived reality for the majority of Americans, and no desperate attempt to reify it will turn it around; families may stay in touch and adapt to changing circumstances, but they have not found ways to bridge distance, divorce, work, and so forth in ways that make it possible to care well for loved ones without some bearing a much heavier burden than others.
- Yet, the ideology of the family, including its responsibilities for private welfare, is ever more entrenched; the failure of the private system is perceived as an individual and not a social failure (Harrington, 1999).
- The often unchosen obligation to give care in a society that elevates free and unfettered choice as the signal marker of autonomous adulthood is simultaneously necessary and anomalous; women who take on this role are subordinate, devalued, and hailed as saints, none of which does much to pay the bills or deepen self-respect.
- The burden falls the heaviest on poor and minority women, because they are the least likely to be able to hire assistance or obtain relief from caregiving responsibilities, or even purchase long-term-care insurance.

In what has become known as the "dependency critique" (Kittay, 1999; Tronto, 1993; West, 2002), the failure of liberal society, particularly our own, to take dependency seriously is systematically confronted. The problem of dependency across generations will not be resolved by the market. Nor will it help to pit the dependent young against the dependent old to ask who are more deserving. That scope is as narrow today as it was in the mid-1980s when the intergenerational equity debate first gained public visibility. We live in a grossly inequitable society, and fighting over who deserves the remnants ought to be beneath us all.

The conditions of our time call for a collective response. Women do ostensibly "choose" the role of caregiver no matter the consequences for their own lives, and the role may reward them with often deep satisfactions; but still, a society imbued with ideals of independence, autonomy, equality, and self-sufficiency should attend to the inability of women who give care to meet these ends for themselves. Enormous inegalitarian consequences, including exploitation, flow from the privatization of care and the prevailing pattern according to which some give care and others do not. Any society, especially one such as ours, which expresses a concern for equality, ought to be concerned about the threats to equality posed by an inequitable distribution of caregiving responsibilities. For this reason, women and others who perform caregiving tasks "ought to have the resources to do so" (Fineman, 1999, p. 29), so as to eliminate or at least reduce the inequality of their social position.

Long-term care must then be "defined as a public responsibility to guarantee a minimal level of services to all citizens as a public good in which all citizens should participate without undue burden" (Hooyman and Gonyea, 1999, p. 165). Care of dependent relatives is socially important work, and so it must be supported with public resources and shared by men and women. It is therefore imperative that we rework the prevailing ethics of autonomy into one that also emphasizes solidarity and the need for a stereoscopic vision that sees the person needing care and the person giving it simultaneously.

But what a struggle we are in. Each day in other parts of my life, I try to balance convictions, personal integrity, and the compromises that are necessary to make small gains in a notoriously parsimonious, indeed miserly, state. Unfortunately, in the political system, even the best argument cannot triumph over the budget, especially if the latter is supported by ideological rather than analytical or empirical, even philosophical, proclivities. In a recent meeting about a vision statement for long-term care in the state of Illinois, I received an almost a blank stare when I suggested that we include acknowledgment that we could not focus just on the older person, that caring for her or him required a set of interlocking interdependencies, that focusing only on what the older person wanted was blind to the many invisible hands that make his or her independence possible.

Caregiving as a Counternarrative

Counternarratives (see Nelson, 2001) allow us to reframe what is taken for granted. In this country the prevailing narrative about independence and autonomy, as well as its corollary in ethics, does not apply to vast numbers of people who need help and those who provide that help. A counternarrative can offer the resources to rethink our fundamental commitments and emphasize other cultural values like connectedness, nurturance, and solidarity. Try to imagine a society in which these values are elevated and so serve as norms for behavior. What would such a change do for public policy, for the distribution of caregiving responsibilities, and for our social attitudes toward those people who do not provide care?

If we recognized our interconnections and mutual dependencies, an alternative vision would uphold moral values that receive too little recognition in the normative visions of the new gerontology. This cultural task challenges contemporary narratives of free and unfettered choice, life—and old age— projects of self-creation, and the realization of personal potential, not because they are bad, but because they are limited and unequally available and because they isolate even further people who give and receive care (Holstein, 1999). New cultural narratives that respectfully integrate the experiences and demands of dependency, frailty, and loss without denying the possibilities of growth and development can begin to create an ethics of solidarity as a counterweight to the ethics of autonomy so that both can be part of society's normative expectations. Ignoring the facts of human contingency, frailty, and dependency does not, unfortunately, make them go away.

Recommendations

What, then, can be done? I wish I had good answers. The possibility that we shall someday support caring activities as we do coronary artery bypass surgery is as unlikely as my walking on the moon. Broad risk-sharing and a response to the dependency critique are not on the horizon. I think we need to keep talking about them, however, and consider research that specifically addresses the larger structural problems that encourage the exploitation of women's labor and deny women the equality that we say we hold so dear. For starters, we ought not abandon the ideal, for without it, we will never know what might be possible. We need to (1) take care seriously, (2) embrace the changing family as a liberal ideal and find ways to support mutual caring activities, (3) make the possibility of equality real for those who give care, whether as a family member or as a paid caregiver, (4) challenge the cultural assumptions that take women for granted, and (5) introduce new normative ideals that focus on solidarity and obligations to others as necessary for human survival and thriving.

Immediately, we might think of how to infuse the system with more money through such possibilities as state income tax increases, an income tax check-off, or a tax on retirement income. We would, of course, have to counter the rhetoric about money belonging in our own pockets—one more version of the individual versus the needs of the commons. Money in someone's pockets often means more free labor from another person; the tax burden is not what most low- or moderate-income women most worry about. Bringing more dedicated money into the system would help, but even that cannot remedy the diversion of resources from women and children to elderly people.

A few simple changes would also help a little. Family leave policies—especially if they can be modified to include some pay—would help to address this problem. Using Medicaid waivers or other housing resources to create different housing options with services is another option. Increasing the asset and income level for community-based and institutional services is also useful. And I think we must find a way somehow to protect some reasonable legacy for the working middle class as we do for the more affluent. Our ability to accumulate resources is not equal; but the wish to leave something behind is a common human wish.

We might also look at models that are in use in other parts of the world. Germany, for example, in 1994 introduced a "landmark national social insurance program for long-term care" (Cuellar and Wiener, 1999, p. 45). Long-term care is supported by a tax on 1.7 percent of salary, shared by employers and employees. The state defines three levels of disability that determine the client's benefit level; there is no means test. Individuals can choose among a cash benefit, services, or a combination of the two. Most have, so far, chosen the cash benefit, which is set at half the value of the service benefit. Seventy-four percent of the care is outside nursing homes. Family members can receive payment for care, but, significantly, they earn pension credits and a four-week vacation each year, with the state paying the costs of replacement care. They also receive special training. The availability of family members does not influence the amount of the benefit; it is based solely on level of disability (Cuellar and Wiener, 2000).

This system achieves certain important ends. The informal caregiver is not taken for granted; nor is a care plan built around her or his availability. Family care is rewarded by cash payments, if that option is chosen, and by vacation time and pension benefits. These elements go a long way toward reducing exploitation. It is beyond the scope of this chapter to consider the actual workings of the system, which are not without concerns (Cuellar and Wiener, 2000), but its broad philosophical underpinnings, based on beliefs that the operating value is solidarity rather than individualism, are worth some attention in this country. And contrary to what some might have expected, the system cost is less than what was projected, perhaps because more people than expected chose the cash option, which is only 60 percent of the service option.

Conclusion

We need to keep talking, to try to get people to understand that obligations flow from relationships of care and dependency. These obligations ought not be a matter of choice that one may accept or reject. Further, those who give care ought to be entitled to "a socially supported situation in which one can give care without the care giving becoming a liability to one's own well-being" (Kittay, 1999, p. 66). As long as large numbers of people are free to ignore the demands of vulnerability, as they are in our autonomy-driven, work-obsessed society, and as long as we fail to recognize collective responsibility for caregiving, we will fail in our goals of being a just and egalitarian society. So I end where I began—with a challenge to those who think like the legislators I opened with. That all of us may need care and some give care is a fact of life. It ought to be acknowledged as the social enterprise that it is. The vision of the autonomous consumer of long-term-care services fails to take that fact into account. If we view society as a set of nested dependencies, as I think we must, then intimate care in the home is a social contribution that calls for reciprocity (Kittay, 1999) and intergenerational solidarity and not, as one of my former colleagues said, sainthood. Few women caregivers crave sainthood.

REFERENCES

Administration on Aging. 2000. America's families care: A report on the needs of America's family caregivers. www.aoa.gov/carenetwork/report.html.
Agich, G. 2003. *Dependence and Autonomy in Old Age.* New York: Cambridge University Press.

Arno, P., Levine, C., and Memmot, M. M. 1999. The economic value of informal care-giving. *Health Affairs* 18(2):182–88.

Baier, A. 1985. *Postures of the Mind: Essays on Mind and Morals.* Minneapolis: University of Minnesota Press.

Brewer, L. 2001. Gender socialization and the cultural construction of elder caregivers. *Journal of Aging Studies* 15(3):217–35.

Bubeck, D. G. 2002. Justice and the labor of care. In E. F. Kittay and E. K. Feder, eds., *The Subject of Care: Feminist Perspectives on Dependency*, pp. 160–85. Lanham, MD: Rowman & Littlefield.

Cole, T., and Holstein, M. 1994. Interpreting the formative literature of gerontology and geriatrics: A view from American cultural history, 1890–1930. In C. Conrad and H-J. von Kondratowitz, eds., *Before and after Modernity: Toward a Cultural History of Aging.* Berlin: DZA.

Cuellar, A., and Wiener, J. 1999. Structuring a universal long-term care program: The experience in Germany. *Generations* 23(2):45–50.

Cuellar, A. E., and Wiener, J. 2000. Can social insurance for long-term care work? The experience of Germany. *Health Affairs* 19(3):8–25.

Family Caregiver Alliance. 2001. *Selected Caregiver Statistics.* San Francisco: Family Caregiver Alliance.

Fineman, M. A. 1999. Cracking the foundational myths: Independence, autonomy, and self-sufficiency. *American University Journal of Gender, Social Policy, and the Law* 8(1):13–29.

Fineman, M. A. 2002. Masking dependency: The political role of family rhetoric. In E. F. Kittay and E. K. Feder, eds., *The Subject of Care: Feminist Perspectives on Dependency*, pp. 215–45. Lanham, MD: Rowman & Littlefield.

Fraser, N. 1989. *Unruly Practices: Power, Discourse, and Gender in Contemporary Social Theory.* Cambridge University: Policy Press; Minneapolis: University of Minnesota Press.

Goodin, R. 1985. *Protecting the Vulnerable: A Reanalysis of our Social Responsibility.* Chicago: University of Chicago Press.

Gordon, M. 2001. A guide to understanding long-term care insurance. *Employee Benefits Journal* 26(3):42–46.

Harrington, M. 1999. *Care and Equality: Inventing a New Family Politics.* New York: Knopf.

Hirschfield, M., and Wikler, D. 2003–4. An ethics perspective on family caregiving worldwide: Justice and society's obligations. *Generations* 27(4):56–60.

Holstein, M. 1998. Commentary: The "new aging": Imagining alternative futures. In K. W. Schaie and J. Hendricks, eds., *The Evolution of the Aging Self: The Societal Impact on the Aging Process*, pp. 319–32. New York: Springer Publishing Co.

Holstein, M. 1999. Home care, women, and aging: A case study of injustice. In M. U. Walker, ed., *Mother Time: Women, Aging, and Ethics*, pp. 227–44. Lanham, MD: Rowman & Littlefield.

Holstein, M., and P. Mitzen. 2004. *Voices of Illinois Elders.* All quotes are from community forums on long-term care. www.hmprg.org.

Hooyman, N., and Gonyea, J. 1995. *Feminist Perspectives on Family Care: Politics for Gender Justice.* Thousand Oaks, CA: Sage.

Hooyman, N., and Gonyea, J. 1999. A feminist model of family care: Practice and policy directions. *Journal of Women and Aging* 11(2–3):149–69.

Kittay, E. F. 1999. *Love's Labor: Essays on Women, Equality, and Dependency.* New York: Routledge.

Lloyd, L. 2004. Mortality, morality, ageing, and the ethics of care. *Ageing and Society* 24(2):235–57.

Marks, N., Lambert, J. D., and Choi, H. 2002. Transitions to caregiving, gender, and psychological well-being: A prospective U.S. national study. *Journal of Marriage and the Family* 64:657–67.

Meiners, M., McKay, H., and Mahoney, K. 2002. Partnership insurance: An innovation to meet long-term care financing needs in an era of federal minimalism. *Journal of Aging and Social Policy* 14(3–4):75–93.

Meyers, D. 1997. *Feminists Rethink the Self.* Boulder, CO: Westview Press.

Montgomery, A., and Holzhausen, E. 2003–4. Caregivers in the United States and the United Kingdom: Different systems, similar challenges. *Generations* 27(4):61–67.

National Alliance for Caregiving and AARP. 2004. *Caregiving in the U.S.* www.caregiving .org/data/04finalreport.pdf.

Nelson, H. L. 2001. *Damaged Identities, Narrative Repair.* Ithaca, NY: Cornell University Press.

Nussbaum, M. 2001. *Women and Human Development: The Capabilities Approach.* Cambridge: University of Cambridge Press.

Nussbaum, M. 2002. The future of feminist liberalism. In E. F. Kittay and E. Feder, eds., *The Subject of Care: Feminist Perspectives on Dependency,* pp. 186–214. Lanham, MD: Rowman & Littlefield.

Rawls, J. 1999. *A Theory of Justice.* Rev. ed. Cambridge, MA: Harvard University Press.

Scheman, N. 1983. Individualism and psychology. In S. Harding and M. Hintikka, eds., *Discovering Reality: Feminist Perspectives on Epistemology, Metaphysics, Methodology, and Philosophy of Science.* Dordrecht, Neth.: Reidel.

Tronto, J. 1993. *Moral Boundaries: A Political Argument for an Ethics of Care.* New York: Routledge.

Verba, S., Schlozman, K. L., and Brady, H. E. 1995. *Voice and Equality: Civic Voluntarism in American Politics.* Cambridge, MA: Harvard University Press.

Walker, M. U. 1998. *Moral Understandings: A Feminist Study in Ethics.* New York: Routledge.

Weinberg, J. 1999. Caregiving, age, and class in the skeleton of the welfare state: "And Jill came tumbling after . . . " In M. Minkler and C. Estes, eds., *Critical Gerontology: Perspectives from Political and Moral Economy,* pp. 257–74. Amityville, NY: Baywood.

West, R. 2002. The right to care. In E. F. Kittay and E. K. Feder, eds., *The Subject of Care: Feminist Perspectives on Dependency,* pp. 88–114. Lanham, MD: Rowman & Littlefield.

Wolgast, E. 1987. *The Grammar of Justice.* Ithaca, NY: Cornell University Press.

CHAPTER SEVEN

Aging, Generational Opposition, and the Future of the Family

H. Rick Moody, Ph.D.

Case Manager's Report on *King Lear*

This is a complex case involving family conflict, dementia, homelessness, and transfer of assets. Mr. Lear suffers from the delusion that he is still "King" despite having divested himself completely of his assets in the kingdom. Lear's initial care plan assumed dependency on two adult daughters (Goneril and Regan), who have now refused to provide support. Probable elder abuse apparent here. Due to mental incompetence, client has a surrogate decision maker (Edgar). Efforts are currently underway to locate estranged youngest daughter (Cordelia). Because Lear's assets were improperly transferred, we recommend vigorous efforts at asset recovery if he is to have access to community-based services needed.

> Respectfully submitted,
> W. Shakespeare

This tongue-in-check "case report" reminds us that ethical dilemmas and struggle between generations are not new to our times. The topic is timeless, treated in literature and arising in every generation. But *King Lear* also reminds us of something else. *Lear* is a play in which Shakespeare, unlike the contemporary case manager, has refused to look at family conflict purely in terms of the family alone. Shakespeare has written a play about the public world and about the way in which the struggle between generations is intertwined with structural elements in the state: Who will govern? How is inheritance to be decided? How are family obligations to be reconciled with the greater good of the commonwealth? In other words, Shakespeare's tragedy has pressed forward a set of normative questions about generational relationships that can be viewed at the level of individuals, the family, and the state. Failure to distinguish what is appropriate at these three different levels can result in a catastrophe, as the aged King Lear learned in the end. The hope is that by thinking more clearly about the future of aging and the family in terms of public policy and responsibility across the generations, we may avoid our own catastrophes in years to come.

Why begin with this invocation of tragedy? Because it is an element that needs to be considered in thinking about aging, the family, and the struggle between generations. I admire the accomplishment of Bengtson, Putney, and Wakeman, who tell us, in Chapter 5, "everything we always wanted to know about the family and aging." Their work is truly a synoptic and dazzling achievement. But it is also a tale of reassurance, a story most reluctant to acknowledge the power of struggle in the world of families and aging. Bengtson and his coauthors do not exactly give us a fairy tale, but they give us a story with a happy ending, the reassurance of "resilience" among the vast variety of families in our aging society. I argue that the ending to this story may not be as happy as they want us to believe it will be.

In this commentary, I want to do two things: first, provide a brief treatment of certain broad social-structural trends that prove decisive for thinking about responsibility across the generations in families; and, second, offer an analytical framework for thinking in more precise terms about the meaning of conflict, ambivalence, and competition among generations, including the much-discussed issue of generational equity.

Changes in the Life Course

Population aging is the dominant, overwhelming force reshaping lives in societies in the twenty-first century. Population aging is a story that unfolds slowly. It is not a dramatic story, like international terrorism, or one that provides clear-cut beacons of progress, like advances in technology. But population aging is a force that reshapes everything in its path, including the lives of families. In thinking about what causes population aging, it is important to note that gains in life expectancy as such (either from birth or from age 65) are less important than lower fertility rates as a factor driving population aging. The big gains in life expectancy came earlier in the twentieth century; later increases have been more modest and incremental, particularly increases in life expectancy beyond age 65.

Perhaps more important than life expectancy alone has been decline in morbidity and disability in later life (Liu, Manton, and Aragon, 2000), a positive trend that has extended the period of active or healthy life into the so-called Third Age (Laslett, 1991). It is this fact, more than longevity per se, that has reshaped our image of the life course, to the point where we can recognize the outlines of something like a "postmodern life course," which includes a more individualized life course with less and less predictability or agreement about age-based normative behavior ("act your age") in both childhood and old age (Powell and Longino, 2001). This fact of postmodernity or late modernity—namely, advancing individualization—is well understood by Bengtson and coauthors and will be important in the discussion that follows as we try to understand the normative challenge that shapes generational opposition.

The advancing power of individualization has far-reaching consequences for normative understanding of family roles. Family roles that might be linked to old age are now more ambiguous than they used to be (e.g., what is the typical age of a grandparent?). There are inner-city neighborhoods where grandparents are in their thirties, whereas among more affluent groups, grandparenthood gets moved to more and more advanced ages as the age of childbearing rises among professional women. This last point underscores the continuing importance of social class and the economy as structural forces shaping aging and the life course, as Bengtson and his coauthors have emphasized.

The Age Structure of Nations

The change in the age structure of nations has brought about shifts in the so-called dependency ratio, a topic subject to continuing debate and interpretation under the label of the "Generational Equity Debate," to which I shall return. Perhaps of more significance is the impact of a shifting dependency ratio *within* families at a time of less stable kinship relations (e.g., high divorce rates). In effect, less predictable kinship structures coexist with diminishing power of norms of loyalty and solidarity in the wider culture. Increasingly, we are living in a world where ideals of autonomy and self-actualization take priority, not only in the economy or the cultural sphere, but also at the level of the family. This long-term shift raises a basic ethical question: can norms of reciprocity and exchange be maintained at the level of the family when all emotional "currencies" of loyalty are being readjusted and shifted? To give a concrete example, what kind of appeal to loyalty or solidarity would serve to underwrite obligations to ex-parents-in-law who need care in old age?

Challenge to the Moral Economy of Caregiving

With longer lives, more and more people are in family networks where they might be in a position to render help to one another. But this purely structural fact does not take account of a changing normative climate. Along with social structure and political economy, we need to consider what has been called the "moral economy" (Minkler and Estes, 1998). The wider availability of intergenerational kinship resources has not been matched by a rise in what we might call "normative resources" (the moral economy) that could sustain sacrifice and transfers across generations and reinforce a sense of interdependence of generations (Robertson, 1997). In our present condition, we have not only blurred kinship structures but also blurred normative structures. Within families, as in other contexts, we are no longer clear about who owes what to whom and with what limits. One example of this problem is ambiguity about the legal role of grandparents caring for grandchildren. Grandparents are increasingly assuming this role, but normative structures (e.g., the legal system) have not kept pace with social change. The practical questions for families are very real: Do grandparents have legal rights in such cases? Should we really assume that a sheer rise in number or range of kin networks (e.g., "fictive kin" in minority communities) will help resolve the problem? Can we believe that these various networks—"problematic, rich and varied," as Bengtson et al. describe them—can compensate for a shortage of traditional family ties or normative structures embodied in law?

This problem is not limited to the context of the family. Robert Putnam, among others, has pointed to a broader decline in social capital and social networks throughout the wider society (Putnam, 2001). In Putnam's view, a major culprit in the decline is not so much a collapse in normative belief as it is the impact of structural factors in the economy and living arrangements—above all, two-earner couples and long commuting times. Whatever the cause, the result has been a shrinking amount of time available in a world where, increasingly, work roles and consumption roles serve to "colonize" the life-world represented by the family (Habermas, 1974). Earlier epochs may have depicted the family as a "haven in a heartless world," but the postmodern family in an aging society is at the center of powerful forces that threaten to disrupt its cohesion.

Change in Governmental Responsibilities

There is a major difference in the ideology of social welfare between Europe and the United States, and this difference has huge consequences for how we think about responsibility across generations and the family. In general, norms of solidarity still count for something in Europe; in western Europe, systems of social welfare protection are stronger than in the United States (ter Meulen, Arts, and Muffels, 2001). Thus, parallel structural trends evoke different responses because of a clear normative difference. For instance, on the structural level, there has been a rising incidence of one-parent families in both the United States and western Europe. But the trend has much more negative consequences in the United States than in Europe because of a weaker social safety net. However, this contrast between Europe and the United States should not be drawn too sharply. The power of the marketplace is gaining ascendancy everywhere as pressures of globalization are felt. In the United States, a trend toward marketization shows up in a variety of ways: for example, in policy proposals for paying family caregivers, in the rise of commodified and privatized long-term care (e.g., assisted living), and in the marketization of care management (e.g., the rise of the profession of private geriatric care managers).

Overriding all these elements are two broad macrotrends: the fiscal crisis of the state and the legitimation crisis of government (Habermas, 1975). In the United States, the electorate has proved resistant to paying higher taxes, even for more popular social welfare programs. Yet, for older persons at least, these programs have not been cut back but have even been expanded, as for instance in the provision of prescription drug benefits under Medicare (2003). The two macrotrends—fiscal crisis and legitimation crisis—are intertwined and have normative dimensions (for example, failure to tell the truth about long-range costs of entitlements and spreading lack of confidence in government or the future of social insurance programs). The Medicare expansion of 2003 was attacked by partisans on the right for failing to acknowledge the true cost of the benefits; the same law was attacked by partisans on the left for betraying consumer interests in favor of pharmaceutical companies (Guglielmo, 2004). On both sides, fiscal crisis and legitimation crisis were intertwined.

Globalization

A dimension of globalization—the migration of the labor supply needed for domestic tasks, including tasks of long-term care, both community-based and in institutions (Wilson, 2002)—deserves much greater attention than it has received. Population aging means a smaller ratio of children to elders, and this trend is recognizable in the family, where the dependency ratio means fewer adult children in a position to care for aging parents. Because of global migration, countries with a more favorable dependency ratio can send their workers to more affluent countries (Massey and Taylor, 2004). Not surprisingly, the migrants have become a key element of the long-term-care labor force. In the United States they come from Mexico, the Caribbean, and Central America; in Europe, they come from North Africa and the Middle East. Historically, this Caribbean and Latin American labor supply has been of greatest importance in states like California, Florida, Texas, and New York. In recent years, the geographic range of low-wage long-term-care labor has expanded throughout the United States. Without this low-wage labor supply, provision of long-term care would not be financially feasible, particularly given constraints on Medicare and Medicaid budgets. Here again, domestic fiscal crisis becomes enmeshed with migration and the global economy.

The phenomenon of "guest workers" in Europe and migrant workers in agriculture and domestic service has long been a familiar part of the labor market and has always raised serious policy problems, problems made more acute by anxiety about immigration since the September 11 events. What is distinctive in the twenty-first century is that future demographic trends ensure that an ever younger developing world will remain juxtaposed with an ever-more-aging population in the advanced industrialized countries. Globalization has created structures of transportation and communication that put these "younger" and "older" societies in even greater proximity, and population aging, along with globalization, fuels a continuing demand for younger workers to meet the long-term-care needs. The normative problems here reach far beyond issues of wages or worker protection. There are, for example, serious questions about the quality of care received by elders when their caregivers do not speak their language or share their cultural background.

Individualization and Risk

In considering normative dimensions of aging and family policy, differences in cohort attitudes toward individual risk are worth noting. According to Putnam, today's elders (members of the World War II generation and the Silent Generation) tend to have attitudes more favorable to solidarity, whereas young cohorts are more supportive of individualization and personal risk. It is therefore not surprising that younger people lack confidence in the future of Social Security and entitlement programs and are more likely to hold favorable attitudes toward individual retirement accounts.

This difference in attitude toward individualization is part of a much broader shift toward a "risk society" (Adam, Beck, and Van Loon, 2000; Hacker, 2006). Individualization and the deinstitutionalization of the life course are driven both by market forces (e.g., erosion of defined benefit pension coverage) and by ideological and normative forces (e.g., the "culture of narcissism" constantly promoted by media). This deinstitutionalization entails less and less predictability in the life course, a trend that may be perceived as good or bad by individuals. Deinstitutionalization evidently represents a trade-off between security and liberty. As family members—under the influence of individualist ideologies—tend to "go their separate ways," the question is inescapable: will aged parents have more or less fear of "being a burden on their children," a worry that they so commonly report? This kind of question is clearly related to the stresses on family members documented by Bengtson and his coauthors.

Opposition among Generations: Some Analytic Distinctions

I want to distinguish three dimensions of generational opposition: (1) conflict, (2) ambivalence, and (3) competition. *Conflict* implies direct antagonism or hostility; metaphors such as a "war between generations" come to mind. *Ambivalence* is not the same as outright conflict but instead is a psychological position that includes elements of affiliation and antagonism, both at the same time. *Competition* arises whenever there is an issue of allocation of scarce resources. Competition may or may not be overt and may or may not be accompanied by conscious attitudes that could be described as either conflict or ambivalence. Competition or allocation is simply a fact about finitude and choices. Finally, let us note that these three dimensions of generational opposition—conflict, ambivalence, and competition—are complementary, not necessarily competing, perspectives about intergenerational relationships (Bengtson et al., 2002).

Let me here distinguish three distinct meanings of the term *generation:* (1) family, (2) age group, and (3) cohort. A generation in a family signifies reciprocal roles such as parent and child. Thus, for example, *grandparent* denotes not an age group but a category within families. A generation at the level of age groups signifies a category such as "older persons" or "people over age 65." A generation in terms of cohort is exemplified by groups such as the baby boomers or Generation X. Note that some commonly used terms, such as *children,* are ambiguous and can refer to either a generation within the family or an age group. Note, too, that individuals do not change their membership in a cohort, but they do move through different chronological ages of life.

With these distinctions in mind, it is possible now to illustrate how the three dimensions of generational opposition can be mapped against the three distinct meanings of generation itself, in the following three-by-three matrix:

	Family	Age Group	Cohort
Conflict			
Ambivalence			
Competition			

Conflict in the family is illustrated by the story of King Lear, which is an archetypal struggle over power and inheritance. Conflict among age groups was displayed in the famous slogan from the sixties, a time marked by a generation gap: "Don't trust anyone over thirty!" Conflict among cohorts is also manifested when members of Generation X show hostility toward baby boomers, who are sometimes accused of monopolizing positions of power. Generational conflict is the stuff of high drama and therefore attracts the most interest. But it is far from characterizing normal relationships in families, among age groups, or between cohorts.

More subdued, and more common, is the dimension of ambivalence, in which both affiliation and antagonism are present. Ambivalence in family relations is manifest in many elder care situations: duty toward aging parents, on the one hand, versus resentment, on the other. Indeed, intergenerational ambivalence is a fact about family life that persists through the whole of the life course (Pillemer and Luscher, 2004). Ambivalence between age groups is seen in attitudes of veterans' groups: Vietnam vets and World War II vets, who have many opinions in common but find themselves in opposition on others. Ambivalence among cohorts is manifest by today's young people who are simultaneously attracted by sixties popular music and irritated by the nostalgia of aging boomers for their youth.

We need to avoid seeing ambivalence in purely psychological terms. On the contrary, Connidis and McMullin (2002) argue that ambivalence needs to be conceptualized as socially structured, that is, as an ingredient of social relationships in which individuals exercise agency through social interaction, by negotiating competing claims. Structure and agency, then, are correlative, not exclusive, categories for thinking about aging and the life course (Tulle, 2004). At the level of the family, this negotiation will certainly be manifest at the level of intergenerational relationships, and the terms of the negotiation may be highly idiosyncratic—recalling Tolstoy's observation that "every happy family is alike but every unhappy family is unhappy in its own way." Further steps in theory and research will have to take more seriously the abiding importance of ambivalence, and the emergence of debates over generational equity only serves to remind us of this point (Luscher, 2002).

Competition in family relations is evidenced when families are faced with simultaneously paying for children's tuition and providing support for aged parents. Competition between age groups is involved when elderly voters reject school spending appropriations at election time. Competition among cohorts is manifested when layoffs affect workers of different ages according to seniority rules; that is, younger workers get fired first (Gullette, 2004). Note again that there is no assumption at all that competition in families, age groups, or cohorts will be accompanied by subjective feelings of either conflict or ambivalence. Competition is simply a fact about allocating scarce resources: there isn't enough of something to go around, so choices must be made. Older voters aren't necessarily hostile to children or their needs: they may just feel frustrated by high property taxes (Ladd and Murray, 2001). Families are not necessarily angry about children or aging relatives: they just don't have enough money to pay for everything they want.

Attitudes are a completely different dimension from the issue of allocation and competition. Public opinion surveys or measurement of attitudes cannot tell us anything at all about competition (e.g., between age groups). We are wrong to look at families and try to make conclusions about wider matters of responsibility across the generations. We are wrong to confuse sentiments about older people with structural issues that demand a response from public policy.

This brings us back to King Lear. What is the cause of the disorder that engulfs the kingdom as a result of Lear's bad choices? At one level, the answer is that Lear is betrayed by his scheming daughters because of his own vanity. Because Lear has chosen retirement and relinquished power, his kingdom falls into chaos and the reign of evil forces. But what is the cause of Lear's bad decisions? We can look at Lear psychologically and characterize his action as narcissism or lack of self-knowledge: as Goneril says about her father, "He hath ever but slenderly known himself." But a purely psychological reading, or even a reading based on family relationships, will miss a larger dimension of the story. Lear has mistakenly blurred the dimensions of family and state, the private and the public worlds. He has asked for assurances of filial piety and received soothing words from his two treacherous daughters, Goneril and Regan, while spurning the truthful expressions of Cordelia. At one level, Lear's mistake is being deluded by his vanity. But at another level, his mistake is a refusal to recognize the necessary tensions—of competition and ambivalence—that arise in relationships across generations. He does not understand that because of structural forces of competition—how to divide a kingdom?—it is not easy for a king to choose retirement (Deats, 1999).

My initial presentation of a "Case Manager's Report" on King Lear is not entirely a joke. There are those who would read Lear's story as an example of elder abuse (Pennant, 2001). But to interpret the story this way is to adopt the language of instrumental reason and social science, which is precisely what Habermas regards as a "colonization of the life-world." The assumption of instrumental reason is that the conflict of generations, in the case of Lear, is a "problem" that can be fixed by appropriate "tools" and "interventions." But to read the story of King Lear in this way is to make a category mistake: to subsume all forms of generational opposition under the category of conflict and to ignore ambivalence and competition, which is precisely Lear's own mistake.

Donow (1994) examined classic works of Western literature dealing with old age and, with respect to generational relationships, he identified themes of intergenerational conflict, cooperation, and continuity. He notes that older people are sometimes depicted as exploiters of youth and as selfishly clinging to power and wealth. At the same time, elders may also be viewed as victims and subject to exploitation by others. Donow argues that in a time of population aging, it is no longer reasonable to depict elders in a simple bipolar way as either victims or victimizers.

For the most part, mainstream gerontology has tended to depict older people as victims: that is, vulnerable people entitled to our collective help. Categorizing older people as especially needy and vulnerable did become widespread—a form of "compassionate ageism," Binstock called it (1985). This picture of age has its political uses in attracting public support for social welfare policies on behalf of the old: elders become the "worthy poor." In recent years, as some policy analysts have pointed to larger numbers of well-to-do elders, it has become fashionable to depict older people as selfish ("Greedy geezers"). The rhetoric of generational equity trades on such images of elders as victimizers.

Conclusion

Let me offer some observations about the subject of generational equity (Williamson, Watts-Roy, and Kingson, 1999). Public discussion of this subject has mostly been a dialogue of the deaf. For the most part, gerontologists have rejected the framework of generational equity, favoring instead something called "intergenerational dependence" (Kingson, Hirshorn, and Cornman, 1986). But why should dependence across or between generations be somehow incompatible with thinking about distributive justice or acknowledging elements of competition or conflict between generations? Management and labor are obviously related through mutual dependence, but one can properly raise questions about distributive justice there, just as one can within families. There are legitimate questions about equity between generations, but one must make careful distinctions about the meaning of *generation:* it is simply a mistake to collapse together the distinct categories of conflict, ambivalence, and competition.

These categories tend to be collapsed in public debates about generational equity, and the result is inflated rhetoric and partisans who talk past each other without engaging in the real arguments at stake (Thau and Roszak, 2001; Hamil-Luker, 2001). For example, two prominent policy analysts issued a monograph under the provocative title *Is War between Generations Inevitable?*

(Gokhale and Kotlikoff, 2001). Their approach to the topic was in the manner that has now become somewhat conventional among proponents of generational equity: namely, looking at financing of public entitlement programs (chiefly Social Security and Medicare) and foreseeing a financial crisis ahead (Peterson, 1999; Longman, 2004). Such forecasts usually cause dismay among mainstream gerontologists, who are more likely to urge an approach like that of Peter Diamond: acknowledgment of financial shortfalls—even recognition of equity problems—but no hysterical invocation of the language of war between generations (Diamond and Orszag, 2004).

In a more recent book, Kotlikoff has invoked a different metaphor, a "storm" between generations, but the rhetoric is much the same (Kotlikoff and Burns, 2004). Consider, for example, whether Gokhale and Kotlikoff (2001) could have made the same argument but under the title *Is Competition between Generations Inevitable?* Or perhaps *Is Ambivalence between Generations Inevitable?* The point is that *war* is a synonym for *conflict*. But in semantic terms, *conflict* is much different in its connotations from *competition* or *ambivalence*. To speak of equity issues, therefore, need not involve the rhetoric of conflict, but it necessarily involves elements of choice: that is, alternative values, options, allocation of resources, and so on. To that extent, any consideration of distributive justice within the family—say, equity in the division of burdens of caregiving—necessarily involves something akin to competition and will entail some of the emotional elements of ambivalence.

Note that ambivalence, understood in any psychodynamically thoughtful way, must distinguish between what people feel and what they say they feel. Partly this is a matter of recognizing that some responses are socially unacceptable. For example, people may respond to public opinion surveys with expressions of racial tolerance. But verbal expression may not capture all the feelings about, say, the affirmative action debate, which itself is stimulated by competition for scarce resources. For reasons of social acceptability, respondents may not be fully truthful with survey researchers. With regard to family feelings about ambivalence, the problem is accentuated by the fact that people may not even consciously experience feelings that actually govern their behavior. That is, they may overtly say things that are contradicted by their manifest behavior. Whether we call this "rationalization" or "the Unconscious" does not matter here. What matters is that ambivalence itself cannot be reduced to verbal expressions captured by survey instruments. Therefore, when advocates for the aging insist that public opinion surveys show no signs of "intergenerational conflict," we need to be suspicious (Silverstein et al., 2000). It is far too easy to dismiss intergenerational warfare as a "myth" and therefore cheerfully avoid any discussion of generational equity (Reinemer, 2001). More thoughtful policy analysts understand that generational equity in relation to aging policy is something that needs to be considered in relation to similar issues of responsibility across generations in fields like taxation and environmental policy (Heller, 2003).

It is understandable that gerontologists are eager to refute hysterical claims about a "war between generations," just as it is understandable that advocates for the old want to insist that there is no necessary conflict between young and old. But we should avoid being seduced by comforting conclusions that exclude questions about justice under the guise of good feelings between age groups. Instead of good feelings, I want to urge a more open debate about the real roots of conflict, ambivalence, and competition. I want to call for a more open acknowledgment of what Hegel called "the tremendous power of the Negative." Failure to recognize this Negative—that is, failure to face the complexity of our human condition—is what led King Lear to his tragedy, both personal and political. Perhaps we can be wiser and thus avoid his fate.

REFERENCES

Adam, B., Beck, U., and Van Loon, J. 2000. *The Risk Society and Beyond: Critical Issues for Social Theory.* Thousand Oaks, CA: Sage.

Bengtson, V., Giarrusso, R., Mabry, J. B., and Silverstein, M. 2002. Solidarity, conflict, and ambivalence: Complementary or competing perspectives on intergenerational relationships? *Journal of Marriage and Family* 64(3):568–76.

Binstock, R. 1985. The oldest-old: A fresh perspective on compassionate ageism revisited. *Milbank Memorial Fund Quarterly* 63:420–51.

Connidis, I. A., and McMullin, J. A. 2002. Sociological ambivalence and family ties: A critical perspective. *Journal of Marriage and Family* 64(3):558–67.

Deats, S. M. 1999. The dialectic of aging in Shakespeare's *King Lear* and *The Tempest.* In S. M. Deats and L. Lenker, eds., *Aging and Identity: A Humanities Perspective.* Westport, CT: Praeger.

Diamond, P., and Orszag, P. 2004. *Saving Social Security: A Balanced Approach.* Washington, DC: Brookings Institution Press.

Donow, H. S. 1994 Two faces of age and the resolution of generational conflict. *Gerontologist* 34(1):73–78.

Gokhale, J., and Kotlikoff, L. J. 2001. *Is War between Generations Inevitable?* Dallas: National Center for Policy Analysis.

Guglielmo, W. 2004. The new Medicare law: Doctors cheer. *Medical Economics* 81:37.

Gullette, M. 2004. *Aged by Culture*. Chicago: University of Chicago Press.

Habermas, J. 1974. *Theory and Practice*. Translated by John Viertel. Boston: Beacon Press.

Habermas, J. 1975. *Legitimation Crisis*. Translated by Thomas McCarthy. Boston: Beacon Press.

Hacker, J. 2006. *The Great Risk Shift*. Oxford: Oxford University Press, 2006.

Hamil-Luker, J. 2001. Prospects of age war: Inequality between (and within) age groups. *Social Science Research* 30(3):386–400.

Heller, P. S. 2003. *Who Will Pay? Coping with Aging Societies, Climate Change, and Other Long-Term Fiscal Challenges*. Washington, DC: International Monetary Fund.

Kingson, E. R., Hirshorn, B. A., and Cornman, J. M. 1986. *Ties That Bind: The Interdependence of Generations: A Report from the Gerontological Society of America*. Washington, DC: Seven Locks Press.

Kotlikoff, L., and Burns, S. 2004. *The Coming Generational Storm: What You Need to Know about America's Economic Future*. Cambridge, MA: MIT Press.

Ladd, H. F., and Murray, S. E. 2001. Intergenerational conflict reconsidered: County demographic structure and the demand for public education. *Economics of Education Review* 20(4):343–57.

Laslett, P. 1991. *A Fresh Map of Life: The Emergence of the Third Age*. Cambridge, MA: Harvard University Press.

Liu, K., Manton, K. G., and Aragon, C. 2000. Changes in home care use by disabled elderly persons, 1982–1994. *Journals of Gerontology: Series B: Psychological Sciences and Social Sciences* 55B(4):S245–53.

Longman, P. 2004. *The Empty Cradle: How Falling Birthrates Threaten World Prosperity and What to Do about It*. New York: Basic Books.

Luscher, K. 2002. Intergenerational ambivalence: Further steps in theory and research. *Journal of Marriage and Family* 64(3):585–93.

Massey, D. S., and Taylor, J. E., eds. 2004. *International Migration: Prospects and Policies in a Global Market*. Oxford: Oxford University Press.

Minkler, M., and Estes, C. L., eds. 1998. *Critical Gerontology: Perspectives from Political and Moral Economy*. Amityville, NY: Baywood.

Pennant, L. 2001. Shakespeare's King Lear: A case study of psychological elder abuse. *Victimization of the Elderly and Disabled* 4(2):22–25.

Peterson, P. G. 1999. *Gray Dawn: How the Coming Age Wave Will Transform America— and the World*. New York: Times Books.

Pillemer, K., and Luscher, K., eds. 2004. *Intergenerational Ambivalences: New Perspectives on Parent-Child Relations in Later Life*. Amsterdam: Elsevier JAI.

Powell, J. L., and Longino, C. F., Jr. 2001. Towards the postmodernization of aging: The body and social theory. *Journal of Aging and Identity* 6(4):199–207.

Putnam, R. 2001. *Bowling Alone: The Collapse and Revival of American Community*. New York: Simon & Schuster.

Reinemer, M. 2001. Intergenerational warfare and other myths: Busted. *Innovations in Aging* 30(1):37–40.

Robertson, A. 1997. Beyond apocalyptic demography: Towards a moral economy of interdependence. *Ageing and Society* 17(4):425–46.

Silverstein, M., Parrott, T. M., Angelelli, J. J., and Cook, F. L. 2000. Solidarity and tension between age-groups in the United States: Challenges for an aging America in the twenty-first century. *International Journal of Social Welfare* 9(4):270–84.

ter Meulen, R., Arts, W., and Muffels, R. 2001. *Solidarity in Health and Social Care in Europe.* Dordrecht, Neth.: Kluwer Academic Publishers.

Thau, R., and Roszak, T. 2001. Are we heading for intergenerational war? *Across the Board,* July–August, pp. 70–78.

Tulle, E. 2004. *Old Age and Agency.* Hauppauge, NY: Nova Science.

Williamson, J. B., Watts-Roy, D. M., and Kingson, E. R., eds. 1999. *The Generational Equity Debate.* New York: Columbia University Press.

Wilson, G. 2002. Globalisation and older people: Effects of markets and migration. *Ageing and Society* 22(5):647–63.

III / Policies and Politics of Generational Responsibility

CHAPTER EIGHT

Minority Elders in the United States

Implications for Public Policy

Kyriakos S. Markides, Ph.D., and Steven P. Wallace, Ph.D.

A demographic revolution is taking place in this country. Gerontologists frequently note that the number of older persons will double in the next 30 years. What is less often recognized is that the number of older African Americans will triple, the number of older Hispanics will quadruple and become the largest group of minority elders, and the number of older Asians and Pacific Islanders will quintuple. As the older population becomes increasingly diverse, it raises a number of issues for public policy and intergenerational ethics. This chapter examines the changing demographic composition of the older population, discusses their health and socioeconomic circumstances, and explores the implications of these impending changes for policy and ethics.

The Diversity of the Older Population

The older population in the United States is less diverse than the younger population, but it will catch up in the next 50 years. In 2005, the population age 65 and older was 81.3 percent non-Hispanic white, compared to 67.1 percent of the total population. The older population in 2005 was 8.4 percent black, 6.2

percent Hispanic, 3.1 percent Asian, and 0.4 percent American Indian and Alaska Native. By 2050, only 61 percent of the older population is projected to be non-Hispanic white. At that time older Hispanics will be the largest minority, comprising 17.5 percent of the elderly population, followed by blacks (12.0%) and Asians (7.8%). The total number of minority elders will grow from 6 million in 2003 to 20 million in 2030 and to 33.5 million in 2050 (Federal Interagency Forum on Aging Related Statistics, 2004; U.S. Census Bureau, 2006). These changing demographics present a challenge for policy and intergenerational ethics because the dramatic growth will be in populations that have not been the focus of past policy and practice.

The changes in the older population become even more complex when we take into account the different subgroups of Hispanics and Asians. In 2004, about half (51.2%) of the 2.1 million older Hispanics were of Mexican origin, 10.8 percent were of Central or South American origin, 12.0 percent were of Puerto Rican origin, 9.6 percent were of other Hispanic origins, and 16.0 percent were of Cuban origin. Because of the low contemporary Cuban migration and the high levels of Mexican and Central American migration, future generations of Hispanic elders will be more heavily Mexican and Central American (U.S. Census Bureau, 2005). The Asian and Pacific Island group is comprised of more than 60 different nationality and language groups. The lumping of these diverse subpopulations into a single category obscures the bimodal nature of health status and other outcomes within the population. Some subgroups of older Asian Americans have good health and wealth profiles, such as Japanese Americans, who are mostly second and third generation U.S. residents. Other subgroups of Asian American elders have poor health and economic profiles, such as Koreans and Vietnamese, who are also more likely to be immigrants (Tanjasiri, Wallace, and Kazue, 1995).

Understanding minority aging now and in the years to come requires a geographical perspective. Today, minority elders are concentrated in specific regions of the country (see Table 8.1), with almost half of all Hispanic elders living in California and Texas. Including Florida, New York, and New Mexico to that base raises the total to more than 75 percent. While the Hispanic population is heavily concentrated in the Southwest, Florida, New York, and New Jersey, Latin American immigrants are now also settling in nontraditional areas such as Georgia and Nevada (Gutierrez, Wallace, and Castaneda, 2004). When that cohort ages, they will present a serious challenge to service systems that have no experience working with Hispanic elders. Asian elders are also highly

Table 8.1. Distribution of Minority Elders by State, 2000

African American (n = 2,619,474)		Asian American (n = 746,657)		Hispanic (n = 1,656,932)	
State	Cumulative Percentage	State	Cumulative Percentage	State	Cumulative Percentage
New York	9	California	45	California	27
California	15	Hawaii	58	Texas	47
Texas	22	New York	67	Florida	63
Florida	28	Illinois	70	New York	73
Illinois	33	Texas	74	New Mexico	76
Georgia	39	New Jersey	77		
North Carolina	44				
Virginia	49				
Michigan	53				
Ohio	57				
Pennsylvania	62				
Louisiana	66				
Alabama	70				
Maryland	74				
South Carolina	77				

Source: Data from U.S. Census Bureau, 2003, Summary File 2.

concentrated, with almost half living in California and more than 75 percent living in six different states. African American elders are the most dispersed, with 15 different states being the residence of three-quarters of the population. California, New York, and Texas are on all three lists and therefore face a complex set of multicultural elders in their service areas.

The pattern of living arrangements of older persons differs widely by race and ethnic group. African American elders are the least likely to be living with a spouse, Hispanic elders are the least likely to be living alone, and non-Hispanic whites are least likely to be living in a household headed by one of their children. Minority elders overall live in larger households than non-Hispanic white elders. This is especially true of Asians and Hispanics (Table 8.2). The larger families of Asians, Hispanics, and African Americans are often thought to provide better social support for the older family members (Johnson 1995; Markides et al., 1997).

Family living arrangements, along with language ability and other cultural values, are shaped by the nativity of the older person (Table 8.2). Three-quarters of Asian American elders are immigrants, and few have parents who

Table 8.2. Socioeconomic Characteristics of Minority Elders, 2003

	African American (%)	Asian American (%)	Hispanic (%)	Non-Hispanic White (%)
Living arrangement				
Married, living with spouse	37.6	54.3	52.7	55.6
Living alone	35.7	35.7	17.5	32.0
Living in child's house	6.7	19.2	13.4	3.2
Living in household with 4				
or more persons	12.2	32.2	22.0	4.2
Nativity				
Foreign born	6.5	75.9	61.3	6.2
U.S. born of U.S.-born parents	91.9	5.8	19.2	77.2
High school graduate	54.6	72.0	38.1	77.4
Poverty rate	23.8	8.4	21.4	8.3
Owns home	72.0	72.7	69.9	85.5

Source: Data from King, Ruggles, and Sobek, 2003.

were both born in the United States. The majority of older Hispanics are also immigrants. Small proportions of both African American and non-Hispanic white elders are foreign born, although fewer non-Hispanic whites have U.S.-born parents, reflecting the large wave of immigrants who arrived in the United States in the early 1900s and whose children now are elderly. Continued immigration of large numbers of persons from Mexico, Central America, and Asia assures that future generations of older persons will continue to contain large numbers of immigrant elders.

The Socioeconomic Situation

Table 8.2 shows a gap in the educational attainment between non-Hispanic white elders and others, especially Hispanics. The high school graduation rate compared to non-Hispanic white elders is almost 40 percent less for Hispanics and more than 20 percent less for African American elders. Future generations of older African Americans will have high school graduation rates similar to those of non-Hispanic whites, because they are similar among current young adults age 25–29. The education gap between Hispanics and others remains 30 percent lower among current young adults, presaging a continued educational disadvantage for the foreseeable future for them.

Educational differences are reflected in economic resource differences as well. Almost one-quarter of African American elders currently live in poverty, as do more than one-fifth of older Hispanics. Home ownership is an indicator of assets, and older minorities are 10–15 percent less likely to own their home compared to non-Hispanic whites (Table 8.2). A lifetime of limited economic opportunities for many minority elders leaves them particularly dependent on Social Security for support in old age. Social Security accounts for 90 percent or more of the total incomes of almost half of minorities (45% of African Americans and 44% of Hispanics), in contrast to 29 percent of whites. The disability and survivor components of Social Security are of special importance to minorities, given their higher and earlier levels of disability and owing to earlier mortality among African Americans. African Americans are twice as likely as whites to be receiving Social Security because of a permanent disability (25% versus 12%) and are three times as likely to be children of deceased workers (10% versus 3%) (Hendley and Bilimoria, 1999).[1] It is unlikely that these differences in economic resources will disappear in the next generation of older minorities, because they are less likely to be covered by a private retirement plan (Verma and Lichtenstein, 2003) and African Americans and Hispanic families have lower incomes in preretirement years. Further, it is likely that the majority of Hispanic immigrants will continue to come from Mexico and to have relatively low educational levels. Thus, while second and later generation Hispanics are likely to show increases in educational and overall socioeconomic attainment, the continued influx of less educated immigrants is likely to assure that the overall socioeconomic standing of the Hispanic population in the United States will be considerably lower than that of the non-Hispanic white population as well as of the rapidly growing Asian-origin population. Poverty rates will likely remain high, especially among older people who today rely on Social Security as their primary source of income. The survival of Social Security as we know it today is thus much more critical for older Hispanics and African Americans, especially Mexican Americans, who will continue to be the largest component of the older Hispanic population.

The Population's Health Status

African American older persons consistently show the worst health status, regardless of the measure considered. The health of older Latinos compared to non-Hispanic whites varies based on the measure of health used, although the evidence is consistent that they have higher levels of disability. The health of older Asian Americans is, overall, favorable compared to older non-Hispanic whites, although there are specific subpopulations and health conditions that remain problematic. Projecting the health status of future cohorts of minority elders is difficult to do. Based on past trends, it is likely that existing health disparities will shrink but not be eliminated.

Mortality

Because of higher mortality rates, the life expectancy of African Americans has historically been shorter than that of whites. When white life expectancy at birth was 47.6 years in 1900, African American life expectancy was only 33.0 years. The gap between the races has shrunk as the life expectancy for both groups has increased, but it remains about five and one-half years lower for African Americans. Even those who survive to age 65 face a differential life expectancy by race, with African Americans at age 65 surviving about one and one-half years less than whites. This gap has been roughly similar for the past 35 years (U.S. National Center for Health Statistics, 2004). Life expectancy is calculated using the observed death rates by age in a population. Figure 8.1 shows the number of deaths per 100,000 older persons for African Americans, Hispanics, and non-Hispanic whites. The trend for the past 20 years shows a decline in deaths among older persons but a continued disparity by race.

Figure 8.1 also highlights the source of considerable debate in the literature about the health status of Hispanics in the United States during the past two decades. Two decades ago, Markides and Coreil (1986) proposed an "epidemiologic paradox" with respect to the health of Mexican Americans: whereas the socioeconomic profile of the population was similar to that of African Americans, their health profile, especially with respect to mortality, was closer to that of the more advantaged non-Hispanic white population (see also Hayes-Bautista, 1992; Vega and Amaro, 1994). The epidemiologic paradox has more recently been applied to all Hispanic-origin groups, and it is commonly referred to as the Hispanic Paradox (see, for example, Franzini, Pibble, and Keddie, 2001). Markides and Coreil (1986) suggested that the relatively good overall health of Mexican Americans could not be explained by traditional risk factors and most likely resulted from a "healthy immigrant" effect.

Hummer and colleagues (1999) employed the National Health Interview Survey / National Death Index linked data set to examine how race/ethnicity and nativity influence mortality in the U.S. population. Foreign-born persons in all major ethnic groups (African Americans, Hispanics, and persons of Asian

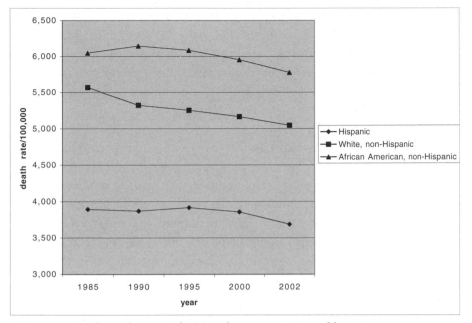

Figure 8.1. Death rate by race/ethnicity of persons age 65 or older, 1985–2002
Source: U.S. National Center for Health Statistics, 2004

origin) had consistently lower mortality rates than native-born persons. Similar findings were obtained with respect to other health indicators by Stephen and colleagues (1994). Markides (2001) noted that studies of the health of immigrants to Western societies suggest that healthy people are more prone to immigrate than less healthy people. Also, Western countries require health screenings of prospective immigrants. Further, because most people immigrate for occupational reasons, they tend to be in relatively good health. Finally, immigrants tend to be people who want to improve their lives and who have a positive outlook on their futures, factors that are consistent with good health (Markides, 2001).

Hummer and colleagues (2004) published an overview of data on racial and ethnic disparities in old age. Official death rates based on vital statistics and population estimates for 1999 show that death rates among Hispanics for each five-year age group beginning at age 65 are considerably lower than death rates for non-Hispanic whites, and the advantage increases with advancing age. It has been estimated, however, that because of misclassification of ethnicity on death certificates, Hispanic mortality rates may be artificially low.

A more accurate source of mortality statistics may be large population surveys linked to mortality follow-up data using the National Death Index. A key advantage of this method is that the ethnicity of the subjects is provided by the subjects themselves or a coresident family member, in contrast to official U.S. data based on vital statistics, where reports of ethnicity are made by funeral directors (Hummer, Benjamins, and Rogers, 2004).

In an analysis of the National Health Interview Survey–Multiple Cause of Death (NHIS-MCD) linked data set, Hummer and colleagues (2004) show that older Hispanics evidence a mortality advantage over older non-Hispanic whites, although the advantage is considerably lower than that based only on vital statistics. At the same time, a potential limitation of this method is that it may miss a significant number of deaths in immigrant populations and may thus underestimate mortality rates among Hispanics, some of whom may return to and die in their country of origin. One analysis of such a "salmon bias" did not find it to account for the relatively low adult mortality rates of Cubans and Puerto Ricans in the United States, who face high barriers to return migration (Cubans) or who are included in U.S. death registrations even if they do return (Puerto Ricans) (Abraido-Lanza et al., 1999). A more recent analysis using different data and a different analytic approach suggested that the mortality differences can indeed be attributed to return migration. The analysis found a mortality advantage independent of socioeconomic status and other characteristics for Mexican immigrants but not foreign-born Puerto Ricans or Cubans (Palloni and Arias, 2004).

An alternative approach to estimating mortality rates for older Hispanics is based on Medicare data linked to application records for Social Security cards maintained in the Social Security Administration's "Numident" (number identification) file. An advantage of this method is that the ethnicity for mortality and for the population comes from one source, avoiding the inconsistencies present in estimates using vital statistics and census data. Elo, Turra, Kestenbaum, and Ferguson (2004) employed the Medicare-Numident data to estimate mortality rates for older (age 65 or older) Hispanics and non-Hispanic whites and compared such estimates to mortality data based on population and vital statistics data. They found the Hispanic advantage to be lower than shown with other data but to exist nonetheless.

Data from other ethnic groups also show evidence of an immigrant mortality advantage. Singh and Siahpush (2002) found a mortality advantage among all major groups of immigrants, including those from Africa, Asia, and

Latin America. While they did not test the extent to which this mortality advantage was the result of return migration (the salmon effect), they did note that health behaviors associated with longevity were more common among immigrants. As noted earlier, the diversity of Asian immigrants can obscure intergroup variation. Nonetheless, a study of mortality among different older Asian American groups (who are primarily immigrants) found that all nationalities exhibited lower mortality rates than whites (Lauderdale and Kestenbaum, 2002). Whether the findings of immigrant mortality advantage is due to return migration before death, healthy immigrant selection, and/or the more healthful behaviors of immigrants, it appears likely that older Hispanics and Asians will continue to have advantageous mortality rates in the near future.

Other Health Indicators

Mortality is an admittedly crude indicator of "health," so it is important to also examine other measures of the health of older minorities. Data from the California Health Interview Survey can provide good comparative information across the major minority groups of elders. Table 8.3 shows that all minority elderly groups have higher rates of diagnosed diabetes than non-Hispanic

Table 8.3. Health Status of Minority Elders, California, 2003

	Hispanic (%)	Asian American (%)	African American (%)	American Indian/ Alaska Native (%)	Non-Hispanic White (%)
Life-threatening condition (ever diagnosed)					
Diabetes	27.7	19.9	26.5	27.8	13.2
Hypertension	55.6	61.2	74.1	69.9	55.3
Heart disease	19.4	18.4	21.6	15.9	26.2
Chronic condition					
Arthritis	53.2	37.6	58.5	65.8	51.9
Incontinent more than once in past 30 days	28.6	11.8	26.0	24.5	20.3
Fell more than once in past year	17.5	7.6	11.1	19.3	11.6
ADL dependence[a]	8.8	4.4	13.4	12.6	6.3
Self-assessed health fair or poor	55.4	48.1	51.1	34.9	27.0

Source: Data from UCLA Center for Health Policy Research, 2003.
[a]Needs special equipment or someone to help with eating, dressing, bathing, getting out of chairs, moving around the house, or using the toilet because of a health problem or condition.

whites. All groups except Hispanics have higher rates of hypertension, which is a risk factor for a variety of disabling conditions including strokes, heart attacks, and kidney failure. Despite the high rate of hypertension, however, all groups show lower rates of diagnosed heart disease than non-Hispanic whites. This could be the result of higher mortality among African Americans (fewer survive heart disease to report it), later diagnosis, the emigration of the sickest elders, or the presence of compensating protective factors in the minority population.

Chronic conditions that are disabling but not often fatal include arthritis, incontinence, and falls. These conditions are also commonly referred to as geriatric syndromes. Asian American elders in California least commonly report all three of these chronic conditions, whereas American Indians and Alaska Natives (AIAN) have the highest rates in two (Table 8.3). Hispanics have particularly high rates of incontinence and falls, but these chronic conditions do not translate into higher rates of ADL dependence (needing special equipment or someone to help with ADLs). African American and AIAN elders have the highest rates of ADL dependence in California. Finally, self-assessed fair or poor health is higher among all minority elders than among whites, with Hispanic and African American elders about twice as likely to report fair/poor health as older non-Hispanic whites.

The diversity of Asian elders is evident in the patterns of subgroups in California. For example, in several indicators Filipino elders report worse health status than the overall Asian group. Among older Filipinos, 55 percent report arthritis and 29 percent report heart disease, levels similar to those of older non-Hispanic whites and substantially higher than the rates for all Asian elders (UCLA Center for Health Policy Research, 2003).

Data based on self-reports of health status are not consistent with the mortality advantage of Hispanics. In national data it has repeatedly been found that, compared to non-Hispanic whites, more older Mexican Americans report their health as being poor (see reviews by Hummer et al., 2004; Markides et al., 1997). National data on activity limitations show that older non-Hispanic whites and Asian Pacific Islanders are less likely to report limitations than other ethnic groups, including Hispanics. Data from the Hispanic Epidemiologic Studies of the Elderly on 3,050 older Mexican Americans from the southwestern United States also show them to report higher disability rates (activities of daily living and instrumental activities of living) than older non-Hispanic whites do (Rudkin, Markides, and Espino, 1997).

Where does the evidence leave us? One possibility is that data based on self-reports are subjective and may not provide a good reflection of the health of older Mexican Americans and other Hispanics. At least one study, for example, suggested that self-ratings of health are less predictive of subsequent mortality among Hispanic immigrants (Finch et al., 2002). Another possibility is that older Mexican Americans (as well as Puerto Ricans) may be more health-pessimistic than other groups and may well report their health to be poorer than it actually is. At the same time, such health reports may be more realistic in that the consequences of chronic conditions and disability for the lives of people from lower socioeconomic backgrounds are greater than they are for those with more economic resources (Markides and Martin, 1983; Markides et al., 1997). The potential interaction of poverty with people's evaluation of their health might also apply to African American and Asian elders as well. But there is also a literature that describes the feeling of "survivorship" that many African American elders express when they live to old age. This outlook may improve self-perceptions of health because having survived in the face of adversity when other family and friends have not can lead to minimizing the importance of medical problems (Becker and Newsom, 2005). Thus, the interaction of adversity, culture, and health conditions may have different outcomes in different groups, with a more pessimistic outlook for Hispanics and a more optimistic one for African Americans.

Finally, there may be good reason to believe that older Mexican Americans live longer than older non-Hispanic whites but live with more disability and in generally poorer health. Data on a variety of health indicators from the Hispanic EPESE paint a rather unfavorable health profile for older Mexican Americans. Their higher disability rates in the community may be explained by the much smaller number of older Mexican Americans in nursing homes and the greater number living in the community (Markides et al., 1996). This factor is unlikely, however, to fully explain away their greater disability rates. Other factors responsible for higher ADL disability are most likely their high rates of diabetes and obesity and their lower rates of physical activity (Markides et al., 1997; Wu et al., 2003). Older Mexican Americans have also been found to have high rates of depressive symptoms (Black, Goodwin, and Markides, 1998). Moreover, high rates of depressive symptoms and depression have been found to exacerbate the negative impact of diabetes on subsequent diabetic complications, physical limitations, disability, and mortality (Black, Markides, and Ray, 2003). Depressive symptoms and depression may exacerbate the negative impact of diabetes by weakening the immune system, by reducing physical and social activity, and by lowering compliance with medication, diet, and self-care efforts to control the disease (Black and Markides, 1999; Black, Markides, and Ray, 2003). At the same time, positive affect, possibly for the opposite reasons, appears to be protective of the development of diabetes-related disability, mortality, and illness incidence in older Mexican Americans (Ostir, Markides, Black, and Goodwin, 2000).

Another disabling condition is cognitive impairment. Using the Mini-Mental Status Examination (MMSE) conventional cut point of 23/24, Black et al. (1999) found that 36.7 percent of older Mexican Americans in the Hispanic EPESE were in the cognitively impaired category. Nguyen et al. (2002) examined changes in the MMSE over a five-year period and found significant declines: 18 percent of older Mexican Americans who had MMSE scores greater than 17 dropped to 17 or below. Older Hispanics with this decline were more likely to be older, less educated, currently unmarried, living with others, and diabetic, to have a history of stroke, and to have near vision impairment at baseline. Data from the Sacramento Area Latino Study of Aging (SALSA) also documented high rates of cognitive impairment in older Mexican Americans and suggested high rates of dementia (Haan et al., 2003). Similarly, African Americans have been found in some studies to have higher rates of Alzheimer disease than whites (Tang et al., 2001) and to be clinically diagnosed at later stages in the disease (Shadlen et al., 1999). Older African Americans are also more likely to have vascular dementias, those caused by small strokes. This finding is related in part to their higher rates of hypertension and diabetes (Demirovic et al., 2003; Kuller et al., 2005).

Researchers have recently started to examine the effect of older persons' neighborhood composition on their health. Because minorities tend to live in segregated neighborhoods, a number of factors might influence the health of minority elders differently than that of non-Hispanic white elders. Although residential segregation is typically associated with poor educational and socioeconomic outcomes (e.g., Massey and Denton, 1993), data from the Hispanic EPESE have uncovered evidence that the health of older Mexican Americans benefits from living in neighborhoods with high concentrations of Hispanics. Multilevel analyses have shown that older Mexican Americans have lower mortality rates (Eschbach et al., 2004), better self-ratings of health (Patel et al., 2003), and lower rates of depressive symptoms than older Mexican Americans living in neighborhoods with lower concentrations of Hispanics.

One explanation for these findings may be that even though neighborhoods that are heavily Hispanic are generally poor, they nevertheless provide supportive environments that promote good physical and mental health.

There does not appear to be a parallel literature for African American or Asian elders, despite their concentration in ethnic neighborhoods. Increased mortality at all ages is associated with more segregated neighborhoods for African Americans (LaVeist, 2003), and decreased health status overall shows the same association (Williams and Collins, 2001). Several studies that examine the neighborhood effects on older African Americans examine the impact of neighborhood socioeconomic status on health, finding that neighborhood socioeconomic status is an important independent predictor of African American elders' health status (e.g., Cagney, Browning, and Wen, 2005). To the extent that older African Americans are overrepresented in low-income neighborhoods, it appears that neighborhood context may work in the opposite direction for older African Americans in comparison to Hispanics. One study identified community effects on the living arrangements of older Koreans. It found that community areas with high concentrations of subsidized housing and Korean stores had the highest rates of living independently (Kim and Lauderdale, 2002). It remains to be seen what the effects of future changes in neighborhoods and communities will be on the health and well-being of older minorities, but existing data suggest that they should not be ignored.

Medical and Long-Term Care

There are clearly differences in the health status of minority elders. There are also significant variations in the access to medical care and use of long-term care by minority elders. This variation is likely to grow as policy encourages older persons to join HMOs, which may offer additional services but can also establish new barriers to service. Table 8.4 provides data on Medicare HMO and fee-for-service (FFS) indicators of the availability of services (travel time less than 30 minutes to the doctor), accessibility of services that are available (insurance coverage and satisfaction with follow-up care), and acceptability of services that are accessed (satisfaction with doctor's concern for overall health) (see also Wallace, 1990). While the vast majority of older persons live relatively close to their doctors, Hispanic and African American elders in fee-for-service practices are more likely than older non-Hispanic whites to live more than 30 minutes from their doctors.

Table 8.4. Access to Health Care Indicators, Medicare Beneficiaries Age 65 or Older, 1996

	Hispanic (%)	African American (%)	Non-Hispanic White (%)
Less than 30 minutes to doctor			
FFS*	82.9	89.5	93.4
HMO	91.3	90.5	94.8
Medicare and Private (FFS)	23.4	37.6	68.8
Medicare and Medicaid	30.1	20.0	4.9
Medicare HMO	20.1	11.2	12.5
Medicare only	23.9	30.5	16.1
Very satisfied with follow-up care			
FFS*	18.1	13.9	24.2
HMO*	17.0	11.5	27.8
Very satisfied with doctor's concern for overall health			
FFS*	16.1	14.4	23.6
HMO*	15.1	14.4	26.5

Source: U.S. National Center for Health Statistics, 2003.
 Notes: FFS = fee-for-service coverage; HMO = managed care coverage.
 *chi-square differences by race/ethnicity significant at $p < .05$

Having a doctor available does not mean that it is easy to access the doctor's care. Financial barriers are a common problem, and the mix of insurance that older persons have influences the level of potential financial barriers. Table 8.4 shows that non-Hispanic whites are two to three times more likely to have a private supplemental insurance plan in addition to Medicare, reducing their immediate out-of-pocket costs when they need to seek medical care. In contrast, Hispanics and African Americans are four to six times more likely to have Medicaid, the program for low-income aged, blind, and disabled persons and for families with children. On the one hand, Medicaid has historically paid for prescription medications when Medicare did not, it pays for long-term care not covered by Medicare, and it assumes the copayments and deductibles in Medicare fee-for-service care. On the other hand, some Medicaid services have limits and other restrictions. Medicare HMOs have been popular with older persons primarily because of their low copayments and coverage of prescription drugs. Older Hispanics have a particularly high coverage by HMOs, likely because of their concentration in California and Florida, where HMO coverage rates are high overall. Most significant is the difference in older persons with only Medicare, meaning that all copayments, deductibles, and uncovered expenses are paid out of pocket. This vulnerable group includes higher proportions of Hispanics and African Americans. In sum, financial accessibility from an insurance perspective is best for older non-Hispanic whites, worse for older Hispanics, and worst for older African Americans (Wallace and Enriquez-Haass, 2001). Another common problem is obtaining follow-up services. Table 8.4 shows the same pattern of non-Hispanic whites in the best situation, followed by Hispanics and then African Americans.

Finally, even if services are available and accessible, the acceptability of the services affects the likelihood that the user will follow the medical advice and return when appropriate for additional care. Satisfaction with the interpersonal process of care is an important aspect of acceptability, and racial/ethnic differences are evident in older persons' satisfaction with their doctor's overall concern for their health (Table 8.4). After controlling for health status, gender, age, education, and other factors, older African Americans still have lower levels of satisfaction with both FFS and HMO care from their doctors than non-Hispanic whites. After controlling for population differences, Hispanics are less satisfied than non-Hispanic whites when in HMOs, but *more* satisfied when in FFS (Wallace and Enriquez-Haass, 2001). These findings emphasize that minority elders encounter different challenges than non-Hispanic whites when seeking medical care for their health problems, independent of their different incomes and educational levels.

Minority elders have historically used nursing homes less than non-Hispanic whites. In 1973, older whites were about twice as likely as older African Americans to be in nursing homes. Since that time, the white utilization rate has dropped about 30 percent while the African American rate has nearly doubled, resulting in a higher nursing home use rate for African Americans than for whites (Ness, Ahmed, and Aronow, 2004). Older Latinos and Asian Americans continue to be institutionalized at much lower rates. In the 2000 census, the institutionalization rate (primarily nursing homes) for persons age 65 or older was 5.4 percent for African Americans, 4.9 percent for non-Hispanic whites, 2.4 percent for Hispanics and for American Indians/Alaska Natives, and 1.6 percent for Asians (U.S. Census Bureau, 2003).

Two factors may help explain the disappearance of the African American–white difference in use of nursing homes. First, the rapid growth in the use of assisted living facilities has been concentrated among the middle-class non-Hispanic white population who can afford to pay privately. While 1.5 million persons live in nursing homes, many of the additional 750,000 persons in assisted living might have otherwise been in nursing homes in earlier times. Second, because disability levels among African Americans are higher than for non-Hispanic whites, it is possible that the growth in moderate-intensity (versus high-intensity) home care services has enabled more non-Hispanic whites than African Americans to remain at home. Comparing African Americans and non-Hispanic whites, a higher proportion of the African American older population is female and widowed or divorced, and thus more dependent on extended family for caregiving, making them particularly sensitive to the availability of home care services (Wallace et al., 2005).

There has been less research on the relation between race and ethnicity and the use of community services. Some studies report that minority elders use community-based care at the same rate as non-Hispanic whites (or at a higher rate) after controlling for need and resources (Wallace, Levy-Storms, and Ferguson, 1995). Other studies find that African Americans and Latinos are less likely to use community services (Wallace, Levy-Storms, et al., 1998; Borrayo et al., 2002). The variation in findings appears to be related to the different populations studied. When only community-dwelling elders are in the sample, long-term care use does not vary often by race. But when both institutional and community elders are analyzed together, racial differences remain. Because African American and non-Hispanic white elders have different patterns and locations of care, it is important to understand racial and ethnic patterns in the entire continuum of care.

Several factors could account for the racial and ethnic differences in use of long-term care. Some studies suggest that minority elders are less knowledgeable than non-Hispanic whites about the types and functions of many community-based services. Others suggest that nursing homes have discriminatory admission policies, that health professionals are less likely to refer minority elders to formal services, and/or that family structure and earlier inception of parenthood result in different use patterns (Wallace et al., 2005). These racial and ethnic variations are typically overlooked by policymakers who design programs for the "average" elder who is non-Hispanic white and middle class (Wallace, Levy-Storms, et al., 1998).

Older Mexican Americans provide a good example of the detailed factors that affect long-term-care use. They remain in the community for as long as possible, although their ability to do so is influenced by economic, geographic, and structural factors, as well as by functional status (Angel and Angel, 1997; Angel et al., 1996). Angel, Angel, and Markides (2000) found that older Mexican Americans who immigrated to the United States later in life are more likely to live with children in the face of diminished health than those immigrating as children or young adults or those who were native born. While options in long-term care and living arrangements are limited by income and other financial resources, it appears that strong cultural values are also related to keeping disabled older Mexican Americans in the community (Angel, Angel, and Markides, 2000). As mentioned earlier (Markides et al., 1996), this results in more disability in the community and greater burdens on Mexican American families, who generally have few financial resources. At the same time, there are higher levels of interdependence between older Mexican Americans who co-reside with their children and these children, because the older generation is typically the one with a steady income (in the form of a Social Security check). The consequences of these interdependencies for both older people and their children are not well understood (Angel et al., 1999; Markides and Black, 1995).

Conclusion

What can we learn from the patterns and trends summarized in this chapter to inform public policy and responsibility across generations? The rapidly increasing numbers of Hispanic, Asian, American Indian / Alaska Native, and African American elders will change the dynamics of policy and intergenerational relationships in coming years because the health status, family composition, socioeconomic status, and long-term-care needs are all different from those of the majority of the current generation of predominately non-Hispanic white elders. Clearly, public policy discussions of ethics and responsibilities across generations and across ethnic groups cannot ignore the special needs as well as talents and contributions of this dynamic segment of the population.

The extent to which we tailor our aging and health policies to address minority health issues is both a political and an ethical issue. If we ignore the variation by race discussed above, we will often design policies that address the needs of the majority non-Hispanic white elders while missing or harming the interests of minority elders. In 2006, for example, Medicare expanded coverage to all outpatient prescription drugs for the first time. One of the policy debates was whether and how to include persons who already had drug coverage under Medicaid (for low-income persons). The ethics debate centered on whether or not Medicare should retain its universal coverage feature; in other words, should all people with Medicare coverage receive the same benefits? The policy debate centered on how the federal government would capture the money that states would save when Medicare (which is funded entirely by the federal government) extended drug coverage to those who also had Medicaid (which states fund up to half of). Lost in that debate was the fact that among Medicare beneficiaries, Medicaid historically paid for one-quarter of African Americans' and one-third of Hispanics' prescription costs but under 10 percent of non-Hispanic whites' (CMS, 2005). This means that any coverage change that may decrease the coverage or scope of benefits for low-income elders will disproportionately affect minority elders. If we ignore this distributional impact, we risk putting the burden of policy changes on those who have experienced lifetimes of disadvantaged circumstances. Ethically, principles of equity and justice would lead us to address long-standing inequalities in the health and medical care of older minorities directly and overtly (Estes and Wallace, 2005). But racial politics at the start of the twenty-first century have been hostile to affirmative action, immigrant rights, and other issues that address racial and ethnic problems. One solution is to be racially aware of the consequences of policy changes but to then construct color-blind need-based policies in ways that implicitly provide services and assistance particularly to the minority groups who are also in the most need (Wallace, Enriquez-Haass, and Markides, 1998).

Because older Hispanics and African Americans often rely on Social Security as their primary source of income, discussions on how to save Social Security also have more meaning for them. Attempts to privatize the system are likely to hurt minority elders more than non-Hispanic whites. Subsequent generations of minority elders are likely to experience increases in their educational, occupational, and financial status. But continuing differences in educational levels, segregation and limited job opportunities, and the continued influx of less educated and less skilled Hispanics and some Asian nationalities are all likely to assure that the minority elderly population as a whole will continue to be socioeconomically disadvantaged for decades to come.

We also owe minority elders a better understanding of their special needs, talents, and contributions in addition to their special health problems. Focusing only on pathologies can stigmatize groups, and we lose insights that could benefit the entire population when we ignore their unique strengths. We saw that the health status of the Mexican American population, in particular, is paradoxical. How can people who have a socioeconomic status similar to that of African Americans have lower mortality rates and higher life expectancies than the considerably advantaged non-Hispanic whites? Is migration selection the primary force behind the Hispanic Paradox or the mortality advantage (and relatively good health) of Hispanics despite their generally lower socioeconomic status? What is the role of selective return migration? Clearly more resources need to be devoted to improving data quality so that we have a better understanding of the true situation. If indeed there is an advantage, can we learn from the population's experience? With their increasing numbers, are we all likely to become a healthier society?

The minority elderly population of the United States is growing and becoming increasingly diverse itself. Mexican Americans in particular are moving out of the Southwest to other parts of the country and are likely to become a truly national minority. Research thus far suggests that older Hispanics, Mexican Americans in particular, enjoy relatively good relations with their families, a situation that may be a cultural holdover from their country of origin and/ or a response to living in an environment that is not as supportive and often hostile. We also saw that living in primarily Hispanic neighborhoods affords health advantages to older Mexican Americans with respect to such important health indicators as perceived health, depressive symptoms, and mortality. With Mexican Americans moving away from the Southwest to other parts of the country, there will be questions regarding the support systems of older Mexican Americans. Will older Mexican Americans left behind become more vulnerable? Will the current reliance on family members jeopardize the financial well-being of Mexican American and other Hispanic women, who often quit their jobs to care for elderly relatives, thus jeopardizing their financial security in old age?

In sum, scholars and policymakers must pay close attention to the growing minority elderly population of the United States. Future research on the overall population's health status and socioeconomic conditions, as well as public policy debates, must take into account the minority population's size and special characteristics.

Acknowledgments

This work was partly supported by grants from the National Institute on Aging (AG-10939 and P30-AG21684) (Resource Centers on Minority Aging Research) and the UTMB Center for Population Health and Health Disparities funded by the National Cancer Institute (IP 50 CA105631). We thank the editors of this book and Soham Al Snih for valuable comments and suggestions.

NOTE

1. Information provided in this article distinguishes non-Hispanic whites from all whites (which includes Hispanics) when possible. Different data sources and articles approach racial and ethnic classifications somewhat differently. Before the 1980s, most official statistics did not include any information on Hispanics, so earlier historical data on mortality and other issues are available only for blacks and whites (which includes Hispanics). Federal data collect Hispanic ancestry separately from race, so some data and research report information on Hispanics (who may be of any race), whites, and blacks (which also includes some Hispanics). When research or data do not separate Hispanics from the white population, we use the term *white*. Because Hispanics are still a relatively small proportion of the white population, data on whites and non-Hispanic whites are nearly the same.

REFERENCES

Abraido-Lanza, A. F., Dohrenwend, B. P., Ng-Mak, D. S., and Turner, J. B. 1999. The Latino mortality paradox: A test of the "Salmon Bias" and healthy migrant hypotheses. *American Journal of Public Health* 89:1543–48.

Angel, J. L., Angel, R. J., and Markides, K. S. 2000. Late life immigration, changes in living arrangements, and headship status among older Mexican-origin individuals. *Social Science Quarterly* 81:389–403.

Angel, J. L., Angel, R. J., McClellan, J. L., and Markides, K. S. 1996. Nativity, declining health, and preferences in living arrangements among elderly Mexican Americans: Implications for long-term care. *Gerontologist* 36(4):464–73.

Angel, R. J., and Angel, J. L. 1997. *Who Will Care for Us? Aging and Long-term Care in Multicultural America.* New York: New York University Press.

Angel, R. J., Angel, J. L., Lee, G. Y., and Markides, K. S. 1999. Age at migration and family dependency among older Mexican immigrants: Recent evidence from the Mexican American EPESE. *Gerontologist* 39(1):59–65.

Becker, G., and Newsom, E. 2005. Resilience in the face of serious illness among chronically ill African Americans in later life. *Journals of Gerontology Series B: Psychological Sciences and Social Sciences* 60(4):S214–23.

Black, S. A., Espino, D. V., Mahurin R., Lichtenstein, M. J., Hazuda, H., Fabrizio, D., Ray, L. A., and Markides, K. S. 1999. The influence of non-cognitive factors on the mini-mental state examination in older Mexican-Americans: Findings from the Hispanic EPESE. *Journal of Clinical Epidemiology* 52(11):1095–1102.

Black, S. A., Goodwin, J. S., and Markides, K. S. 1998. The association between chronic diseases and depressive symptomatology in older Mexican Americans. *Journal of Gerontology: Medical Sciences* 53(3):M188–94.

Black, S. A., and Markides, K. S. 1999. Depressive symptoms and mortality in older Mexican Americans. *Annals of Epidemiology* 9(1):45–52.

Black, S. A., Markides, K. S., and Ray, L. A. 2003. Depression predicts increased incidence of adverse health outcomes in older Mexican Americans with Type 2 diabetes. *Diabetes Care* 26(10):2822–28.

Borrayo, E. A., Salmon, J. R., Polivka, L., and Dunlop, B. D. 2002. Utilization across the continuum of long-term care services. *Gerontologist* 42(5):603–12.

Cagney, K. A., Browning, C. R., and Wen, M. 2005. Racial disparities in self-rated health at older ages: What difference does the neighborhood make? *Journals of Gerontology, Series B, Psychological Sciences and Social Sciences* 60(4):S181–90.

CMS (Centers for Medicare & Medicaid Services). 2005. *Health and Health Care of the Medicare Population,* table 4.6. Available at www.cms.hhs.gov/apps/mcbs/MCBSsrc/2001/01cb3d.pdf.

Demirovic, J., Prineas, R., Loewenstein, D., Bean, J., Duara, R., Sevush, S., and Szapocznik, J. 2003. Prevalence of dementia in three ethnic groups: The South Florida program on aging and health. *Annals of Epidemiology* 13(6):472–78.

Elo, I. T., Turra, C. M., Kestenbaum, B., and Ferguson, R. F. 2004. Mortality among elderly Hispanics in the United States: Past evidence and new results. *Demography* 41:109–28.

Eschbach, K., Ostir, G. V., Patel, K. V., Markides, K. S., and Goodwin, J. S. 2004. Neighborhood environment and mortality among older Mexican Americans: Is there a barrio advantage? *American Journal of Public Health* 44:1807–12.

Estes, C. L., and Wallace, S. P. 2005. Older people. In B. S. Levy and V. W. Sidel, eds., *Social Injustice and Public Health,* pp. 113–29. New York: Oxford University Press.

Federal Interagency Forum on Aging Related Statistics. 2004. *Older Americans, 2004: Key Indicators of Well-Being.* Washington, DC: U.S. Government Printing Office.

Finch, B. K., Hummer, R. A., Reindl, M., and Vega, W. A. 2002. Validity of self-rated health among Latino(a)s. *American Journal of Epidemiology* 155:755–59.

Franzini, L., Ribble, J. C., and Keddie, A. M. 2001. Understanding the Hispanic paradox. *Ethnicity and Disease* 11:496–518.

Gutierrez, V. F., Wallace, S. P., and Castaneda, X. 2004. *Demographic Profile of Mexican Immigrants in the United States.* UCLA Center for Health Policy Research. Available at www.healthpolicy.ucla.edu/pubs/publication.asp?pubID=102.

Haan, M. N., Mungas, D. M., Gonzalez, H. M., et al. 2003. Prevalence of dementia in older Latinos: The influence of Type 2 diabetes mellitus, stroke, and genetic factors. *Journal of the American Geriatrics Society* 51:169–77.

Hayes-Bautista, D. 1992. Latino health indicators and the underclass model: From paradox to new policy models. In A. Furino, ed., *Health Policy and the Hispanic,* pp. 32–47. Boulder, CO: Westview Press.

Hendley, A. A., and Bilimoria, N. F. 1999. Minorities and Social Security: An analysis of racial and ethnic differences in the current program. *Social Security Bulletin* 62(2):59–64.

Hummer, R. A., Benjamins, M. R., and Rogers, R. G. 2004. Racial and ethnic disparities in health and mortality among the U.S. elderly. In R. A. Bulatao and N. B. Anderson, eds., *Understanding Racial and Ethnic Differences in Health in Late Life: A Research Agenda.* Washington, DC: National Academy Press.

Hummer, R. A., Rogers, R. G., Nam, C. B., and LeClere, F. B. 1999. Race/ethnicity, nativity, and U.S. adult mortality. *Social Science Quarterly* 80:136–53.

Johnson, C. L. 1995. Cultural diversity in the late-life family. In R. Blieszner and V. H. Bedford, eds., *Handbook of Aging and the Family,* pp. 307–31. Westport, CT: Greenwood Press.

Kim, J., and Lauderdale, D. S. 2002. The role of community context in immigrant elderly living arrangements: Korean American elderly. *Research on Aging* 24(6):630–53.

King, M., Ruggles, S., and Sobek, M. 2003. *Integrated Public Use Microdata Series, Current Population Survey: Preliminary Version 0.1.* Minneapolis: Minnesota Population Center, University of Minnesota. www.ipums.org/cps.

Kuller, L. H., Lopez, O. L., Jagust, W. J., Becker, J. T., DeKosky, S. T., Lyketsos, C., Kawas, C., Breitner, J. C., Fitzpatrick, A., and Dulberg, C. 2005. Determinants of vascular dementia in the Cardiovascular Health Cognition Study. *Neurology* 64(9):1548–52.

Lauderdale, D. S., and Kestenbaum, B. 2002. Mortality rates of elderly Asian American populations based on Medicare and Social Security data. *Demography* 39(3):529–40.

LaVeist, T. A. 2003. Racial segregation and longevity among African Americans: An individual-level analysis. *Health Services Research* 38(6):S1719–33.

Markides, K. S. 2001. Migration and health. In P. Baltes and N. J. Smelser, eds., *International Encyclopedia of the Social and Behavioral Sciences,* pp. 9799–9803. New York: Elsevier.

Markides, K. S., and Black, S. A. 1995. Race, ethnicity, and aging: The impact of inequality. In R. H. Binstock and L. K. George, eds., *Handbook of Aging and the Social Sciences.* San Diego: Academic Press.

Markides, K. S., and Coreil, J. 1986. The health of southwestern Hispanics: An epidemiologic paradox. *Public Health Reports* 101:253–65.

Markides, K. S., and Martin, H. W. 1983. *Older Mexican Americans: A Study in an Urban Barrio.* Austin: University of Texas Press.

Markides, K. S., Rudkin, L., Angel, R. J., and Espino, D. V. 1997. Health status of Hispanic elderly in the United States. In L. G. Martin and B. Hess, eds., *Racial and Ethnic Differences in the Health of Older Americans,* pp. 285–300. Washington, DC: National Academy Press.

Markides, K. S., Stroup-Benham, C. A., Goodwin, J. S., Perkowski, L. C., Lichtenstein, M., and Ray, L. A. 1996. The effect of medical conditions on the functional limitations of Mexican American elderly. *Annals of Epidemiology* 6:386–473.

Massey, D. S., and Denton, N. A. 1993. *American Apartheid: Segregation and the Making of the Underclass.* Cambridge, MA: Harvard University Press.

Ness, J., Ahmed, A., and Aronow, W. S. 2004. Demographics and payment characteristics of nursing home residents in the United States: A 23-year trend. *Journal of Gerontology: Medical Sciences* 59A(11):1213–17.

Nguyen, H. T., Black, S. A., Ray, L. A., Espino, D. V., and Markides, K. S. 2002. Predictions of decline in MMSE scores among older Mexican Americans. *Journal of Gerontology: Medical Sciences* 57(3):M181–85.

Ostir, G. V., Markides, K. S., Black, S. A., and Goodwin, J. S. 2000. Emotional well-being predicts subsequent functional independence and survival. *Journal of the American Geriatrics Society* 48(5):473–78.

Palloni, A., and Arias, E. 2004. Paradox lost: Explaining the Hispanic adult mortality advantage. *Demography* 41:385–415.

Patel, K. V., Eschbach, K., Rudkin, L. L., Peek, M. K., and Markides, K. S. 2003. Neighborhood context of self-rated health in older Mexican Americans. *Annals of Epidemiology* 37:1197–1202.

Rudkin, L., Markides, K. S., and Espino, D. V. 1997. Functional disability in older Mexican Americans. *Topics in Geriatric Rehabilitation* 12:38–46.

Shadlen, M. F., Larson, E. B., Gibbons, L., McCormick, W. C., and Teri, L. 1999. Alzheimer's disease symptom severity in blacks and whites. *Journal of the American Geriatrics Society* 47(4):482–86.

Singh, G. K., and Siahpush, M. 2002. Ethnic-immigrant differentials in health behaviors, morbidity, and cause-specific mortality in the United States: An analysis of two national data bases. *Human Biology* 74(1):83–109.

Stephen, E. H., Foote, K., Hendershot, G. E., and Schoenborn, C. A. 1994. Health of the foreign-born population: United States, 1989–90. *Advance Data* 241:1–12.

Tang, M. X., Cross, P., Andrews, H., Jacobs, D. M., Small, S., Bell, K., Merchant, C., Lantigua, R., Costa, R., Stern, Y., and Mayeux R. 2001. Incidence of AD in African-Americans, Caribbean Hispanics, and Caucasians in northern Manhattan. *Neurology* 56:49–56.

Tanjasiri, S. P., Wallace, S. P., and Kazue, S. 1995. Picture imperfect: Hidden problems among Asian Pacific Islander elderly. *Gerontologist* 35:753–60.

UCLA Center for Health Policy Research. 2003. California Health Interview Survey, 2003. Accessed at www.chis.ucla.edu/main/default.asp (site discontinued; last accessed March 15, 2004).

U.S. Census Bureau. 2003. *2000 Census of Population and Housing.* Summary file 2. Accessed at factfinder.census.gov/servlet/DatasetMainPageServlet?_lang=en.

U.S. Census Bureau. 2005. Population by sex, age, and Hispanic origin type: 2004, table 1.2. In *Current Population Survey, Annual Social and Economic Supplement, 2004,* Ethnicity and Ancestry Statistics Branch, Population Division. Accessed at www.census.gov/population/socdemo/hispanic/ASEC2004/2004CPS_tab1.2a.pdf.

U.S. Census Bureau. 2006. *Current Population Survey, Annual Social and Economic Supplement, 2005.* CPS Table Generator. Last revised March 9, 2006. Accessed at www.census.gov/hhes/www/cpstc/cps_table_creator.html.

U.S. National Center for Health Statistics. 2003. *Health, United States, 2003.* Hyattsville, MD: NCHS.

U.S. National Center for Health Statistics. 2004. *Health, United States, 2004.* Hyattsville, MD: NCHS.

Vega, W. A., and Amaro, H. L. 1994. Latino outlook: Good health, uncertain prognosis. *Annual Review of Public Health* 15:39–67.

Verma, S., and Lichtenstein, J. 2003. Retirement plan coverage of baby boomers and retired workers: Analysis of 1998 SIPP data. Pub ID: 2003-10. Washington, DC: AARP Public Policy Institute.

Wallace, S. P. 1990. The no care zone: Availability, accessibility, and acceptability in community-based long-term care. *Gerontologist* 30(2):254–61.

Wallace, S. P., Abel, E., Pourat, N., and Delp, L. 2005. Long-term care and the elderly population. In R. Andersen, T. Rice, and G. Kominski, eds., *Changing the U.S. Health Care System,* 3rd ed. San Francisco: Jossey-Bass.

Wallace, S. P., and Enriquez-Haass, V. 2001. Availability, accessibility, and acceptability in the evolving health care system for older adults in the United States of America. *Pan American Journal of Public Health* 10(1):18–28.

Wallace, S. P., Enriquez-Haass, V., and Markides, K. 1998. The consequences of color-blind health policy for older racial and ethnic minorities. *Stanford Law and Policy Review* 9(2):329–46.

Wallace, S. P., Levy-Storms, L., and Ferguson, L. R. 1995. Access to paid in-home assistance among disabled elderly people: Do Latinos differ from non-Latino whites? *American Journal of Public Health* 85:970–75.

Wallace, S. P., Levy-Storms, L., Kington, R. S., and Andersen, R. M. 1998. The persistence of race and ethnicity in the use of long-term care. *Journals of Gerontology, Series B, Psychological Sciences and Social Sciences* 53(2):S104–12.

Williams, D. R., and Collins, C. 2001. Racial residential segregation: A fundamental cause of racial disparities in health. *Public Health Reports* 116(5):404–16.

Wu, J. H., Haan, M. N., Liang, J., et al. 2003. Diabetes as a predictor of change in functional status among older Mexican Americans: A population-based cohort study. *Diabetes Care* 26:314–19.

CHAPTER NINE

Allocating Resources for Lifelong Learning for Older Adults

Ronald J. Manheimer, Ph.D.

Forty or fifty years ago, only a tiny fraction of the older population, the wealthy and healthy, could enjoy a robust retirement-age period. Now that segment of the life course has become both lengthened and democratized, giving millions of ordinary citizens more choices than they had ever dreamed of. For British sociologist Peter Laslett (1991), who focused his research on the post-industrial societies of Britain and the United States, the retirement-age generation of the late 1950s to early 1960s was the first to possess the discretionary time, good health, and sufficient funds to determine how its members would occupy themselves in a continuing active stage, or Third Age (dependency typically demarcating the Fourth Age). As a result, millions of older people now participate in leisure activities such as travel, gardening, sports, and outdoor recreation. And they volunteer in record numbers. Because rising rates of high school and college completion are also attributes of senior adults, and because prior education is the chief determinant of demand for continued learning in the later years (Snyder, Hoffman, and Geddes, 1997), people in the Third Age represent a significant growth area for lifelong learning.

Since the 1970s, educational participation rates for people 55 or older have climbed steadily. More recently, according to the National Household Education Surveys, during the 1990s the percentage of people in the United States ages 66–74 who took at least one adult education class in the previous year more than doubled—from 8.4 percent in 1991 to 19.9 percent in 1999. The biggest growth in participation of individuals ages 55–74 was in community-provided, nonformal education. This includes not-for-credit courses, workshops, and seminars offered by churches, libraries, department stores, senior centers, and so on, where the rate went from 4.6 in 1991 to 11.6 in 1999. About 5.5 percent took courses in a school or university in 1991; the figure rose to 8.6 percent in 1999. The increase among the "young-old" (ages 66–74) surpassed that of any other age group (Hamil-Luker and Uhlenberg, 2002).

Access to and public support of learning opportunities for older adults may not seem particularly controversial, especially when compared to ideologically driven debates in the United States over how to pay for social entitlement programs such as Medicare and Social Security. Though far less audibly, similar debates do occur over policies and rationales related to funding for and support of lifelong-learning programs for older adults. While there is general consensus that adequate health care is an important social good in which all generations should benefit fairly, there is less agreement on the value and necessity of lifelong learning. So when opportunities arise for mature citizens to share the resources of college campuses, questions about generational equity also come to the surface. And when programs include young undergraduates and mature adults sharing the same classroom by participating in intergenerational learning opportunities, college administrators and program leaders are further challenged to articulate rationales incorporating principles of distributive justice and fair exchange of time, money, and resources.

In this chapter, I look at some of the ethical issues that arise relative to the evolution of lifelong-learning programs, particularly in the United States but with reference to developments in other countries. I find it helpful not only to make a quick survey of the linkages between rationales for older learner programs, theories of aging, and public policy, but also to take particular situations (and voices) as case studies that introduce concerned leaders and scholars to the multiple dimensions of lifelong learning for older adults, to intergenerational education, and to questions about who should pay and who gets the most benefit. A particularly useful theory of distributive justice drawn from the arena of health care, the "prudential lifespan account" (Daniels, 1988), will be contrasted to another approach that uses exchange theory—a sociological and economic notion of behavior based on perceived fair value (Cook, 1987).

Lifelong Learning, Theories of Aging, and Social Policy

Until about 35 years ago, nonvocationally related educational programs for individuals nearing or in their retirement years hardly existed. Echoing the so-called disengagement theory of aging (Cumming and Henry, 1961), the then-prevailing view implied that it was developmentally inappropriate for mature adults to try to learn new skills and adopt new ideas because to be old meant to engage in a process of gradual withdrawal from society as one turned inward in preparation for death. Moreover, few representatives of the older population expressed strong need or demand for organized lifelong-learning programs. Then came a change. Advocates for older adults proclaimed the "activity theory" of aging. Seniors needed to remain involved in social activities and stay informed in order to function as good citizens. Laslett's Third Age individuals became politically savvy and recognized their importance as a growing percentage of the population. Over the past three decades, a sea change in attitudes about aging, retirement, and the creative use of leisure time has led to dramatic expansion of programs for learners age 50 or older in the United States, Canada, Europe, Latin America, China, and elsewhere. In the United States, providers include senior centers, libraries, museums, banks, unions, colleges, department stores, for-profit and nonprofit travel-learning companies, and a host of self-organized special interest organizations (Manheimer, 2003).

Most of the growth of older-learner programs has come at the grassroots level. Elderhostel, for example, was a tiny experiment in short-term college residencies started in 1975 at the University of New Hampshire by a visionary activist, Marty Knowlton. His goal was to make an inexpensive college-like experience available to middle- and low-income seniors who had never been to college. That was an admirable goal, but Elderhostel tended to attract a somewhat more affluent and typically college-educated clientele, and it grew into a household name, annually enrolling more than 200,000 individuals in both domestic and international programs (Ruffenach, 2004). Likewise, Lifelong Learning Institutes, once a scattering of participant-organized and -led groups, sprang up on college campuses in the mid-1970s, the idea spreading by word of mouth, and by 2006 there were more than 350 such organizations in the United

States and Canada. The schools shared some funding and space as part of their public service mission, and the seniors supplied the balance with volunteers and modest fees.

On the public-sector side, in the mid-1970s, some 39 state governments enacted legislation entitling people over age 62 or 65 (varying by state) to enroll in public colleges and universities tuition-free on a space-available basis. While community colleges enrolled thousands of seniors, for whom they were reimbursed through state funding, university host institutions received no additional funding for taking on this responsibility. Consequently, they did comparatively little to publicize these opportunities. Nevertheless, legislators could pat themselves on the back for doing something for elderly people. There are other instances of state support for education in the later years, including generous funding from the National Endowment for the Humanities and the National Endowment for the Arts, but these sources have been episodic and have done little to create sustained infrastructures for ongoing programs. As a consequence, by the 1990s most programs required participants to help underwrite the cost of their education; they received some assistance, usually in the form of in-kind services and resources, from host institutions.

Today, we could say that older adult education in the United States is mainly a consumer-driven market. For the healthy, well off, and well educated, prospects for the future look great. For the less privileged, the prospects are poorer. Opportunities for continued learning in the later years are viewed by American society as optional, not necessary. This is in contrast to public policies in Scandinavia, where learning throughout the life course is deemed an important social good that benefits both the individual and society as a whole. State funding for evening schools, annual public forums, residential community colleges, and other forms of lifelong learning have been commonplace in countries like Denmark and Sweden for more than 130 years. No doubt there is a close link between nationally supported lifelong learning in Scandinavian countries and their long-established national health care insurance policies. This latter is a type of social welfare legislation that U.S. citizens have supported in fragmentary fashion (e.g., Social Security, Medicare, Medicaid, Section 8 housing) and with less cultural consensus and social solidarity.

In a sense, the U.S. government bears a certain amount of responsibility for the rise in demand for continued learning in later life. The GI Bill enabled millions of World War II and Korean War veterans to become first-generation college grads. They carried the value of education with them into their retirement years. Because prior education is the chief predictor of desire for continuing education, when the veterans entered retirement in the 1970s, they started knocking on the doors of various possible hosts for educational programs. Since then, participation rates for learners 50 or older have grown in direct relationship to the percentage of college graduates—11.1 percent of people over 65 in 1989 and almost 20 percent (projected) by the year 2010 (Manheimer, Snodgrass, and Moskow-McKenzie, 1995).

With the coming of an aging society, the role played by education in the later years is increasingly in the public eye. Stories about "seniors" going back to school proliferate in September newspaper columns while awestruck reporters write about 70- and 80-year-olds graduating from law school or winning fiction prizes in grad school. The question in relation to expenditure of public dollars on the education of older adults is similar to one asked about health care: is education a right or a privilege? Who should pay? Why should society invest in the education of older people, who are primarily consumers, not producers? Why should institutions such as colleges and universities share scarce resources such as classroom and parking spaces, library resources, and even college fitness centers with older people? Might this not pose a detriment to the young?

The most frequently articulated institutional rationale supporting increased access to education for older learners in this period of programmatic expansion was the notion that seniors "deserved" these opportunities. The pendulum swing from the disengagement theory to the activity theory of aging paralleled this idea of rewarding older adults with educational opportunities. However, as the economic condition of the majority of seniors continued to improve through the 1980s and 1990s, the socially perceived "deserving" elderly population turned into either "greedy geezers," were portrayed as overreaching their fair share of public entitlements, or, in a more positive light, "successful agers," able, thanks to social entitlements, national health care insurance, public and private pension funds, and better health care and self-care, to lead lives of unprecedented productivity and social contribution.

One consequence of the success story of Third Age individuals around the world is a challenge to the assumption of public entitlements based mainly on chronological age (e.g., for the United States, Medicare, Social Security, and college tuition waivers) rather than a condition of need. Decades ago Bernice Neugarten anticipated the question of whether age or need should determine the distribution of social welfare dollars. She coined the term the "age-irrelevant society" to stimulate debate as to whether chronological age was still the best determinant of how social goods should be distributed (Neugarten, 1982). Dramatically increasing older populations and rising health care costs have exacerbated this dispute in recent years.

Countries across the world, from dramatically "graying" Japan, Sweden, Germany, Italy, and Greece to more slowly "aging societies" like the United States and Canada, are facing economic and social issues of enormous proportion. Each is challenged to establish principles of equitable justice between generations while searching for visions of how to create truly "age-integrated" societies in which strong bonds of mutual care and nurture exist between generations. Governments and social institutions at all levels are compelled to identify the principles of social justice that will guide them in decision making about the fair allocation of resources and opportunities. At the more concrete level, rational cost-benefit analyses of social exchange tend to emerge almost spontaneously from ideological shifts influenced by changing demographics. For example, several states have repealed their tuition-free-for-seniors policies, having determined that many of those who most benefit are also among the most affluent in their age group. Similarly, the once idealistically motivated Elderhostel is experiencing strong competition from dozens of more expensive and luxurious travel-learning programs. Elderhostel has repositioned itself in the market by offering more tailored, adventuresome, and upscale travel programs (Ruffenach, 2004). And a whole new market niche of high-end university-linked retirement communities has cropped up in college towns around the United States, their residents clamoring to use campus recreation facilities and libraries (Manheimer, 2003).

Our tale of Dave Rosen's redemption unfolds into the mid-arc of this pendulum swing in the perception and condition of what might be called neo-elderly people (Manheimer, 2005). Sometimes by looking at a single case, we more readily grasp the competing assumptions that underlie institutional policies and both culturally shared and disputed sentiments. Our case study will prompt us to examine the changing nature of obligations between the generations in the context of the exchange of knowledge and experience that lifelong learning has become.

Dave Rosen's Redemption: A Representative Anecdote

Not everyone in Asheville knew Dave Rosen by name, but a great many recognized the trim, fast-paced figure in jeans and a college sweatshirt, his tanned, smiling face shaded by the visor of a New York Yankees baseball cap from under which a few strands of gray hair might protrude. The Yankees? Here in the South? The guy had some nerve.

Dave and his wife, Dorothy, moved from Brooklyn to Asheville, North Carolina, in the early 1990s. Dave retired from the highly competitive business world of women's fashion and Dorothy from professional choreography. They became involved in the NC Center for Creative Retirement (NCCCR), a lifelong-learning, leadership, and community service program of the University of North Carolina at Asheville (for which this author serves as director). Dorothy started off taking peer-led courses and then decided to offer tap dancing. Her class was a big hit, and soon "Rosen's Rascals," her tap dance troupe, was performing at nursing homes, senior centers, and outdoor festivals. Dave had once considered a career in journalism but was deterred at college registration. "I'd just gotten out of the army and even though it was the GI Bill, I still wasn't going to stand in any more long lines." Instead, he chose the shorter line, signing up for NYU's School of Business. Now, forty years later in retirement, he signed up to take those writing courses in a lifelong-learning program.

Dave achieved three important goals within the few years after he and Dorothy arrived in Asheville. First, claiming he identified with the disenfranchised, he volunteered to serve on the board working to organize an annual Native American festival called Kituah. Second, he became a Big Brother, taking on eleven-year old Chris, who lived with his grandparents and was reading at a second-grade level. And third, he eventually wrote a play about his experiences with Chris.

Of Kituah he said, "I learned that if I kept my mouth shut and stopped trying to be number one, eventually they would call on me for advice." Of his little brother, Chris, he said: "Helping Chris with school, Dorothy and I tutoring him in reading, and taking him to minor league ball games, gave me a chance to do for him what I hadn't done for my own kids." And of his play, which he hoped to see produced, he said: "I finally got back to creative writing, my first love."

Though he was raised in the Jewish tradition, Dave was not observant. Yet his unselfconscious quest to embrace humility, redo the mistakes of earlier parenting, and give literary shape to his new life with Chris exhibit what might be called a pattern of "secular redemption" (Manheimer, 1989). Dave Rosen took advantage of learning opportunities in later life to redeem past mistakes and omissions and make his life whole. He used education as the vehicle of self-change.

Though Dave Rosen paid modest fees to enroll in NCCCR's College for Seniors courses, such fees only partially supported the cost of this educational enterprise. Other people helped to ensure that the program could use campus office and classroom space, and to cover administrative costs that supported continued operations, year after year. North Carolina taxpayers helped to underwrite Dave Rosen's redemption, just as taxpayers in other states partially supported their residents' lifelong-learning ventures.

Dave Rosen's story is an example of what in less dramatic form occurs daily in lifelong-learning programs for older adults across the United States, Canada, and other countries. Such programs, which only emerged in significant numbers since the mid-1980s, are typically precariously perched on the farthest branches of college and university organizational charts. Most operate with minimal budgets and even lesser campus political power. Members of the lifelong-learning institutes, with the help of some paid staff, usually run them. They are part of a broad international movement of educational programs for older learners. And their future depends in part on how we, as taxpayers in a democratic society, regard the fair distribution of limited resources across age groups and generations.

We can tease out the issues of social justice between the generations and explore approaches that enhance solidarity between younger and older generations by focusing on this question: Who should pay for Dave Rosen's redemption? To frame the issue, we turn to a similar debate in the health care arena.

Equity in Health Care and Lifelong Learning

Bioethicist Norman Daniels advanced the notion of the "prudential lifespan account" (Daniels, 1988) as part of an ethically imaginative way to frame dilemmas about the fair distribution of scarce health care resource across age cohorts and the stages of life. His premise, based on John Rawls's theory of distributive justice (Rawls, 1971), depends on our ability to envisage the whole life course and, as a corollary, the overlapping cycle of generations as the total realm of our concern. Through powers of empathy, anticipation, and recollection, we may attain the perspective that nineteenth-century German philosopher Arthur Schopenhauer (1890) reserved for old age: the capacity to see life as a complete cycle. In this way we can transcend narrow life-stage interests or value biases related to generational affinities. We should, argues Daniels, drawing on Rawls's metaphor, imagine that we stand behind a "veil of ignorance," setting aside our own age, stage, or time of life. Our goal is to view the life course flowing like a river with various generational cohorts—past, present, and future— sailing along toward the open sea beyond.

Given his approach, we no longer look at age equity issues in the here and now as competition between age groups; instead, we view them with dynamic understanding—we will all eventually be old, will have traversed this life course. Daniels uses this approach to justify rationing of health care by age and regards this as a more just and equitable approach than is currently in place in the United States. He wants to identify a set of age-relevant priorities for how health care resources are distributed (Daniels, 1988). As one ages, one draws down the pool of available health care dollars, and so in later life a person has less claim on limited resources than younger people. In countries with national health care systems, the rationing of expensive, life sustaining medical interventions seems to follow a principle such as Daniels sets out. In the United States, where public and private insurance coverage frequently overlap and where dispensers of health care fear costly litigation for failure to do everything to sustain a life, no such principles are consistently followed.

The same could be said of lifelong learning. Some states, such as Maine, have invested millions of dollars in encouraging the proliferation of lifelong-learning opportunities, especially as an aspect of inducing retirement migration that promotes economic development. Other states, such as California, have reduced or eliminated funding for older adult education. And the federal government plays little or no role despite periodic recommendations coming from White House Conferences on Aging.

Institutionally supported education is a limited resource on which our society spends a great deal of money, especially for people in the earlier part of life, childhood through young adulthood. Most forms of education are state supported and dollars are highly limited. In higher education, the public share of funding continues to decline and the private share rises as legislators and citizens increasingly view college education as a commodity that primarily benefits the individual (future earning power) and only secondarily society (informed citizenship, international competition, and security). Continuing education, especially career-related, is an expanding field. For some universities and colleges, it is a proverbial "cash cow."

One might argue that education in later life is hardly equivalent to health care. Is education a life-and-death issue such that restriction and limited access would seriously impair or shorten one's life? At first glance, it would hardly seem so. But in recent years an abundance of research (Rowe and Kahn, 1998; Nussbaum, 2003; Cohen, 2004) has shown that continued intellectual stimulation and social connections made possible, in part, by education, actually help to delay the onset of dementia, counteract depression and social isolation, and promote the growth of new brain cells and connectivity (dendritic growth). While we should not exaggerate the positive health benefits of continued learning in later life, we do not want to underestimate its relevance to our discussion.

The problem with drawing the parallel between access to health care and to education is that medical interventions to help us survive a stroke or heart attack, live with less pain, overcome disabilities, or manage chronic illnesses are unquestionable goods, whereas attending a yoga or T'ai Chi class, a lively reading and discussion group, or a current events seminar seem a lesser good. While living quantitatively longer is a questionable good that has been the subject of continuing debate over the cost-benefit balance of life-extending medical intervention, unplugging someone from an inspiring educational seminar has generally not provoked similar debate.

We cannot easily claim that education in the latter years has the significance of medical intervention in life-and-death situations, but the broader epidemiology of health care and wellness (including disease prevention) for the young and the middle aged does compare with the value of lifelong learning for those in the post-50 decades (to choose an arbitrary threshold). We want to keep in mind that psychosomatic illnesses are the likeliest cause for office visits to doctors. In this perspective, we can seriously consider the mental and physical health benefits (and related dollar savings) of continued learning.

Education in the Later Years

Justifications or rationales for education in the later years span a wide gamut of virtues. The most frequently cited benefits of continued learning in later life are these: promoting a knowledgeable citizenship, enabling people to make new friends, helping to offset depression and isolation, providing a sense of purpose and meaning, filling leisure time, helping people keep physically and mentally fit, helping older people gain skills that may make them both more independent and socially more valued, keeping people connected to society, and increasing self-esteem.

In addition to all these pragmatic values, one could argue that education is also an intrinsic good, self-satisfying, an "end in itself," to echo the famous words of Cardinal Newman.

Now supposing we draw on Daniels's "prudential lifespan account" as a framework for considering the fair distribution and generational equity of this topic. Let's first try the veil of ignorance. Let us pretend we do not know how old we are when asked: "Is the opportunity for continued publicly supported learning a good that should be provided after the age of, say, 50 or 60, even when it is not part of vocational enhancement?" Do we, as taxpayers, use up our allocation of publicly supported education once we graduate from high school or college? Will some age cohorts have gained more than others from lifelong-learning opportunities?

Whereas in earlier years, society sought to ensure opportunities for education for the young but not the old, now the old are beginning to receive a small but growing share. One might say we are living in a lifelong-learning society, because half of all adults engage in some form of educational programming every year (Belanger, 1999). Of course, elderly people are part of that rising tide. And Daniels himself says that we have to "shed the outdated view that education is just a matter for youth." Granted, but who should pay? Should those advantaged by prior education and ample discretionary funds get what they want and need by paying while those less well off in money and education, who may not even know what they're missing, do not? Or is there justification for intervention in terms of public policy to ensure that all older citizens gain benefit from education? Should state governments or Congress enact something like a social insurance plan for lifelong learning—"Educare" and "Educaid"?

The latter argument was often made in grant applications for arts and humanities funds from federal and state endowments in the 1970s and 80s when elderly people were first being "discovered" as a deserving, previously neglected, special interest group. Celebration of the nation's bicentennial helped to raise the country's historical consciousness, catalyze the historical preservation movement, and generate considerable interest in oral history. By association, elderly people were recognized as a rich repository of knowledge, wisdom, lore, and expertise. Older adults were untapped or underused human capital in the form of narratives that needed to be passed on to younger generations.

However truthful, this often-sentimental attitude peaked in the mid-80s and then began to wane as older persons' collective successes led to the view that elderly people were receiving their fair share, perhaps to the detriment of disadvantaged children and youths. Concurrently, in the mid-1980s, the Americans for Generational Equity (AGE), got started on the theme that younger age groups were feeling resentful of all the entitlements being lavished on older people, thus diminishing their part of the pie. Public opinion surveys failed to confirm this sentiment, but that did not deter those who perceived an age equity imbalance from beating the drum for their viewpoint and warning about the "gray peril."

Given this bit of history concerning social attitudes about aging and lifelong learning, suppose we use Daniels's method to understand our present situation. Let's say that from a prudential life-span account, as a general principle, it makes good sense to ensure equal access to education throughout life. We will want to treat the young differently, because we recognize that education in the earlier part of life is the foundation for what comes later and will probably not be critical in the same way in one's later years. We will want to say that this should be true for all generations, not just the elderly people. Ideally, continued learning opportunities should be open to all, regardless of ability to pay. But because that goal seems impractical in our society, and we do not have the collective commitment to lifelong learning that is traditional for Scandinavian countries, it is probably more prudent to allow that some part of lifelong learning should be consumer-driven, paid for privately, and perhaps consumer-led (e.g., Lifelong Learning Institutes). That would still leave room for a government role in partially supporting learning opportunities for underserved seniors.

If education adds to quality of life, then everyone should have some of it. If it helps people to become better-educated voters and serves as a catalyst to channel them into either for-pay jobs (postretirement careers or bridge jobs) or socially beneficial volunteering, so much the better. Perhaps intergenerational education, young and old learning together and from one another, is another valued form because it will help young people become more aware of the aging process and of the needs for goods and services of a large, growing segment of society. Indeed, in 20 years, one of every five Americans will be over age 65 and probably one of every four over age 55. That means today's undergraduates will be serving a large older clientele in their future vocations and professions. Through such intergenerational learning ventures, elderly people will experience greater understanding and solidarity with younger people, whom they have come to know in the classroom. As a consequence, seniors may be more inclined to financially support schools either directly out of their own pockets or indirectly by voting in favor of school bonds and increased higher-education appropriations. And, reciprocally, younger generations will be sensitive to the needs, strengths, and weaknesses, and contributive power of older generations.

A Case for Intergenerational Equity: Personalizing the Account

Suppose now that I am addressing my colleagues and fellow administrators at UNC Asheville, where the program I direct, NC Center for Creative Retirement, is located. My program does receive some state support: 30 percent of our annual budget. It was allocated by the North Carolina General Assembly some 19 years ago, after our local legislative delegation lobbied for it on the basis that such a center would be good for the local economy. In fact, our program does attract migrant retirees from other states, and they do bring their investments, Social Security, pension checks, and a good deal of volunteer service into the local economy. Recently, NCCCR members helped to raise $4.5 million (donating half that amount themselves) to build Reuter Center, a dedicated classroom and conference center on the University of North Carolina, Asheville, campus that serves as the program's headquarters (the UNCA Board of Trustees granted NCCCR the use of 5.5 acres of campus property). Center members, mainly retirement-aged individuals, help run the center, teach on a volunteer basis, provide service to the campus and community, and pay for many of the goods they receive through their affiliation (see NCCCR's Web site, www.unca.edu/ncccr/). These goods include intergenerational courses.

The center offers intergenerational courses through the UNCA honors program, through several academic departments, and through freshmen colloquia (a type of "first-year experience" offered at many liberal arts universities). In earlier years, we let the state policy apply, so that those over 65 received free tuition but had to pay the "student fee" portion for three credit hours; those under 65 had to pay the full regular student fee to enroll. The cost then was about $100 for those over 65 and $200 for those under 65. Not particularly expensive as far as higher education is concerned. Usually, I taught the classes, and because that is not a required part of my job description, it did not cost the university added salary money, nor were seats lost that undergraduates would otherwise have filled (we reserved about 10 seats for the older students and 10 for the younger). I could always find enough older students willing to pay the fee and take on 16 weeks of course work and assignments. Also, we could provide a few partial scholarships for those who could not afford the full price. Dave Rosen was a student in my first foray into intergenerational honors, a course called "1946: the Meaning of a Year." The year 1946 was when Dave came home to Brooklyn from the battlefields of Europe, a boy become a man.

As the price of tuition has increased to offset declining state dollars, it now costs our members about $390 for the under-65 age group and about $190 for the over-65 group. That price tag created a ceiling that was deterring most of our members. So I petitioned the vice chancellor for academic affairs to let me sign up seniors for $100 each (some scholarship money was also available), though they would not be officially registered (not that credit or grades was an issue). He gave provisional approval, noting that this was a fair exchange of my time for participation of older adults. But what if I was not the only one offering an intergenerational class? Then a colleague would be devoting some of his or her state-paid time to teaching older people who were not paying their state-mandated fair share, and some seats would be lost that might have been filled by undergraduates. This administrator and, indeed, our chancellor wanted to see the number of intergenerational courses expand because they believed the presence of mature adults added value to an undergraduate's education. But how could we justify to our colleagues the apparent inequity? Why were some older adults getting special treatment?

This question was the tip of an iceberg because, when the center was first established in 1987, many UNCA faculty members complained: "What do old people have to do with the mission of a public liberal arts university?" An easy answer was that as part of its threefold mission, UNCA was supposed to carry out "community service" (in addition to teaching and research). But everyone knew that community service was something of a public relations ploy—good, if the university could afford it, for improving the school's image among the townspeople. Some few genuinely believed in the merits of community service and, indeed, today's service-learning initiatives have raised the importance of community service to a new level. But in the late 1980s, the community-service rationale didn't carry much weight, certainly not enough to justify giving the center a classroom and some tiny offices, which were then in short supply.

While the development staff spoke of cultivating potential donors among the retiree crowd, and then-chancellor David Brown pointed to the potential of free expertise that could be drawn into the classroom, these arguments fell on my colleagues' deaf ears. Moreover, these trade-offs or pragmatic rationales just didn't add up to a vision of the intergenerational campus or the ideal of learning across the life course. When it came to dealing with the highly specific matter of special fees for intergenerational classes, all the earlier issues, which had largely faded away as the center prospered and brought the campus excellent national and local press, might be resurrected. All it would take was an email protest launched by an irate faculty member. A more convincing rationale was needed.

One proposed solution echoed principles of exchange theory. The case might be made that because members of the center volunteer for a variety of types of campus service (e.g., helping students with resumes, conducting mock interviews in the campus Career Center, and giving special invitation lectures), wouldn't it be fair for other seniors to reap the benefit of an exchange of goods? We might even be able to put a dollar sign on the two sides of this exchange equation. We could tally up the number of volunteer hours and calculate their financial worth, and we could tally the income lost if undergraduates had enrolled to help pay the salary of the instructor. This might function like Edgar Cahn's "Time/Dollar" bartering system (1992).

What would be wrong with this calculative approach to fairness as equal exchange? It wasn't necessarily inconsistent with principles of distributive justice; it just added an element of mutuality—seniors giving as well as getting in relation to other generations. I suspect we will encounter a great deal of this type of duty-based, exchange theory ethics in the coming years. Currently a public relations campaign is under way to persuade baby boomers to do their part as volunteers, not to slack off or succumb to the unfortunate trait (read: stereotype) of the self-indulgent generation (Harvard School of Public Health, 2004).

In certain institutional contexts, older people are going to have to prove their worth. Many books and articles have appeared that highlight the contributive role of older adults to society. Merely staying fit and enjoying life do not seem adequate to justify social investments in older citizens. There is an unspoken ethos that seniors ought to remain productive down to their last days. In the case of older learners, especially those who are retired, they will have an obligation to do their part to continue to serve society in whatever ways they can manage. Politically speaking, programs for older learners will have to show social benefit as well as individual enhancement. Older adults, whether or not they care to be so categorized, will have to demonstrate their social value if younger generations are going to be willing to help support them. Not only the undifferentiated young, but the younger African Americans, Latinos, and Asian Americans, who will make up a near majority of the future workforce and who are already overrepresented in low-income jobs in nursing homes and assisted living facilities and as home chore service providers and health aides. Will these younger minority people be inclined to project themselves into old age or to view the life course as an integral whole, when the old-age group they serve is mainly Caucasian?

Ironically, the justification for older learner programs based on exchange theory is exactly in line with the rhetoric of value supporting the more than 20,000 "universities for old people" that have been established in China since the 1980s. Personal enrichment is balanced by the exhortation to serve others. China's elders are invited to learn traditional cultural forms like flower arrangement, calligraphy, and herbal medicine, while they are also taught dietary improvement, better hygiene, and physical fitness. Older learners in China are expected to use their knowledge to benefit others and to take better care of themselves so as to save the state unnecessary health care expenditures. China's older learners have a "sacred duty" to learn and to serve (Herzhong, 1997).

"From those who have received much, much is due," goes the old adage. But how, in a loosely knit democracy and pluralistic society like the United States, can one impose a duty-oriented ethics that presupposes a basic sense of social solidarity and shared history? And in a country where public higher education receives increasingly smaller percentages of state government funding each year, almost blurring the distinction between public and private colleges and universities, how can one insist that, for our older citizens, education should be a right, not a privilege?

Taking the Search on the Road

I was attracted to but uneasy with the exchange-theory approach, because it put unfair burdens on older people to remain productive regardless of circumstances, and it judged their worth mainly in extrinsic or utilitarian terms. I decided to take the problem with me as I made a number of presentations at conferences that included younger and middle-aged audiences. Did they have ideas about how to fashion a rationale for older-adult participation in public-funded lifelong-learning programs? I heard a wide range of responses. Some earnestly protested that older people should in fact not be granted equal access to lifelong-learning opportunities, and certainly not if it could mean displacement of traditional-age undergraduates. Others felt it was unfair that only privileged elderly people had access to lifelong learning, but they weren't sure what could be done about it. In a few instances, I heard the type of response that Daniels might approve—to wit, the woman who said: "When I'm that age, I want those kinds of programs to be there for me." This young woman could project herself forward in time. She did not live exclusively in the selfish me-now. But she did not say, "I want those opportunities to be there for *us*."

I heard another approach voiced at Virginia's James Madison University in a seminar with college juniors studying economics. One student suggested reconceptualizing the role that older class participants would play. Instead of students, they would become "resource associates." He reasoned that their presence would provide an enrichment of the curriculum. Older students would be sharing their knowledge, experiences, and expertise with younger students. Nothing makes historical understanding more vivid than the story of someone who was part of a great battle, political upheaval, tough economic time, scientific discovery, momentous cultural event, or social movement. So these older adults would no longer be only fellow learners; they would function like faculty assistants. In fact, admission to this status of resource associate might depend on what the older person could bring to the seminar table, not only life experience but also knowledge and expertise appropriate to the subject matter of the course. Contributive capability could be a principle of selection, that they would have something to offer as part of the intellectual exchange process. I thought this formulation was ingenious and wished I had thought of it myself.

For the moment, this is our solution. The vice chancellor for academic affairs liked this reformulation that helped distinguish the role and responsibility of the resource associate. What this version adds to Daniels's "prudential lifespan account" is a way to put value back into your life-span account after you've subtracted education credits over the years. You, the older person, are not just a needy recipient; you're a contributor to learning drawing from your accumulated experience, expertise, heritage, and possibly wisdom. In this sense, the parallel to health care collapses. As we age, we will only have more need for health care, not less. And we cannot replenish our heath care debits except with money (such as through personal health care accounts) or by taking the best possible care of ourselves. We could choose preemptive suicide to save health care dollars in our last years, and some may feel the burden to do so, especially as health care costs are increasingly being borne by individuals and families.

Does this refinement—the exchange-theory approach suggested by the resource associates policy—make a greater contribution to resolving the dilemma of equitable distribution of lifelong learning as a social good? I can hear my colleagues in Europe (Findsen, 2005) complaining that once again we've let the state off the hook and only underscored the lengths we have to go to in order to justify even a small modicum of public support for lifelong access to learning. But we are in an era of increasing emphasis on self-responsibility, privatization, and the demise of the social welfare state (even in Scandinavia, where funding for adult education has been sharply curtailed). While government has not played a leadership role (except, as noted, in China and, we should add, in France, where the universities of the Third Age are based at publicly supported universities), the grassroots initiatives have exhibited a degree of innovation and ingenuity that may surpass anything that might have come from governmental efforts. Moreover, having seniors play a major role in helping to run their own programs suggests a significant element of emancipation that programs run strictly by professional educators and public administrators do not. Nevertheless, the lifelong-learning quandary about who deserves what remains.

Dave Rosen Revisited

"Dave, I think I may have failed you."

"No, Ron. That's all right. You've made a good point about what we old-timers have to offer. But all this business of exchange theory and resource associates. I'm afraid we're going to lose sight of something equally important."

"What's that, Dave?"

"Friendship. Fellowship. That's what makes it fun. We get to know each other a little better. I want to know whom I'm leaving this country to. And I want these young students to make me think a little harder. You know how we tend to get a little closed-minded, a little more timid, more conservative as our hair turns gray and falls out."

"Yeah, that's what Aristotle said about impulsive youth and timid old age."

"Aristotle? Gee. I didn't know he was that smart."

"But Dave, I'm still disappointed. I think Daniels was on the right track. If we're going to have a society that sees the interdependence of generations and age groups, we need a vision of the complete life course."

"See ourselves as part of a larger whole?"

"Right."

"That's hard to do, Ron. It's taken me a whole lifetime to grow up. Even now I still find it hard to get the big picture."

"So, for now, I guess we just have to figure out what's a fair exchange."

"For now. Yes."

Dave Rosen died in the summer of 1997 and was buried in the Veterans Cemetery in Black Mountain, North Carolina. Only a few months stood between the diagnosis of pancreatic cancer and his death. Dave was a young 72, so the brevity of his retirement life made his late-life accomplishments all the more poignant. It was as if he knew time was short and he had much to do to earn his redemption. Dave was a great lifelong learner and friend. And the undergraduates whose lives he touched will not quickly forget him.

Conclusion

In most developed countries, the new longevity and relative security of the retirement-age population has transformed older citizens into a new and dramatically growing consumer group. Following this overarching trend, access to continued learning opportunities has similarly become a matter of the marketplace. Opportunities for the adult-education business sector to expand are seen everywhere, from upscale travel-learning programs to corporate retiree retraining seminars at prestigious universities. An earlier rationale, providing education to "deserving" elderly people, has largely faded from public discourse. The dramatic rise of the healthy and financially secure Third Ager has also led to widespread availability of new, fee-driven (though sometimes partially publicly supported) educational programs of surprising variety. The good news here is that such programs can create the infrastructure necessary for stability and sustainability, whereas earlier efforts floundered when the private or public foundation grants that paid the bills expired and the organizations folded or ceased their adult-education efforts.

How, then, should equity be understood in the context of lifelong learning? Should the marketplace determine who gains access to continuing education, or could this laissez-faire ideology be balanced by public interest in ensuring that the broadest range of mature adults have a chance to continue learning? Is it not in a society's best interest to encourage mental stimulation, intellectual and cultural enhancement, and the enlightenment of its older citizens, if for no other reason than health promotion and disease prevention—proven indirect benefits of continued learning? And what of intergenerational exchange promoted by colleges and universities that encourage young and old to study and learn together and from one another? What is needed, as Normal Daniels, Arthur Schopenhauer, Erik Erikson, Lawrence Kohlberg, and others have pointed out, is a vision of the whole of the life course. Only then can citizens and decision makers step outside of their particular age, stage, and interest group perspective to support what is good from one generation to another. In the absence of such a unifying vision, we fall back on a cost-benefit balance sheet of fair exchange of social goods.

REFERENCES

Belanger, P., ed. 1999. *The Silent Revolution of Adult Learning Societies: Who Participates in Adult Learning?* New York: Elsevier Science.
Cahn, E. 1992. *Time Dollars: The New Currency That Enables Americans to Turn Their Hidden Resource—Time—into Personal Security and Community Renewal.* Emmaus, PA: Rodale Press.
Cohen, G. 2004. *The Creative Age: Awakening Human Potential in the Second Half of Life.* New York: HarperCollins.
Cook, K. 1987. *Social Exchange Theory.* Beverly Hills, CA: Sage.
Cumming, E., and Henry, W. 1961. *Growing Old: The Process of Disengagement.* New York: Basic Books.
Daniels, N. 1988. *Am I My Parents' Keeper?* New York: Oxford University Press.
Findsen, B. 2005. *Learning Later.* Malabar, FL: Krieger Publishing.
Hamil-Luker, J., and Uhlenberg, P. 2002. Later life education in the 1990s: Increasing involvement and continuing disparity. *Journal of Gerontology* 57B:6.
Harvard School of Public Health, Center for Health Communications. 2004. *Reinventing Aging: Baby Boomers and Civic Engagement.* Boston: Harvard School of Public Health.
Herzhong, L. 1997. The university for old people in China. *Third Age Learning International Studies* 7:91–96.
Laslett, P. 1991. *A Fresh Map of Life: The Emergence of the Third Age.* Cambridge, MA: Harvard University Press.
Manheimer, R. J. 1989. The narrative quest in qualitative gerontology. *Journal of Aging Studies* 3:231–52.
Manheimer, R. J. 2003. Education of older adults in the United States: Present and fu-

ture prospects. In L. A. Vitt, ed., *Encyclopedia of Retirement and Finance.* Westport, CT: Greenwood Press.

Manheimer, R. J. 2005. The older learner's journey to an ageless society: Lifelong learning on the brink of a crisis. *Journal of Transformative Education* 3(3):198–220.

Manheimer, R. J., Snodgrass, D., and Moskow-McKenzie, D. 1995. *Older Adult Education: A Guide to Research, Programs, and Policies.* Westport, CT: Greenwood Press.

Neugarten, B. 1982. *Age or Need?* Beverly Hills, CA: Sage.

Nussbaum, P. 2003. *Brain Health and Wellness.* Tarentum, PA: Word Association.

Rawls, J. 1971. *A Theory of Justice.* Cambridge, MA: Harvard University Press.

Rowe, J. W., and Kahn, R. L. 1998. *Successful Aging.* New York: Pantheon.

Ruffenach, G. 2004. Road scholars: A new travel program tries to take some of the "elder" out of Elderhostel. *Wall Street Journal,* February 23, p. R-6.

Schopenhauer, A. 1890. The ages of life. In *Counsels and Maxims,* translated by T. B. Saunders. London: Swan Sonnenschein.

Snyder, T. D., Hoffman, C. M., and Geddes, C. M. 1997. *Digest of Educational Statistics, 1997.* Washington, DC: U.S. Department of Education, National Center for Educational Statistics.

CHAPTER TEN

Transforming Age-Based Policies to Meet Fluid Life-Course Needs

W. Andrew Achenbaum, Ph.D.,
and Thomas R. Cole, Ph.D.

Elie Metchnikoff coined the term *gerontology* in *The Nature of Man: Studies in Optimistic Philosophy* (1908, pp. 289, 297–98): "How can we try to transform to a normal and physiological condition old age, at present utterly pathological, unless we first understand the most intimate details of its mechanism? . . . I think it is extremely probable that the scientific study of old age and of death, two branches of science that may be called *gerontology* and *thanalogy,* will bring about great modifications in the course of the last period of life."

The Nobel laureate was optimistic about the powers of science to transform "the morbid nature of old age," especially precocious aging and premature death (Metchnikoff, 1908, p. 285). Once researchers understood the basic mechanisms that caused degeneration in late life, argued Metchnikoff, older people could be rehabilitated so that they would become productive and integral to societal well-being. Policymakers then would have the opportunity to design measures to capitalize on the wisdom of age and would not be limited to assuaging its vicissitudes.

Gerontologists no longer subscribe to all of Metchnikoff's assumptions about the nature of old age, much less follow his recommendation that older people eat yogurt to rectify its pathological nature. Investigators doubt that old age is an "infectious disease." Anti-aging enthusiasts notwithstanding, few nowadays seek an "elixir of life" (Binstock, 2003). While modern-day gerontologists generally share Metchnikoff's hope that applying basic science will improve the lives of ordinary older people, they also recognize how the fundamental policy decisions—for instance, how the National Institute on Aging allocates research dollars—affect the scientific priorities in gerontology and geriatrics. Scientists currently play an important, but not an exclusive, role in policymaking.

At least one of Metchnikoff's ideas about how to study old age persisted for decades—i.e., most gerontologists, until recently, considered men and women over the age of 65 to be their subject matter. Even those who declaimed that 65 no longer marked *the* onset of old age typically relied on data sets that included only those 65 and over. Researchers who focus on late life typically defer to other specialists to illuminate the parameters of childhood, youth, and middle age. Recent collections on midlife development (Lachman, 2004) support an increased interest in middle age.

The extraordinary prolongation of the human life course during the twentieth century has affected images not only of older people but of all age groups. Demography demands a reconsideration of old-age policies in the context of population aging. In 1974, the National Council on Aging (NCOA) joined Lou Harris in publishing *The Myth and Reality of Aging in America*. Whereas most Americans viewed senior citizens as poor, ill, and isolated, the survey documented that men and women over 65 reported a more salutary situation—though these men and women suspected that their good fortune was exceptional. The 2002 NCOA/Harris report, *American Perceptions of Aging*, laid to rest many ageist assumptions about 65-year-olds. It complemented surveys finding that at least a significant minority of people over 85 are healthier, wealthier, and more socially connected than people in the same age group were a generation ago. Meanwhile, AARP claims in some of its publications that "60 is the new 30." The meanings and experiences ascribed to late life have undergone a dramatic change within the careers of most of today's gerontologists.

Yet it is not just the last years of life that have changed with increasing longevity. Just as "childhood" was discovered in the early modern period, and "adolescence" in the latter part of the nineteenth century, so too there have been important shifts in the earlier periods of the life course, especially during the last half century. Puberty for boys and especially for girls commences several years earlier than it used to. That 20-year-olds are increasingly inclined to return home after college prolongs youth in the other direction. Marriages (and the way laws define them) are postponed until people are in their 30s. Divorce is more likely than death to dissolve marriages in adulthood. In short, it is hard to talk any more about "stages of life." Gender, race, income, and a host of other variables affect options at every age. Chronological age per se is a poor predictor of activities at later stages of life—nor is it a reliable guide to how younger people live. The life course has become more fluid and variegated as it has become more elongated.

Because of alterations in the map of life, it is difficult to study continuities and changes in late life without paying attention to prior developments. Doctors now claim that because of Americans' penchant for fast food, the propensity for coronaries begins at age 5, not at age 50. Youth with disabilities enjoy greater educational and career opportunities thanks to policy interventions and changing public perceptions. Because women are likely on average to live longer than men, gender-specific differences at various ages have a cumulative effect on the quality of late life. Few Americans can rely on the extended family networks common in nineteenth-century rural America. Kin ties now resemble a four-generational string bean (Bengtson, Biblarz, and Roberts, 2002), with interchangeable sets of elders and siblings interacting with one another. Gerontologists concerned about designing and refining age-related policies must focus on *aging* from womb to tomb.

None of this is news, of course. Bernice Neugarten (1982) proposed decades ago that we think more in terms of needs-based than age-based policies. The paradox underlying Neugarten's recommendation—that Americans create age-graded institutions to deal with various sorts of dependency in an age-irrelevant society—remains valid. Our policy system seems to prefer the neutrality afforded by "age" as an eligibility criterion rather than to take a broader look at people's real conditions, preferences, and access to service. Our policies could induce better outcomes if age were not the primary factor animating them.

Gerontologists will have to do more contextually to help policymakers think and rethink the relative importance of age in designing social programs. Most research focuses on individuals or collections of subjects. A few scholars have developed "big" theories—the moral/political economy of aging and dependency theory of Fennell, Phillipson, and Evers (1988) and Estes (1979) to name two research teams—but these rarely delve into that "middle" ground where societal values and structural contexts are actualized in particular policies. Splendid monographs are available on individual policies such as Medicare (Marmor, 1970; Pratt, 1976), yet they focus on senior citizens, rarely citing policies that affect younger age groups. Academic specialization predisposes researchers to think about age-specific policies and structures. Unwittingly or not, such compartmentalization segments people at particular stages of life.

In speeches for nonspecialists, as well as in conceptualizing policies, gerontologists often talk about the salience of "the three boxes of life"—getting an education, going to work and earning a living, and living in retirement. The framework was fashioned by John Bolles (1978) in a best seller by that title. Noting that the first and last segments were getting longer as people extend or delay movement from one box to another, Bolles argued that "these periods have become more and more isolated from each other" (p. 6). While acknowledging that public policies could be altered to provide "systemic" routes out of these boxes, *The Three Boxes of Life* paid little attention to institutional reform. Bolles explained: "In dealing with the problem of the three boxes of life, and how to get out of them, it is not my intention to dismiss the importance of systemic change. . . . But this is intended to be a book dealing with individual approaches: a kind of *What to Do until Systemic Change Arrives*. Or a kind of *How to Bring in Systemic Change by Each of Us Taking Responsibility for What Happens in Our Own Life, Now*. This is a book of Tools for the Individual" (p. 25). Of course, Bolles had every right to focus on individual solutions and to eschew an analysis of institutions and policies. Our task here is to focus on what he ignored; we begin by calling into question Bolles's framework. One of our main points is that the three boxes of life are not isolated. Education, work, and leisure have never been compartmentalized by age.

We will illustrate this point with historical examples. We contend that educational policies, disability programs, and retirement mechanisms, which would appear to fit into Bolles's tripartite sequence, have always been transgenerational. Being able to work matters to Americans of all ages. We prepare for it in school. Most of us expect to work in some paid or volunteer capacity until we die. Although women and men in their prime are expected to be gainfully employed, mental and physical impairments often preclude their engagement in the labor force. We focus disability policy to underscore its intimate connection to the country's privileged work ethic. Similarly, leisure in late life was a luxury engaged in only by the rich until the spread of Social Security coverage. And, as we shall see, even the notion of retirement has changed as older Americans opt for part-time positions to supplement their pensions.

We do not have to reinvent the wheel to adapt existing policies and institutions to the new map of life. Incremental changes can accommodate the extension of the life course as it shapes the opportunities and desires of the "new old." At the same time, current policies can be adapted for younger Americans who can expect to live longer than their grandparents. To do so, we must think outside of the boxes.

Education

Current U.S. educational statistics clearly demonstrate that the first box of life—educational institutions—caters primarily to children and youth. The percentage of 6- to 17-year-olds enrolled in American elementary and secondary schools between 1970 and 1998 fluctuated between 97.9 and 98.5 percent. During the same period, the number of 18- to 24-year-olds enrolled in postsecondary educational institutions in this country rose from 25.7 to 36.5 percent. The greatest increase in educational enrollments has occurred at the preprimary level: in 1970, 37.5 percent of all 3- to 5-year-olds were enrolled in prekindergarten or kindergarten; the proportion had increased to 64.5 percent by 1998 (U.S. Department of Education, 2000, p. 114).

The infrastructure of today's first box of life was already taking shape by the time of the Revolution. In keeping with European traditions, families settling in the New World played a key role in teaching their children practical skills, rudimentary reading and writing, and basics of faith. The Boston Latin School (1635) was the first town-supported school in the British colonies; three years later, the Dutch Reformed Church opened the first religious-based school in New Amsterdam. Schooling beyond elementary levels became available in the eighteenth century, first in grammar schools and then in private academies. Anglican, Baptist, Congregational, Dutch Reformed, and Presbyterian churches established nine colleges between 1636 and 1769. The Philadelphia Academy (1751), later named the University of Pennsylvania, was the first nonsectarian college in the British colonies. Several other institutions (the University of Delaware; Dickinson College; St. John's College, Annapolis, Maryland; and Washington and Lee University) began as secondary schools before the Revolution; they recreated themselves as colleges considerably later. Some Quaker and Anglican missionaries taught Native Americans, African Americans, and poor whites to read and write English (Geiger, 1991, p. 321).

After the founding of the republic, the federal government and various states reinforced private educational initiatives. The Northwest Ordinance of 1787 required townships on the frontier to set aside land for schools: "Religion, morality, and knowledge being necessary to good government and the happiness of mankind, schools and the means of education shall forever be encouraged" (article 3). Most institutions provided primary education; the first high school funded with taxes was created in 1824 (Collins, 2004). As states established boards of education in the 1830s and 1840s, public officials set minimum standards for school attendance. Connecticut in 1842 permitted no child under the age of 15 to work without proof that the child had gone to school for at least three months. Massachusetts a decade later became the first state to impose compulsory education: children between the ages of 8 and 14 had to attend school for at least three months, half of this period consecutively. An 1875 case upheld the right of Kalamazoo, Michigan, to collect public funds to maintain a village high school (Grocke, 2004; Wright, 2004).

School attendance for white boys and girls rose during the period (Geiger, 1991, p. 315). Roughly one-third of those between the ages of 5 and 19 enrolled in schools in 1830; the proportion rose to half of that age group by 1850, and to 61 percent by 1870. (Public schooling existed in the South, but it was not widely available until the end of the century.) Typically one teacher taught 30–40 students in a one-room schoolhouse. As more and more children attended school, students were clustered according to subjects and levels of knowledge attainment. In due course, school boards directed elementary and secondary schools to be age-graded; middle schools were added decades later.

Architects of U.S. primary and secondary education during the nineteenth century targeted subsets of the younger population who were not afforded equal opportunities for education. Results were mixed. Based on the theories of Friedrich Froebel, who thought that children needed to play in order to learn, Margarethe Schurz established a kindergarten in Wisconsin in 1856; by 1872, the program was endorsed by the National Education Association, the country's first professional interest group for teachers. U.S. educators were less successful in convincing the 1 million Roman Catholics who came to America between 1830 and 1850 to enroll their children in public schools. The Church's decision to erect parochial schools, where the Douay Bible instead of the King James Version might be read, provoked riots and other acts of violence.

Young women took advantage of learning opportunities in the public sector. By 1870, the majority of high school graduates were female. They served as a talent pool for white-collar jobs in the new bureaucratic order. Attempts to afford ladies postsecondary educational opportunities evolved more slowly. Arguably the most important vehicles were "normal schools," established by Horace Mann in 1839 in Massachusetts, to train female teachers (Cheek, 2004). The sex ratio of instructors shifted—the percent of male teachers declined 44 percent between the 1830s and 1880s. Salaries fell commensurately. To provide instruction similar to that offered in colleges attended by men, "female seminaries" were established by Emma Willard in Troy (1821) and Catherine Beecher in Hartford (1823). Mary Lyon's seminary, which became Mount Holyoke College in 1837, served as a model for women's colleges founded after the Civil War. In 1837 Oberlin College accepted female students, becoming the country's first private coeducational college; the University of Michigan allowed women to attend classes and gave them "special degrees" (Woloch, 1991, p. 326).

The Freedmen's Bureau, established at the end of the Civil War, was the nineteenth century's most ambitious effort to extend literacy to African Americans. By 1869 it had established nearly 3,000 schools; it contributed to the growth of institutions such as Howard University, Tuskegee Institute, and Spelman College. In 1870, however, the Bureau curtailed its educational programs. Over the next quarter century, Jim Crow laws doomed blacks to inferior facilities and second-rate instruction. A racial bias pervaded pre-elementary to postsecondary education with few exceptions: some public and private colleges matriculated members of "The Talented Tenth." And the dispute between Booker T. Washington, who stressed practical learning in racially separate facilities, and W. E. B. Du Bois, who equated integrated schools with equality, underscored a basic dilemma in the American system: could the country accommodate diversity while assuring minimal standards of competency required in the workplace?

This dilemma was also manifest during the second wave of immigration to the United States. Those who feared the foreigners would pollute the nation's racial stock wanted schools to "Americanize" students, inculcating the "proper" set of skills, hygiene, and values. States mandated more stringent compulsory attendance and child labor laws, but regulations often were defied by families who needed their children's earnings. Resistance came as well from the Roman Catholic Church, which was denied public funds because of its insistence on running parochial schools as it saw fit, independent of the public school system.

At least two innovations sought to broaden education's reach in the last quarter of the nineteenth century. First, Calvin Woodward opened the Manual Training School for boys in St. Louis in 1879 to teach the value of manual labor. Because vocational education was not viewed as a replacement for traditional learning, it was incorporated by 1900 as a track in 100 municipal high schools (Westerink, 2004). Second, Jane Addams's Hull House (1889) became a proto-type for more than 100 settlement houses designed to teach mothers domestic skills and to provide their children with vocational and citizenship skills.

While the U.S. educational infrastructure was being adapted to address gaps based on gender, race, ethnicity, and class, native-born reformers were con-structing new theories about childhood and youth. John Dewey, for instance, stressed the importance of communicational skills. He viewed education as a societal process that began in childhood and continued through maturity. G. Stanley Hall's *Adolescence* (1903) defined a new stage of the human life course, which affected how youth were trained. High school enrollments grew 650 percent between 1900 and 1930. Within the walls of high schools, adolescents created a milieu based on "peer relations." In contrast, the Commission on the Reorganization of Secondary Education (1918) stressed the importance of teaching basic, health, vocation, civic education, and leisure in high schools (Scherer, 2004; Fass, 1977, p. 124). Into this mix was added Lewis Terman's Stanford-Benet Intelligence Test (1916) as well as Edward Thorndike's princi-ples of "scientific education," which set into practice a series of psychological tests to be used in classrooms.

Meanwhile, religious denominations continued to found colleges; most were small and financially poor. By 1860, there were 217 colleges, mainly in the Midwest, designed to lure prospective settlers to their meccas of culture. After the Civil War, several factors transformed higher education. First, the Morrill Act (1862) gave land to states to sell, so that they could create endowments for public institutions primarily offering instruction in "applied" studies. Second, following the lead of Harvard and Johns Hopkins, elite institutes and new uni-versities joined other places of higher learning in recruiting faculty to do "sci-entific" research. Classical education became discipline-specific as specializa-tion supplanted general studies. Medical, law, and other professional schools were founded. Third, college enrollments increased tenfold between 1890 and 1940. The GI Bill (1944) made college education accessible to veterans eager to climb the employment ladder. Finally, large-scale federal funding during the cold war reconfigured higher-education budgets. Various agencies underwrote large research projects. As the baby boom generation came of age, student enrollments doubled in the 1960s, largely in state universities and community colleges (Geiger, 1991, p. 323; Lightcap, 2004; Baylis-Heerschop, 2004).

The federal government intervened in primary and secondary education in other ways. African Americans worked through the courts to integrate universities and professional schools; *Brown v. Board of Education* (1954), which challenged segregation in primary schools, was a major victory in the civil rights movement (Collins, 2004). Gerald Ford lobbied for Public Law 94-142, which provided that disabled persons between the ages of 3 and 21 be educated in the "least-restrictive environment" and provided special education programs. Every president since Ronald Reagan has created blue-ribbon panels to upgrade the quality of primary and secondary education, by emphasizing basic skills and by setting guidelines to prepare students for careers in a global economy (Scherer, 2004).

A mixture of public and private interventions at the federal, state, and local levels constitutes today's tripartite division of education centers—primary and secondary schools and institutions of higher learning. Current networks are far more bureaucratic and complex than those that existed two centuries ago. Educators wrestle with competing priorities, special interests, and ill-defined outcomes. The quality of education afforded in suburban school districts, for example, surpasses that offered in the inner cities and remote areas. Why? Just as the Founding Generation was willing to support education—but not too generously—America's present educational network lacks the funds necessary to provide students from age 3 to age 24 equal access to learning experiences preparing them for work, citizenship, and lifelong learning.

The U.S. educational infrastructure has been designed first and foremost to serve children and youth, but it has not ignored the needs of older Americans. Indeed, the origins of continuing and adult education also date back to the pre-Revolutionary era. Over time, a variety of private and public agencies at the federal, state, and local levels have offered vocational and cultural programs aimed at mature students.

Benjamin Franklin was the father of adult education for the masses and the elite. In 1727, he established the Junto, which provided working men in Philadelphia a course of study in politics, philosophy, and other topics of useful knowledge to broaden their intellectual horizons. Four years later, he helped to charter the first public library in the British colonies, to which adults could subscribe on a system of fees and fines. Franklin was one of the founders of the

American Philosophical Society (1743), which remains a magnet for scholars and scientists aspiring to "multiply the conveniences and pleasures of life" (Martin et al., 2001, p. 86). *Poor Richard's Almanac,* which was published from 1733 to 1758, entertained ordinary people with its aphorisms and practical information.

Adults in every period organized their own intellectual activities. Two nineteenth-century ventures stand out. Josiah Holbrook created the Lyceum movement, which invited speakers such as Ralph Waldo Emerson to travel the country to enlighten residents of small towns and to sponsor debates on religion, politics, and other current events. Before it dissolved in the late 1830s, there were more than 3,000 Lyceum centers in the country (Bode, 1968). In 1874, an industrialist and a Methodist minister launched the Chautauqua movement in upstate New York, a summer camp for Sunday School teachers. Chautauqua was a magnet for students of all ages and educational levels. Over time it provided a platform for U.S. presidents and other luminaries to address the issues of the day. Within the decade, Chautauqua began to send out speakers and programs to nearly 10,000 communities. The Depression and the invention of the radio ended the circuit in the 1930s, but the original site remains a popular destination for those who seek intellectual stimulation and exposure to the arts on their vacations (Simpson, 1999).

The federal government became involved in adult education during the twentieth century. Starting with the Smith Act (1914), Washington provided funds for training in agriculture, home economics, and other practical vocations. New Dealers enacted the Works Projects Administration in part to train adults for reemployment. This strategy was reincarnated during the Great Society in various manpower acts to make unemployed adults more marketable in the labor force (Scott, 2004). The Economic Employment Act (1964) earmarked dollars for adult basic education, for those who were illiterate or who had not completed high school. Within a year, nearly 38,000 Americans enrolled in the program. The Adult Education Act (1998) has been amended more than a dozen times since its inception to focus on the special needs of Native Americans, prisoners, elderly people, and refugees from south of the Equator; to provide courses in bilingual education and workforce literacy; and to assist states and private agencies in developing community programs. An illustration from the present is that Area Agencies on Aging often teach the basics of computer literacy in senior citizen centers.

In recent decades, the private sector has filled important gaps in lifelong learning. Founded in 1975, Elderhostel is a nonprofit institution that now offers roughly 200,000 men and women over age 55 10,000 programs in 90 countries. Elderhostel attracts people who wish to share adventures and ideas with their peers and faculty (Elderhostel, 2004).

Institutions of higher education provide opportunities for enrichment and practical skills for older learners. People over 30 constitute a significant proportion of those who enroll in community college courses. Educators rely on new technologies to deliver their subject matter. Distance education courses taught by faculty in many private colleges and public universities are available on television or video; senior citizens usually are given discounts or pay no tuition. In 1976, the University of Phoenix became the first accredited institution of higher learning to offer degree programs over the Internet. With more than 17,000 instructors and 128 campuses worldwide, the university has granted degrees to more than 171,000 working people, and it cooperates with business and industry to develop curricula (University of Phoenix, 2004).

Corporate America operates its own training programs to upgrade the skills of employees. Following the lead of General Motors and McDonald's, companies have established more than 2,200 in-house "universities," through which they reach more older adults than do institutions of higher education. Employers spent $57 billion on their "learning-by-doing" training in 2003. (They took as their model the case-based curricula used by medical, law, and business schools for more than a century.) Amid projections that there will be fewer qualified younger people entering the workforce in coming decades, business is putting an unprecedented "premium on human capital" that exists among its midcareer and mature workers (Tech, 2002).

In sum, the first box of life caters primarily to children and youth, but since colonial times there has also been a genuine effort to attend to the educational desires and needs of men and women beyond the first quarter of life. Population aging and the constant need to facilitate workers' efforts to keep abreast of organizational and technological changes in the marketplace will put added pressure on public and private agencies to develop continuing education programs and to allocate resources to benefit older workers. The importance of education does not end when the young exit the first box of life. It persists over the life course.

Disability

Because we broadly view "work" (that is, paid or volunteer productive activities) as a transgenerational activity, we have opted to discuss disability programs for two reasons. First, most people who are disabled are middle-aged. Second, disability programs were designed specifically for people who are willing but unable to work.

Disability policy in the United States is a complicated maze of state and federal, public and private programs. These programs were born in different historical eras, often use different definitions of disability, and sometimes work at cross-purposes with one another. At first glance, disability policies serve only the needs of middle-aged workers forced out of employment by accident or disease. In actuality, disability policies are closely intertwined programs for retired workers and the indigent, as well as children and nonworking spouses.

Disability policies fall into two basic categories: income maintenance and rehabilitation services. The vast majority of funds go to cash payments for income maintenance and health benefits. Federal payments to disabled people come from two basic programs: Social Security Disability Insurance (SSDI) and Supplemental Security Income (SSI). Federal disability insurance (SSDI) is one of three basic insurance protections—along with Old Age Insurance and Survivors Insurance—provided by the Social Security Administration. People who are unable to work or who are impoverished because of disability may also qualify for welfare benefits under the Supplemental Security Income program (SSI).

In 2001, approximately 6.8 million people received public insurance disability benefits under SSDI, at a cost of $52.8 billion (AARP, 2003). Of these recipients, 76 percent were disabled workers and 24 percent were family members of disabled workers. In January 2004, approximately 7 million people received welfare benefits under SSI; blind and disabled people made up 82 percent of these recipients. Among all recipients of SSI, 14 percent were under 18, 57 percent were 18–64, and 29 percent were 65+ (Social Security Administration, 2004b). The poverty rate for families with a disabled worker is more than double that for families without a disabled worker: 18.5 percent compared with 9 percent. Without Social Security benefits, the poverty rate for families with a disabled worker would increase from 18.5 percent to 55 percent (AARP, 2003).

Modern disability policies and programs arose in three historical eras: state industrial accident laws passed early in the twentieth century; Social Security programs developed during the New Deal; and the extension of disability policies during the civil rights advocacy of the 1970s. Because of this complex historical accretion, terms such as *functional limitation, impairment,* and *handicapped* have no uniform usage. Even the term *disability* can mean different things in different contexts. As Edward Berkowitz put it, "In the workers' compensation program and the courts, disability means the damages that one person collects from another as a result of an insult or injury. In the Social Security Disability Insurance program, disability refers to a condition that links ill health and unemployment. And in the context of civil rights laws, disability connotes ' handicap'" (Berkowitz, 1987, p. 5).

Before the twentieth century, public policymakers did not single out individuals disabled by birth, accident, or disease. Rather, the disabled were lumped together with other dependents. Throughout the colonial period and into the first third of the nineteenth century, welfare functions were largely carried out under the aegis of local towns and parishes, working essentially in the tradition of Elizabethan poor laws. Beginning in the 1820s and 1830s, states established a system of almshouses or asylums, inspired initially by a vision of returning individuals to work. By the second half of the nineteenth century, almshouses had essentially become custodial institutions, though specialized asylums were created for groups like elderly or insane people (Rothman, 1971, 1980).

The first modern disability programs emerged in the Progressive Era, when states responded to the plight of workers injured in industrial accidents. In 1911, Wisconsin and New Jersey passed the first workers' compensation laws, which tried to avoid litigation by transferring control over payments, health care, and other services to state governments. By 1948, all states had workers' compensation laws designed to end struggles between employer and employee by equating a specific injury with a specific compensation (Berkowitz 1987, chapter 1).

Workers' compensation laws originally exempted several categories of employment (agricultural, domestic, railroad, nonhazardous). Coverage was gradually expanded until by 1995, 92 percent of the nation's wages and salary payments were covered. Likewise, coverage for occupational diseases was gradually adopted; by the 1980s all states had some form of coverage. Throughout the 1950s and 1960s, underfunding, inadequate administration, and gross state disparities led to many calls for the federalization of workers' compensation, which was a distinct possibility when Congress passed the Occupational Safety and Health Act (OSHA) in 1970. OSHA appointed a national commission to study state workers' compensation laws. The commission left the state system in place but provided specific recommendations and incentives for states to set higher benefit levels (Berkowitz, 1987, pp. 38–39). Hence, a series of amendments to state laws sharply increased the maximum weekly benefit payments during the 1970s.

By 1995, disability payments amounted to almost 80 percent—and health care benefits amounted to more than 50 percent—of wages and salaries covered under workers' compensation. Although states establish basic rules, individual companies have the freedom to choose private insurance carriers, government-sponsored insurance funds, or self-insurance to cover their compensation responsibilities (Fishback, 2001). Today, workers' compensation programs provide more adequate benefits but remain plagued by problems of their original structure. Litigation remains an unresolved problem, and the program still sees benefits as a reflection of damages. As a result, many states provide benefits based on impairment rather than lost wages or reduced ability to work. The program still does not take adequate account of medical improvements or provide incentives for rehabilitation (Berkowitz, 1987, p. 40).

Planners in the Social Security Administration began conceptualizing disability insurance in 1936, amid strong skepticism and opposition. In order to mitigate opposition and distinguish clearly between unemployment and disability, they wrote a stringent definition of disability as "an impairment of mind or body which continuously renders it impossible for the disabled person to follow any substantial gainful occupation" and was likely to last "for the rest of a person's life" (Berkowitz, 2000).

Congress did not look seriously at Social Security Disability Insurance until 1949, when the United States had clearly emerged from depression and war (which had given birth to rehabilitation medicine). Until 1950, aid to the blind and to disabled children, part of the original Social Security Act, were the only programs that reached people with disabilities. Congress in that year added Aid to the Permanently and Totally Disabled as a public assistance measure. Opponents of SSDI argued that Congress should provide recipients with rehabilitation services, rather than cash benefits that allowed them to retire from the labor force for life.

The Eisenhower administration's approach to disability was articulated by Roswell Perkins, who argued that "the first line of attack on disability should be rehabilitation, in order that people be restored to useful and productive lives" (Berkowitz, 2000). Compromise measures in 1952 and 1954 smoothed the way for final passage of SSDI in 1956. The 1956 bill was itself a compromise between the House disability insurance measure and the opposition of the Senate Finance Committee, along with the American Medical Association and the insurance industry. In order to gain enough votes to ensure passage, proponents of the legislation limited benefits to those over age 50, excluded benefits for dependents of disabled workers, and allowed states to make eligibility determinations.

This compromise meant that in its formative years, SSDI was essentially a retirement program. Because older workers were considered the worst candidates for rehabilitation, the program never developed a strong connection with vocational rehabilitation. And caseloads were disproportionately filled with illnesses affecting older workers (e.g., heart disease and arthritis) rather than impairments more common among younger workers, especially mental illness.

The stringent definition needed to guarantee passage of SSDI generated paradoxical and volatile effects. Pressure from the courts and Congress led to rapidly expanding rolls in the 1970s. Attempts to stop this growth followed in the 1980s, and those efforts again generated pressure that led to a rise in the rolls in the later 1980s and early 1990s.

Supplemental Security Income—the other pillar of the U.S. disability system—emerged unexpectedly from the welfare reform initiated by President Nixon in 1969. When Nixon's plan to transform child welfare failed to pass Congress, policymakers turned to adult welfare categories. The administration decided to federalize Aid to the Blind, Aid to the Permanently and Totally Disabled, and Old-Age Assistance and to continue to administer these newly combined programs through the Social Security Administration.

The Social Security Amendments of 1972 created the Supplemental Security Income (SSI) program, which relieved families from the financial responsibility of caring for their adult disabled children and also consolidated existing federal programs for disabled people who were ineligible for SSDI. Welfare beneficiaries were assigned to the same administrative apparatus that handled SSDI benefits. States made the initial eligibility determination, and both programs used a common definition of disability.

Social Security officials projected that the new program would serve primarily those elderly people who were already receiving Social Security benefits but had still not emerged from poverty. When SSI benefits started flowing in 1975, blind and disabled adults and children represented 42 percent of the caseload. But when Congress established SSI, it also increased Social Security benefits by 20 percent and indexed them to inflation. As a result, fewer older people needed SSI; by 1994, blind or disabled adults and children made up two-thirds of the caseload (Berkowitz, 2000).

In contemporary America, there is a one in seven chance that a worker will become disabled for five years or more. Although SSDI is the primary source of disability insurance, approximately 25 percent of nongovernmental workers have long-term disability (LTD) insurance through their employers, while an unknown number of others buy coverage in the private market (Brackey, 2002). About half of all private pension plans contain a disability clause, allowing qualification for a disability retirement, usually based on the employee's age and years of service. Most LTD policies require the disabled worker to apply for Social Security as a condition of receiving benefits. If the worker qualifies for Social Security, private benefits are "integrated"—the amount due from the LTD policy is reduced by the payment from Social Security.

The first policy to pay for lost wages due to illness was written in 1850 by the Franklin Health Assurance Company of Massachusetts. By 1864, 47 other insurance companies wrote policies for virtually any type of loss. Despite availability, a 2001 survey by the Consumer Federation of America and the American Council of Life Issues found that 82 percent of workers had no LTD coverage or had inadequate coverage. In 1996, the National Academy of Social Insurance estimated the cost of the average policy at $1,271 per year—simply beyond the means of most workers (Mashaw and Reno, 1996).

Along with income-maintenance programs, vocational rehabilitation, employment of disabled persons, and independent living have played a role—though less prominent—in U.S. disability policies. State vocational rehabilitation programs originated in 1920. Initially, vocational rehabilitation offices anticipated that their caseload would come from state workers' compensation programs, because both equated disability with the inability to work in one's accustomed occupation. But a smooth working relationship between compensation and rehabilitation never took hold.

Workers' compensation programs became attached to state "labor" bureaucracies, concerned with wages, hours, and safe working conditions. Vocational rehabilitation, in contrast, was framed as a training operation. It was therefore linked to the state chief education officer, whose primary concerns were public schools and vocational training (Berkowitz, 1987, pp. 155–56). Vocational rehabilitation has also been fragmented by the separate rehabilitation programs maintained for the blind and for veterans.

Despite the appeal of rehabilitation as a source of hope for independence rather than a form of welfare dependency, the program was never effectively linked to workers' compensation or Social Security Disability Insurance. Throughout the 1960s, federal funding increased substantially, and what began as an effort to rehabilitate workers' compensation clients developed into a major social program (Berkowitz, 1987, p. 174). Funding declined in the 1970s, after a congressional mandate required vocational rehabilitation programs to serve the severely disabled, which raised costs per person and reduced effectiveness.

The vocational rehabilitation bill passed in 1973 transformed disabled clients into consumers, and professional rehabilitation counselors regretted their inability to practice a clinical model of rehabilitation. Tensions arose between a newly active disabled community (which believed it possessed inherent rights) and professional counselors (who valued their professional autonomy).

Disability policies in the 1970s were also shaped by the emergence of the independent living movement, led by disabled individuals aiming to become integrated into the social and economic mainstream. By 1978, the Carter administration supported legislation that provided grants to state vocational rehabilitation agencies to fund comprehensive independent living services. States received funds to establish and operate independent living centers.

The 1973 rehabilitation act contained a provision that states: "No otherwise qualified handicapped individual in the United States shall, solely by reason of his handicap, be excluded from participation in, be denied the benefits of, or be subjected to discrimination under any program or activity conducted by an Executive agency or by the United States Postal Service" (Berkowitz, 1987, p. 212). This provision, known as Section 504, became the basis of lawsuits against institutions inaccessible to disabled people. In 1977, Health, Education and Welfare secretary Joseph A. Califano Jr. signed regulations (applying to all hospitals, schools, local governments, or other institutions receiving HEW funds) requiring that all new buildings be barrier-free, all activities be made accessible to people with disabilities, all disabled children receive a free public education, and all colleges and universities make modifications allowing disabled persons to participate.

Independent living centers and Section 504 were fundamental additions to U.S. disability policies, aiming at mainstream participation rather than retirement and at independence rather than professional control. These advances by a newly energized minority group have been primarily useful to the young and to those with impaired mobility. They are welcome as an alternative to dependency but can become burdensome pressures on older or demoralized workers who wish to retire.

Despite numerous attempts to reduce the number of people who receive SSDI, disability benefits were paid to more than 6.8 million people in 2003, with benefits totaling about $66 billion (Social Security Administration, 2004a). Thus, even though amendments were made to the program—making it more difficult for alien residents to qualify for SSDI and eliminating drug and alcohol addiction from the medical listing—these changes had little or no effect on the overall utilization rates. What has changed significantly is the percentage of overall income that beneficiaries receive from SSDI payments. In 1984, SSDI accounted for an average of 71.4 percent of a beneficiary's income. By 1999 that proportion decreased to 57.5 percent (Martin and Davies, 2003–4). Likewise, the total number of applications for SSDI has continued to grow, especially from 1990 through 1994. There was a slight dip in applicants from 1996 to 1997, but since then the total has continued to climb. Similarly, the ratio of awards to applications has continued to hover around 41 percent, fluctuating up and down year after year (Kennedy, 1999). Thus, one could conclude that despite attempts to decrease use, the SSDI program continues to grow. The significant change, if any, is that beneficiaries as a group are less dependent on SSDI and have other sources of income.

Social Security

The continual effort to move people off public disability rolls underscores the transgenerational nature of work. Americans don't like "deadbeats." And if they feel that people are malingering or trying to beat the system, policymakers will tighten eligibility criteria and limit benefits to those truly in need. Bolles describes "leisure" as the main focus of the third box of life. In contemporary America, this means that people have reached an age at which they can retire. Because the foundation of their retirement income is Social Security, we focus here on that policy.

According to the 2003 Old Age, Survivors, and Disability Insurance (OASDI) Trustees Report, one out of every six Americans receives Social Security. Nearly one-quarter of all U.S. households collect benefits. Most of the recipients are older people. Of the 46.4 million Social Security beneficiaries, 29.2 million (constituting 63% of the total) are retired workers. Another 10 percent are the

4.6 million widows, widowers, or parents over the age of 62 who are receiving survivors' benefits. Social Security, moreover, has been remarkably successful in reducing late-life poverty. Except for the richest quintile of older Americans, Social Security is the largest single source of income for senior citizens. It provides more than half the income received by two-thirds of program beneficiaries; the incomes of most older women would fall below the official poverty line, were OASDI benefits reduced drastically or curtailed (Hill and Reno, 2003). Such data reinforce the notion that retirement under Social Security—the third box of life—primarily serves the nation's elderly population.

It was not inevitable that Social Security should have become America's chief weapon against old-age dependency. Reform-minded citizens rarely intervened throughout U.S. history to assure the well-being of aged people. It was not a major concern, because few Americans survived to old age. Furthermore, a piecemeal approach to dealing with the elderly population's individual and collective needs seemed to suffice. Creating institutional networks to promote the health, education, and welfare of children and youth was a far greater priority since colonial times.

To avoid the poorhouse, aged people worked as long as possible and relied on family and friends to help them make ends meet. Local communities sometimes provided "worthy" elders with food and shelter. Around 1900, private old-age homes and charitable relief programs supported about 5 percent of individuals over 65. Retirement pensions were available to some municipal workers, teachers, military personnel, and federal civil servants; about 15 percent of the U.S. labor force were eligible for private-sector pensions in 1930 (Achenbaum, 1986, pp. 14–15). Military pensions were the predominant source of support in late life: 82 percent of all recipients of public or private pensions were aging veterans or survivors of various wars; 80 percent of all traceable funds transferred to senior citizens came from this source alone (Achenbaum, 1978, p. 124; Skocpol, 1992). Despite their generosity to old soldiers, their widows, and orphans, few public officials or private citizens drew an analogy between military veterans and veterans of industrialization. On the eve of the Great Depression, old-age dependency was perceived as a growing "problem" but not yet deemed a major concern.

The financial crash ripped older people's safety net. The elderly population had higher unemployment rates than any other age cohort, lost their savings, and did not receive pensions (which corporate America viewed as "gratuities" to be awarded in good times). Increasing numbers depended on their families, themselves often in dire straits. Followers of Dr. Francis Townsend's Revolving Old Age Pension plan, among others, demanded immediate relief for the old. But Franklin Delano Roosevelt, who had signed key welfare legislation as governor of New York, concentrated on reconstructing various sectors of the economy, reforming the commercial arena, and relieving the needs of rural Americans and segments of the middle class before he turned his attention to the plight of senior citizens.

In June 1934, President Roosevelt declared to Congress that he was in favor of legislation to provide "security against several of the great disturbing factors in life—especially those which relate to unemployment and old age" (Breaking soil, 1934). His chief advisers on the Committee of Economic Security expected FDR to make unemployment compensation the centerpiece. Indeed, in November 1934, the president told a National Conference on Social Security that he was unsure whether the time was ripe for any federal legislation on old-age security. The public's outcry was negative, the media's reaction swift. FDR got the message: when he submitted his legislative proposals to Congress two months later, a solution for reducing old-age dependency was given top billing.

The 1935 Social Security Act mounted a two-pronged attack on late-life poverty. Title I offered assistance, financed with federal and state funds, to anyone over 65 who met residency requirements and needs tests. To reduce the cost of such support in the future, Title II created an old-age insurance program, whereby employers and their employees contributed 1 percent of a worker's wage (up to $3,000). Contributors could draw a retirement pension at age 65, beginning in 1942. Originally, 9.4 million workers were excluded from the program, because FDR was more concerned about establishing a precedent: "We put those payroll contributions there so as to give the contributors a legal, moral, and political right to collect their pensions and unemployment benefits. With those taxes in there, no damn politician can ever scrap my social security program" (Schlesinger, 1958, pp. 308–9).

The 1935 measure addressed other needs of other age groups. Congress enacted an unemployment compensation program through a federal-state partnership. Nearly $25 million initially was allocated to provide "aid to dependent children," and another $3 million was earmarked for the blind. Under Title V, "Grants to States for Maternal and Child Welfare," Congress appropriated funds for crippled children, rural public health services, and vocational rehabilitation; in addition, the Public Health Services received funds for training personnel and investigating disease. Social Security, in short, was an omnibus piece of legislation with provisions intended to relieve the burden on middle-aged taxpayers.

Signing Social Security into law on August 14, 1935, the president opined that "we can never insure one hundred percent of the population against one hundred percent of the hazards and vicissitudes of life" (Rosenman, 1969, p. 324). Nonetheless, over the next fifty years, lawmakers filled gaps. Older Americans were the prime beneficiaries. In 1939, even before the first Social Security check was issued, Congress radically amended Title II: checks became payable in 1940; the benefit formula was changed to reflect average rather than total earnings; older people who earned up to $14.99 per month could still collect retirement pensions. Most important of all was the provision to establish monthly payments for survivors of both active and retired employees and dependents of retired workers (Achenbaum, 1986, p. 32). "We shall make the most orderly progress," FDR declared at a Teamsters convention in 1940, "if we look upon social security as a development toward a goal rather than a finished product" (Rosenman, 1969, p. 79).

As envisioned, Social Security became the foundation for old-age security. During the 1950s and 1960s, compulsory coverage was extended to agricultural and domestic workers, military personnel, and the self-employed. Local, state, and federal government employees could elect to contribute to Title II. As the program expanded and matured, the system approached universal coverage. Congress enacted early retirement benefits (with actuarial reduction) for women in 1956 and for men in 1961, giving older workers more options in planning for retirement. A permanent disability insurance plan (1956) for all Americans over 50 was justified as an early-retirement measure; as soon as beneficiaries became entitled to Title II benefits, they were removed from the disability rolls (Berkowitz and McQuaid, 1988, p. 187). In the heyday of the Great Society, Lyndon Baines Johnson shepherded Medicare and Medicaid into law. Only Social Security beneficiaries over 65 were eligible for Medicare hospital benefits. Although Medicaid was to assist poor people of all ages, its architects anticipated that it largely would be used to cover nursing home costs for aged dependents.

Old-age insurance programs dwarfed all other Social Security provisions. In 1965, for instance, welfare provisions to children, the blind, and others who met means-tested criteria amounted to $3 billion in federal outlays; the social insurance programs cost $16.6 billion (Berkowitz and McQuaid, 1988, p. 194). In 1972, Richard Nixon approved a 20 percent increase in Social Security benefits and allowed automatic Cost of Living Adjustments (COLAs) to future benefits. And, as noted earlier, Congress combined certain assistance measures into the Supplemental Security Income program. Little effort was made to reconcile the overlap between the minimum benefits afforded by welfare and insurance programs (Achenbaum, 1986, pp. 72–73). Eyes remained fixed on increasing Title II benefits.

Interest in old-age economic security concurrently spurred initiatives in the private sector. More individuals bought policies from insurance companies and, as wages increased, set aside retirement savings. A 1948 National Labor Relations Board ruling and other court decisions made pension plans subject to collective bargaining. The United Auto Workers and United Steel Workers were the pacesetters. By 1970, more than one-third of the civilian workforce was covered by business and industrial pension plans; funds invested to pay for workers' retirement benefits constituted one of the chief sources of financial power in the nation (Drucker, 1976).

Ironically, Social Security became a victim of its own success. Thanks to incremental changes in benefit coverage and entitlements, the incidence of poverty among older Americans fell precipitously. By 1984, there were more children living in poverty than senior citizens. Neoconservatives decried the generational inequities that they said were built into the system. Older people, once depicted as deserving sympathy and support, were featured in periodicals as "Greedy Geezers," squandering public funds in a self-indulgent manner that would leave their children and grandchildren with a bankrupt Social Security system and few private resources for their own old age.

From the mid-1970s to the present, the biggest challenge facing Social Security has been its solvency. During the 1970s—after benefits had been indexed to inflation—the growth of inflation and the decline in real wages strained the system's ability to pay benefits beyond 1982. A bipartisan compromise was reached that aimed to keep Social Security solvent through the baby boomers' retirement (Schieber and Shoven, 1999). The 1983 amendments increased the age for receiving benefits from 65 to 67 by 2007 and made Social Security benefits taxable. In 1986, Social Security was extended to all new federal employees. Thus, the system saw an increase in revenues through taxation and additional participants and will experience a slowing down of liabilities when the age to receive benefits increases to 67. These changes notwithstanding, the system is still under financial constraints, and proposals for privatization are circulating (see Chapter 15 in this volume). Because of the program's popularity, however, we foresee no major modification of either eligibility requirements or benefit levels and only incremental changes to the system during the retirement of the baby boomers.

There is a heated debate over privatization, fueled by fears that there will be more older Americans making claims on fewer resources. But no one challenges the importance of Social Security in providing a floor for the truly vulnerable. Nor do Americans question the right of the middle class to get back what they contributed. Social Security remains the cornerstone of the American welfare state.

Conclusion

Even this cursory overview of the history of education, disability policies, and retirement programs should suffice to demonstrate that "the three boxes of life" have never exclusively circumscribed specific age groups. Since colonial times, preparing young people to be good citizen workers has been a major educational priority; concurrently, public and private institutions were established to enrich the cultural lives of adults, even those in their later years. Many middle-aged workers had accidents in rural settings toward the end of the nineteenth century. In addition, industrial accidents threatened men's ability to remain productive. But special institutions were also created during the period for the blind, for the deaf, and for crippled children (Rothman, 1971); similarly, a bit later, policies were established for those who had chronic ailments in the second half of life. Finally, although older persons come to mind when we talk about the benefits and funding crises associated with Social Security, the original legislation targeted the blind and rural citizens; since 1939, children and middle-aged widows have benefited from survivors' benefits. Just as gerontologists have grown skeptical about stage theories based on chronological segmentations of the life course, so too they should acknowledge that even public policies that seem quite age-specific actually affect segments of the population of all ages.

That this is the case is no historical accident: policymakers have tinkered with educational, health care, social service, and poverty programs in an incremental manner throughout our nation's history. Some programs come and go, but the three we have examined in this chapter have endured long enough to develop in distinctive ways. Institutions age, though not in ways analogous to human aging. Except for those with sunset provisions, the institutions rarely are ascribed a life expectancy at the moment of their creation. When programs falter or decline, it is usually because they fail to serve their constituencies or are underfunded. People who advocate on behalf of educational initiatives, interventions for disability, and welfare provisions seek innovative ways to expand the purview of their specific programs.

It is essential that demographers pay attention to population aging. Social scientists must continue to take the pulse of social, political, economic, and cultural trends as they affect elderly people in the world's oldest republic. But the time has come for researchers of aging to keep track of structural trends and lags (Riley, Kahn, and Foner, 1994) in the "middle range": we must take account of how the aging of institutions affects people over the life course. In short, we must envision the big picture by disentangling and reintegrating continuities and changes in individual and population aging, as well as in institutional and societal developments.

From these observations, we draw at least two conclusions. First, we are more convinced than ever about the wisdom of Neugarten's preference for age-irrelevant policies: we should think less in terms of how specific age groups should be entitled to certain benefits. Instead, we should pay greater attention to the specific needs of men and women who lack access to existing programs that might improve their lives, thereby enhancing their capacity to contribute to a productive society. Second, neither human longevity nor the graying of the United States demands radical policy changes, as has been documented for decades (Hudson, 1978). Instead, we call for modifications that would increase institutional flexibility across the public and private sectors, to better serve all age groups.

Insofar as lifelong learning requires a lifelong investment, education should be accessible and affordable to the entire population. Needs and levels of training vary by age, though they tend to be cumulative in nature. Younger people (from first grade through graduate school) must be taught to write. Human resource managers invariably complain that their new hires cannot spell or construct a meaningful two-page memo.

Great strides have been made in developing continuing education programs and in affording opportunities for distance learning. More can be done in linking courses to activities in the voluntary sector. Teaching public speaking and learning foreign languages, for instance, merit higher priority. These are skills most workers did not need earlier in this nation's history. Now, in a global economy and an increasingly multicultural society, whites, blacks, browns, yellows, and other segments of the population find it necessary to communicate with people unlike themselves if they are to participate in community affairs.

Most institutions of higher education increasingly resemble corporations in their strategic planning (Kirp, 2003), yet few colleges and universities have entered into meaningful partnerships with businesses in their vicinity to train middle-aged workers. Both sides could gain from such cooperation: corporations would benefit from the pedagogical expertise of faculty members who have discovered how to inspire teachable moments among adult learners; academic deans facing budget cuts could benefit from the revenues generated from firms.

The changing faces of retirement, in turn, demand a fundamental reexamination of what opportunities should be offered to workers in their late forties and fifties. Most employees know they must set aside funds for "rainy days," but few are willing to take the risk of "repotting." Most workers would rather watch the clock and perform the predictable, routine tasks of a boring job. Starting over is too daunting a prospect for many mature workers. It entails risks. Yet, given anticipated shortages of younger workers as baby boomers approach their seventh decade, it makes sense to energize employees who may be burning out or who have disabilities that preclude their continuance at their current jobs.

The educational needs of elderly workers offer a variation on this theme. Given the likelihood that there will be greater part-time, flexible opportunities for those who are "unretired," it makes sense to offer senior citizens practical courses so that they too may retool and acquire greater technological competency. Corporations and institutions of higher learning might also seize on the wisdom of age by offering select employees an opportunity to mentor younger workers.

The histories of both SSDI and SSI reveal that disability programs initially designed for elderly people or those soon to retire quickly came to serve the needs of children and young adults. Chronic illnesses and disabling birth defects stalk humans at all ages, yet one of the enduring flaws in state and federal disability policies has been their poor coordination of income maintenance and rehabilitation.

Thanks to advances in medical technology and the reduced marginalization of people with disabilities, it makes increasing sense to invest in rehabilitation programs. A nation concerned about capitalizing on its human resources should be ready to adopt policies that make it possible for men and women to return to the workplace if they do not need to rely entirely on cash benefits to compensate for their maladies. Many disabled people cannot travel to a work-place. For them, there should be greater use of technologies that link the home-bound to their place of employment. Finally, policymakers should confront the stigma of mental illness, which demoralizes the person with mental illness who might otherwise seek productive employment. Mental illness strikes all age groups, not only frail elderly people. Accordingly, more funds should be allo-cated to provide treatment and rehabilitation opportunities so that mentally ill people, like physically disabled people, might share their talents in a dynamic economy.

While Social Security remains the cornerstone of retirement planning, it is important to remember that FDR's advisers envisioned private savings and cor-porate pensions as part of the package. We recommend that younger people spend less time worrying about the system's long-term solvency and devote more energy to investing beyond options afforded by IRAs and bonuses. In our opinion, continuing education is one of the best investments younger workers can make. Not only do they realize greater incomes than those with less educa-tion, but also they prepare themselves for job transitions in the middle and lat-ter phases of their careers, which might prove more lucrative than staying put. We acknowledge that few workers relish the prospect of a three-hour account-ing class after putting in a ten-hour day. But if there were incentives, from the employer as well as from the policy world, then such a commitment might be more attractive. For instance, Social Security contributors might borrow against part of their retirement accounts to pay for their training and education.

Incentives are needed in other areas. It is time to revisit the proposal that So-cial Security credits be given to those who care for the needy at both ends of the life course and the disabled in between. To the extent that we wish to en-courage family members to assist their own kin, such a policy initiative would prove a step in the right direction. And it would provide an additional source of income for women, who are more likely than men to be dependent at ad-vanced ages.

In short, note how far we have come in policy terms from Bolles's three boxes of life. Rather than viewing education initiatives, disability programs, and re-tirement policies as discrete, independent entities, we assert that they affect all age groups in a direct manner. Education policies make it possible for disabled people to earn a living and for elderly people to continue to be productive (as well as to ripen and to nurture young people) to the extent to which they de-sire. Disability programs designed to enable men and women to engage in civic life can be readily adapted across generational lines to cultivate a diverse communal milieu that some critics claim has been lost in the United States (Putnam, 2000). And since retirement as a social institution no longer begins at age 65 and rarely signals the end of growth, personal and otherwise, we need to pay more attention to ways to use education and remedial programs, as well as self-empowering measures, to make the extra years of life as vital as possible.

By coordinating the policies we have, and interconnecting them across the human life course, we are bound to increase the prospects of all age groups to make contributions to our nation's future. One of the legacies of American history has been the continuing struggle to reconsider the potential assets of those who were forgotten or marginalized and then to deploy such individual talents in effective ways. As a nation we have grown richer and more productive by creating policies that remedy flaws in the system. Generally that has entailed opening doors, not compartmentalizing segments of the population on the basis of race, ethnicity, gender, or age.

The challenge facing change makers in the policy arena—lawyers, elected officials, lobbyists, and ordinary citizens—is not what Michael Ignatieff identified as the problem of the heath, that "vast, grey space of state confinement . . . where needs are met, but souls are dishonoured" (1984, p. 50). The United States has made much progress in enclosing the heath, by embracing deserving others, by including those we tend to marginalize (Ignatieff, 1984). Rather, we remain confounded by what Garrett Hardin (1968) called the "tragedy of the commons." Hardin claimed that "the problem for years ahead is to work out an acceptable theory of weighting synergistic effects." How we reallocate finite, limited institutional resources to maximize human potentials in ways that benefit society at large will be messy but ultimately more synergistic than building silos on the basis of a three-box conception of life. It will pit legitimate interests against legitimate interests. But as the life course expands and people of all ages see fit to act in age-irrelevant ways, nurturing the future health of the commons takes on fresh urgency.

REFERENCES

AARP. 2003. *Social Security Disability Insurance: Some Facts.* Publication FS92, February. Available at http://research.aarp.org/econ/fs92_ssdi.html.

Achenbaum, W. A. 1978. *Old Age in the New Land*. Baltimore: Johns Hopkins University Press.

Achenbaum, W. A. 1986. *Social Security*. New York: Cambridge University Press.

Adult Education Act. 1998. Federal response to adult illiteracy. National Adult Education Professional Development Consortium, Inc. Available at www.naepdc.org/issues/AEA Histort.htm.

Baylis-Heerschop, C. 2004. Federal aid to education. University of Notre Dame. Available at www.nd.edu/~rbarger/www7/fedaid.html.

Bengtson, V., Biblarz, T. L., and Roberts, R. E. L. 2002. *How Families Matter*. New York: Cambridge University Press.

Berkowitz, E. D. 1987. *Disabled Policy: America's Programs for the Handicapped*. Cambridge: Cambridge University Press.

Berkowitz, E. D. 2000. Disability policy and history. Social Security On-line, statement before the Subcommittee on Social Security of the Committee on Ways and Means, July 13. Available at www.ssa.gov/history/edberkdib.html.

Berkowitz, E. D., and McQuaid, K. 1988. *Creating the Welfare State*. 2nd ed. New York: Praeger.

Binstock, R. H. 2003. The war on "anti-aging medicine." *Gerontologist* 43:4–14.

Bode, C. 1968. *The American Lyceum Movement*. Carbondale: Southern Illinois University Press.

Bolles, J. 1978. *The Three Boxes of Life*. Berkeley: Ten Speed Press.

Brackey, H. J. 2002. Many workers find the cost of disability insurance crippling. *Miami Herald*, November 18.

Breaking soil. 1934. *Time Magazine*, November 26. www.time.com/time/magazine/article/0,9171,882302–1,00.html.

Cheek, K. 2004. The normal school. University of Notre Dame. Available at www.nd.edu/~rbarger/www7/normal.html.

Collins, B. 2004. The rise of high school. University of Notre Dame. Available at www.nd.edu/~rbarger/www7/riseofhs.html.

Drucker, P. 1976. *The Unseen Revolution*. New York: Harper & Row.

Elderhostel. 2004. What is Elderhostel? Available at www.elderhostel.org/about/what_is.asp.

Estes, C. L. 1979. *Aging Enterprise: A Critical Examination of Social Policies and Services for the Aged*. San Francisco: Jossey-Bass.

Fass, P. 1977. *The Damned and the Beautiful*. New York: Oxford University Press.

Fennell, G., Phillipson, C., and Evers, H. 1988. *Sociology of Old Age*. Philadelphia: Open University Press.

Fishback, P. V. 2001. Workers' compensation. In EH.Net Encyclopedia of Economic and Business History, edited by R. Whaples. August 15. Available at www.eh.net/encyclopedia.

Geiger, R. 1991. Higher education. In *The Reader's Companion to American History*, ed. E. Foner and J. A. Garraty. Boston: Houghton Mifflin.

Grocke, V. 2004. Compulsory education. University of Notre Dame. Available at www.nd.edu/~rbarger/www7/compulso.html.

Hall, G. S. 1903. *Adolescence*. New York: D. Appleton.

Hardin, G. 1968. The tragedy of the commons. *Science* 162:1243–48. www.sciencemag.org/cgi/content/full/162/3859/1243.

Hill, C., and Reno, V. 2003. *Social Security Finances: Findings of the 2003 Trustees Report.* Social Security Brief 15. Washington, DC: National Academy of Social Insurance.

Hudson, R. B. 1978. The "graying" of the federal budget and its consequences for aging policy. *Gerontologist* 18:428–40.

Ignatieff, M. 1984. *The Needs of Strangers.* New York: Vintage/Ebury.

Kennedy, L. D. 1999. SSI at its twenty-fifth year. *Social Security Bulletin* 62:52–58.

Kirp, D. L. 2003. *Shakespeare, Einstein, and the Bottom Line.* Cambridge, MA: Harvard University Press.

Lachman, M. E. 2004. Development in midlife. *Annual Review of Psychology* 55:305–31.

Lightcap, B. 2004. The Morrill Act of 1862. University of Notre Dame. Available at www.nd.edu/~rbarger/www7/morrill.html.

Marmor, T. R. 1970. *The Politics of Medicare.* Chicago: Aldine.

Martin, J. K., et al. 2001. *America and Its Peoples.* 4th ed. New York: Addison, Wesley, Longman.

Martin, T., and Davies, P. S. 2003–4. Changes in the demographic and economic characteristics of SSI and DI beneficiaries between 1984 and 1999. *Social Security Bulletin* 65:1–13.

Mashaw, J. L., and V. P. Reno, eds. 1996. *The Environment of Disability Income Policy and Programs, People, History, and Context.* Washington, DC: National Academy of Social Insurance.

Metchnikoff, E. 1908. *The Nature of Man.* New York: Putnam's Sons.

National Council on the Aging. 1974. *The Myth and Reality of Aging in America.* Washington, DC: National Council on the Aging.

National Council on the Aging. 2002. *American Perceptions of the Aging.* Washington, DC: National Council on the Aging.

Neugarten, B. L., ed. 1982. *Age versus Need.* Beverly Hills, CA: Sage.

Pratt, H. J. 1976. *Gray Lobby.* Chicago: University of Chicago Press.

Putnam, R. D. 2000. *Bowling Alone.* New York: Simon & Schuster.

Riley, M. W., Kahn, R. L., and Foner, A. 1994. *Age and Structural Lag.* New York: John Wiley.

Rosenman, S., ed. 1969. *The Public Papers and Addresses of Franklin Delano Roosevelt.* New York: Russell & Russell.

Rothman, D. 1971. *The Discovery of the Asylum: Social Order and Disorder in the New Republic.* Boston: Little, Brown.

Rothman, D. 1980. *Conscience and Convenience: The Asylum and Its Alternatives in Progressive America.* Boston: Little, Brown.

Scherer, M. 2004. The cardinal principles of secondary education. University of Notre Dame. Available at www.nd.edu/~rbarger/www7/cardprin.html.

Schieber, S. J., and Shoven, J. B. 1999. *The Real Deal: The History and Future of Social Security.* New Haven, CT: Yale University Press.

Schlesinger, A. M., Jr. 1958. *The Coming of the New Deal.* Boston: Houghton Mifflin.

Scott, P. A. 2004. The adult education movement. University of Notre Dame. Available at www.nd.edu/~rbarger/www7/adult-ed.html.

Simpson, J. 1999. *Chautauqua: An American Utopia.* New York: Abrams.

Skocpol, T. 1992. *Protecting Soldiers and Mothers.* Cambridge, MA: Harvard University Press.

Social Security Act. 1935. Crippled children, secs. 511–15. Social Security Administration. Available at www.ssa.gov/history/1935chart9.html.

Social Security Administration. 2004a. *Annual Statistical Report on Social Security Disability Insurance Program, 2003.* Available at www.ssa.gov/policy/docs/statcomps/di_asr/2003/ (accessed December 4, 2006.

Social Security Administration. 2004b. Supplemental security record, 100 percent data, January. Available at www.ssa.gov/policy/docs/statcomps/ssi_monthly/2004–01/table2.html (site discontinued).

Tech: Online courses the rage in corporate training. 2002. *USA Today,* April 29. Available at www.usatoday.com/tech/news/2002/04/30/online-training.htm.

U.S. Department of Education, National Center for Education Statistics. 2000. *The Condition of Education, 2000.* Washington, DC: U.S. Government Printing Office.

University of Phoenix: The nation's leading online university. 2004. University of Phoenix. Available at http://online.phoenix.edu.

Westerink, D. 2004. Manual training movement. University of Notre Dame. Available at www.nd.edu/~rbarger/www7/manualtr.html.

Woloch, N. 1991. Women's education. In *The Reader's Companion to American History,* ed. E. Foner and J. A. Garraty, s.v. Boston: Houghton Mifflin.

Wright, S. 2004. The Kalamazoo case. University of Notre Dame. Available at www.nd.edu/~rbarger/www7/kalamazo.html.

CHAPTER ELEVEN

The Political Paradoxes of Thinking Outside the Life-Cycle Boxes

Robert B. Hudson, Ph.D.

Two developments—one economic and one political—have transformed aging policy in the United States over the past half century. The first was the aggregate improvement in well-being among older people that began in the 1960s and grew dramatically in the ensuing years. The second was the rise of conservative thought in the 1970s, culminating in the election of Ronald Reagan in 1980 and in the continuing dominance of the Republican party in American politics through the 2004 election. The dramatic improvement in living standards of older people helped transform them from a marginal and residual population to one enjoying full legitimate "life course" status, embodied principally by the institutionalization of retirement. In turn, the economic improvements—resulting principally from growth in and liberalization of Social Security—generated a presence for older people in modern politics that did not exist 40 years ago. In social policy terms, these economic and political developments are essentially tectonic. They have bedrock implications for the future well-being of older people, the nature of relations among the generations, and the respective roles of public, private, and personal sectors in promoting individual and social welfare.

Political Perspectives on the Life Cycle

These developments have direct implications for the types of policy suggestions raised in Chapter 10 by Andrew Achenbaum and Tom Cole. Those authors would like us to think outside of the traditional life-cycle "boxes" when it comes to the usual segmentation of education, disability, and Social Security policy. In their recommendations for generationally related policy changes, Achenbaum and Cole would ease or break this life-cycle connection. While there is a strong philosophical case to be made for moving in this direction, my analysis here suggests that, in thinking outside of these boxes, we must not lose track of the likely political and policy consequences of so doing.

Regarding *education,* Achenbaum and Cole locate historical efforts to educate middle-aged and older people even during the time when most educational activity was directed at young people. They go on to urge that education be made more accessible and affordable to people of all ages, including the training of workers in their 40s and 50s and the development of flexible and part-time educational opportunities for older people. In the case of *disability,* Achenbaum and Cole emphasize how programs long associated with middle age and aging have more recently centered on younger people. Beyond loosening the disability/retirement linkage, this evolution has been energized by a rights emphasis, with individuals heretofore understood as clients now participating in program implementation as consumers. The degree to which older people will be part of this process and share in its success remains an open question to Achenbaum and Cole. Finally, in calling for *Social Security* to be more relevant across the life span, they would like preoccupation with the system's long-term viability to be at least partially supplanted by innovative thinking centered on preparation for retirement. Specifically, they would place greater emphasis on the need for education tied to what can be expected in one's later years and to crediting people of middle age for the nonmonetized care they provide to both the old and the young.

The following pages review, first, how politics past have shaped America's approaches to education, work/disability, and retirement/leisure questions and, second, how the more recent political realities centered on age-based policy will impinge on the directions Achenbaum and Cole might take us. Their emphasis on productivity fits with much contemporary thinking, but the potential political and policy costs of moves in that direction need to be explored.

Traditional Policy Developments

In a voluminous literature addressing social policy developments in the United States, much attention has been paid to questions of eligibility, benefits, and administration. In comparison to the experience of other nations, the American response has been more variegated because of "exceptionalist" views about the role of government and the bases on which government benefits should be bestowed. In the Continental European and Scandinavian experiences, a more accepted role for the public sector and a more corporatist understanding of claimants' social and economic status has led to more integrated responses.

Education

As noted by Achenbaum and Cole and documented by many other commentators, the United States took an early and highly democratic view of education. The authors point out that the first tax-funded high school was created in 1824 and that mandatory attendance became widely established by the 1840s. It is, of course, essential to recall that the lion's share of this governmental involvement was at the state and local level; federal funding and regulation came many years later. Even today, the federal government pays only 7 percent of the nation's K-12 school budget.

The place of education in the United States is remarkable on two counts: (1) how early it occurred, and (2) why the focus was on education rather than on other arenas of social policy. In comparative perspective, an equally interesting observation is that the United States fostered broad-based public education decades before European nations, where government involvement in activities of all sorts was well established. As Heidenheimer, Heclo, and Adams (1983, p. 30) observe, "What distinguished American education policy making in the mid-nineteenth to mid-twentieth centuries from that in most European nations was the greater attention paid to demands from the middling parts of the population. School and college opportunities became so plentiful that even some poorer American youth could make their way to college." Indeed, these authors found that while educational opportunities were expanding for American youth, such opportunities for most European youth declined in the nineteenth century, where emerging central government bureaucracies were concentrating their efforts on governmental and other political elites.

The development of education stands in stark contrast to the well-known "Europe leads; America lags" pattern found in most other social welfare policy arenas. Although this long-standing depiction has come under some critique in recent analyses (Orloff, 1988; Skocpol, 1992), there is no question that non-military old-age pensions, welfare payments, and rudimentary health care benefits came into existence in Europe at an earlier time and in a more broad-based fashion than they did in the United States. Explanations for the discrepancy vary, but most address questions of both class (Myles, 1984; Esping-Andersen, 1985) and culture (Rimlinger, 1971; Kaim-Caudle, 1973), each finding the American experience different from the European. Both class consciousness and class-based institutions such as unions and political parties were more salient in Europe, leading to ideologically structured debates around questions of social welfare. The contrasting American focus on individualism, morality, and ethnic identification inhibited similar social welfare developments.

Nowhere is the separation between the two experiences more observable than in education. It can be seen most clearly through the famous lens of T. H. Marshall (1964) in contrasting the development of civil rights (freedom of speech, religion, and movement), political rights (freedom of assembly and organization for public purposes), and social rights (the right to substantive social benefits such as income, health care, and housing). In historical terms, the United States was a leader in the first two arenas, whereas in the third, it is widely viewed as falling far behind. However, a glaring exception is found in the case of education, where mandatory, publicly supported, and generally revenue-funded schooling made education a social right in the United States long before it was a right elsewhere.

It is also true that Americans usually categorize education separately from other arenas constituting social welfare (income, health care, employment, housing, and social services). This separation of education can be seen in the formal policy dimensions along which policies are organized and compared: eligibility (overwhelmingly the young), benefit structure (a highly separated and distinct set of services), administration (local school boards operating with considerable discretion), and financing (heavily local and state dollars).

On historical, ideological, substantive, and fiscal grounds, moving education in a meaningfully intergenerational direction would require extraordinary efforts. The implications of population aging contribute to a reasonable case for investing more educational resources in middle-aged and older people, but this initial review makes clear just how much would have to be done.

Disability

The policies of disability, as compared with education policies, lend themselves much more to a mainstream political symbiosis with aging. As Achenbaum and Cole observe, there is a historical connection between the two, and contemporary policy developments have brought them even closer together.

Early disability policy in the United States dates to the late nineteenth century and is tied to intersecting questions of law and morality of that era. Again as Achenbaum and Cole note, policy interventions related to disability centered on state industrial accident laws. As with education, we are first reminded that early social policy was conducted largely at the subnational level (including "national" Civil War pensions, which often became the currency of local political patronage and graft [Skocpol, 1992]). However, these disability laws differed from the education scene in that they broke with longstanding moral strictures proclaiming that individuals alone are responsible for their own betterment.

As recounted by Theodore Lowi (1990, p. 28) in discussing the evolution of risk and responsibility in the United States, the tenets underlying insurance were long resisted. About life's activities in general and about industrial life in particular, it was long held: "take your risks and accept responsibility for your negligence." To socialize risk—which is what all forms of insurance do—was to eliminate blame, the moral consequence for bad deeds. Under this regime, the rise in the number and severity of industrial accidents proved costly to companies in both monetary and worker-retention terms. To contain and regularize these costs, businesses gradually moved to limit their liability while providing benefits to injured workers. State-based industrial accident laws were the codification of this movement, although, as Lowi (p. 28) notes, court verdicts consistently favoring entrepreneurs and risk takers "would leave a lot of widows and orphans dependent on the community."

The shift from blame to risk is a critical one for the development of modern social policy. It is a recognition that social and economic factors beyond individual control should be recognized and accommodated when they lead to negative occurrences. Disability has now long been seen as one of those events that, in probabilistic rather than moral terms, can be viewed as highly contingent. And, in both historical and epidemiological terms, old age has been closely linked to disability, long rendering older people the comorbid poster children of welfare state development.

In moving their disability discussion to the passage of Disability Insurance under Social Security in 1956, Achenbaum and Cole make this clear. Until 1960, eligibility for DI was confined to workers age 50 or older. It served, in effect, as an early retirement program for many workers who had spent long years in physically arduous labor and were largely without income until their full Social Security retirement benefits kicked in at age 65 (or early retirement benefits at age 62 for women after 1956 and for men after 1962).

The authors' third disability policy episode centers on the passage and evolution of the Supplemental Security Income (SSI) program, enacted in 1972. Passed in the wake of Richard Nixon's failed Family Assistance Plan, which was intended to radically reform the Aid to Families with Dependent Children (AFDC) program, SSI emerged as a face-saving piece of welfare legislation (Burke and Burke, 1974). SSI, directed at the so-called adult categories, federalized benefit levels under the earlier welfare titles serving the poor old, blind, and disabled. Unlike the young mothers enrolled under AFDC, these impoverished adults were not expected to work and could thus be assisted without controversy. And, in light of SSI's evolution over the years, Achenbaum and Cole make the important and often lost point that it was the poor old who were the principal targets of the original legislation. In the years since SSI's enactment, the proportion of people rendered eligible by reason of age has fallen from nearly 60 percent to less than one-third. However, concerning the early impetus for the legislation, it was a clear intent that poor elders who could not work should be given a supplement to their meager or nonexistent Social Security benefits.

More recent developments in the world of disability may have less sanguine effects on older people seeking to retire. Achenbaum and Cole speak briefly of the "rights movement" that has been strongly associated with the disability community; it has generated a paradigmatic shift in understandings of eligibility, from client-based to consumer-based. These efforts, legally associated with Section 504 of the Vocational Rehabilitation Act of 1974, have generated political pressure around the right to accommodations and the right to work.

A separate law arising from a separate set of politics yielded an analogous outcome for older people during this period as well. Eliminating the upper age limit for protections under the Age Discrimination in Employment Act resulted in the historic elimination of mandatory retirement and established older people's "right" to work. One argues against these rights at his or her own peril, but Achenbaum and Cole make the important observation that these advances could "become burdensome pressures on older or demoralized workers who wish to retire." The "right" to productive aging through new retirement disincentives may come at the expense of some who may legitimately prefer substantive benefits to procedural safeguards. Martha Holstein (2005, p. 28) makes a similar cautionary statement, noting that "this heralding of 'successful' aging, though well-intentioned, can also serve to threaten the self-esteem of people who cannot or choose not to live up to those new norms."

Social Security

Social Security underpins leisure, the "third box of life" in Achenbaum and Cole's presentation. Their discussion emphasizes the degree to which Social Security—principally Old Age and Survivors Insurance—and later Medicare have been very much about aged people. They note that older people were featured during Social Security's enactment in 1935 and have become its principal beneficiaries. Indeed, they add a more controversial note, opining that Social Security has become "a victim of its own success" with the rise of a large older population many of whom are in reasonable or better economic circumstances.

Truncated as their discussion is, Achenbaum and Cole have a good handle on the centrality of old age. In the absence of class-based politics, in the absence of any commitment to "social rights," and in the presence of benefits only for "the deserving," older people came to have a prominent place in the development of the American welfare state. Old Age Assistance and Old Age Insurance served as Titles I and II of the original Social Security Act; Medicare as originally enacted was only for the old; and, as indicated, SSI was exclusively about the old and other deserving populations deemed unable to work. Subsequent liberalization and indexing of benefits under these programs has led to a point where roughly 30 percent of the federal budget is today directed at persons age 65 and over. That the United States has what amounts to an old-age welfare state is beyond controversy.

This said, it is not axiomatic that this weighting ought to be reworked. Unlike observers on the right of the political spectrum who would cut or privatize old-age benefits, Achenbaum and Cole make more modest suggestions, centered on promoting education about what awaits people in old age, providing incentives for younger workers to prepare for retirement through career enhancement, and crediting middle-aged individuals for caring for the young and for the old.

In an engagingly original analysis, Achenbaum and Cole place great reliance on educational opportunities and strategies. Going beyond intrinsic rewards of "adult education," they emphasize the social and economic results that flow from educational opportunity and accomplishment. For people in their middle years, education is critical to maximizing human potential; for people in their latter years, educational, and even remedial, programs can contribute to the remarkable quantity and quality of life that now remains beyond the traditional retirement age of 65.

Contemporary Policy Developments

Three lenses are useful in assessing Achenbaum and Cole's thoughts about future directions for a public policy more adept at bridging life-cycle stages: life-course distinctions, generational relations, and ideological divisions. We can look at each of these in turn.

Life-Course Boxes and Policy Boxes

Achenbaum and Cole contribute to a growing literature either documenting or calling for a reworking of life stages as they have traditionally been viewed: education, work, leisure. In particular, Riley and Riley (1994), invoking the construct of "structural lag," highlight growing discontinuities in roles and expectations associated with these boxes. Education can and should occur throughout life; work and labor force patterns increasingly vary by economic, gender, racial, and age profiles; and leisure remains problematic for many in old age while blissfully enjoyed by many younger people of substantial means.

In an iterative fashion, public policy has built on but, more importantly, has contributed to the twentieth-century evolution of assumptions around education/work/leisure and the life cycle. At least in the K-12 years, governmental support and mandates lie at the heart of education for the young. Whether the young learn more readily than the old can be debated, but, as Achenbaum and Cole nicely recount, education of the young has long been considered an essential public investment in human capital. Public spending by state and local governments for K-12 education totaled $373 billion in 2000 (with federal education spending for children totaling only an additional $20 billion [Congressional Budget Office, 2004]). At the other end of the life span, federal spending on the old totaled $615 billion in 2001 (principally Social Security and Medicare), constituting the vast majority of non–Civil Service public-sector old-age expenditures. Education for the young and economic support for the old remain highly segmented in our federal system.

It is hard to overstate the role public policy played in old age's emergence as the third element of today's conventional life-cycle triad. Social Security was the largest single factor in the formal creation of old age as an institutionalized life stage, to the degree that it is uniquely responsible for the reification of age 65 as marking the beginning of old age. Studies across all industrial countries (Kohli et al., 1991; Quinn and Burkhauser, 1990) demonstrate that the retirement age established by national pension systems is by far the best predictor of the timing of older workers' labor force exit. And studies by political scientists, most notably Campbell (2003, 2004) in the United States, find Social Security and Medicare to be the principal factors in the creation of age-based political consciousness among older Americans.

The most central question in age-related social policy debates today is whether age 65 (or 62 or 67) is an appropriate point at which to settle into the leisure "box." Some would raise the age; some would lower it; some would grade it by race and gender; and some would eliminate age altogether as a stand-alone retirement criterion. O'Rand (2005, p. 7) makes the critical observation that "*old age is a variably emergent*, not a fixed, status that reflects the cumulative impact of several interrelated factors over time" (italics in original).

The prospects for Achenbaum and Cole's principal inference pattern—that age-based distinctions throughout the life cycle should be reduced—hold up differentially. The strongest centers around disability, where incidence, advocacy, and policy *are* reducing age-based distinctions. As the authors cogently point out, the young and the middle-aged are receiving benefits once targeted disproportionately, if not exclusively, to the old. However, for the nation's investment in education to move notably up the age range seems much more problematic. Apart from ingrained patterns and understandings, one need not look much beyond recent rounds of welfare reform, where the efforts of liberals to make education and training count against recipients' mandated work hours are currently being held up by Republican majorities in Congress (Pear and Hernandez, 2004).

The movement to modify chronological boundaries around old age itself may be less about softening than about simply elevating (i.e., raising the effective [public] definition of when old age begins). That may well force an "enhancement" of work and other "productive" activities for so-called young-old individuals. Whether it might also bring increased leisure to individuals in their middle years—as a call for moving outside the life-cycle boxes requires—seems much less certain. Given growing concern about pending labor shortages associated with population aging (Nyce and Schieber, 2004), prospects for governmental support for greater midlife leisure, if not necessarily education, seem fairly remote. A nation that cannot provide paid leave through the Family Medical Leave Act seems unlikely to promote breaks from the labor force under far less stringent conditions.

Generational Distinctions

As Achenbaum and Cole make clear, there is a strong case to be made for breaking down the tripartite barriers traditionally marking the life cycle. But taking a one-point-in-time snapshot of these relations is focusing on three age groupings each at a different point in their life-course experience. If we also think about each of these generations at multiple points in time, our willingness and ability to move boxes may shift in important ways.

Such discussions these days usually focus on the baby boom generation, since it is seen as the "pig moving through the (demographic) python": double shifts in elementary school, constrained job opportunities, and threatened Social Security benefits. In this formulation, boomers' chances to optimize their experience at any stage of life are compromised in comparison to those of other generations. (Recent analysis by Alicia Munnell [2004], however, highlights the larger historical or period effect currently at work, namely, that the entire population is aging; that is to say, the python itself is moving!)

The generational contrast is made most strikingly by historian David Thomson (1989), extolling the cross-national experiences of the generation born roughly between the two World Wars. Referring to members of this cohort as a "welfare generation," he points to how they had to the good fortune to "age" along with the welfare state itself: when they were young, the nascent welfare state tended to provide education and housing benefits; later they became the beneficiaries of the pension and health benefits that have constitute the lion's share of the contemporary welfare state. The story is a complicated one (both wars contributed to major education and housing expenditures on behalf of young veterans, e.g., the G.I. Bill in the United States), but the cohort and program trajectories are parallel.

The question for our purposes becomes how to recalibrate what different generations may owe each other and whether they owe it at one point in time or over time. On the matter of pensions, Diamond and Orszag (2003) would impose a "legacy tax" to acknowledge the good but inevitable break that Thomson's welfare generation received. Looking to the future, John Myles (2005) struggles with how to acknowledge the claims of workers and retirees at different points in time. Invoking Richard Musgrave's "rule" that in times of generational imbalance, one can justify neither "fixed replacement rates" (favoring the baby boomers in old age at the expense of today's workers) or "fixed contribution rates" (favoring today's workers at the expense of aged boomers), he calls for a "fixed relative position model" that would establish an equitable ratio among current earners and pension recipients.

And what is to become of the young in all this? Demographic profiles suggest some hope for Generation Xers (born from the mid-1960s to the mid-1980s); indeed, there is concern in corporate America that there may be a leadership gap resulting from a shortage in workers in the critical late-30s to early-50s age groups (Dychtwald, Erickson, and Morison, 2004). Of those yet younger, one is struck by the aphorism that their student loans are the equivalent of their parents' mortgages.

The point here is that notions of generational justice, reciprocity, and opportunity will color society's ability to alter life-course expectations. In the case of the old, the issue will probably emerge as whether and for whom "leisure" is an option. As always, class will trump age and generation, but innovative and hopeful talk about "productive aging" may ring truer for those for whom it is an option than for those now coming along for whom it will be an obligation.

Ideology

Perhaps the most intriguing political aspect of Achenbaum and Cole's call for greater policy flexibility in roles across the life cycle—and especially their emphasis on education and exploration—is its implicit ideological underpinning. They favor greater flexibility in four arenas: (1) thinking "less in terms of how specific age groups should be entitled to certain benefits"; (2) fostering the ability of individuals to enhance "their capacity to contribute to a productive society"; (3) having "colleges and universities [enter] into meaningful partnerships with businesses in their vicinity to train middle-aged workers"; and (4) providing formal credits "to encourage family members to assist their own kin."

Social policy developments over the past quarter century have emphasized a renewed reliance on informal over formal care mechanisms, local over cen-tralized delivery systems, and the use of private-sector entities in lieu of public-sector ones. Much of this, of course, results from a neoconservative effort to decentralize, individualize, and privatize initiatives (Hudson, 1991), under-taken or contemplated by the federal government. In boldest terms, these ac-tivities are directed at nothing less than "starving the [federal] beast." But at the microeconomic and micropolitical level, these efforts rest on what Marmor, Mashaw, and Harvey (1990) refer to as the "new behaviorism." People in all cir-cumstances—certainly those who are recipients of governmental largesse—must be held to standards of individual accountability. Thus, one of welfare re-form's principal architects, Lawrence Mead (1986), speaks of the need to move from entitlement to "the obligations of citizenship," to the need for welfare to be understood as a contract wherein benefits are received in exchange for stay-ing in school, working, remaining drug-free, or not becoming pregnant. Paul Starobin (1998) frames this reformulation as a shift from "the nanny state" to "the daddy state."

The degree to which the tenets of the new behaviorism will (or should) affect aging policy is a question of enormous importance, and Cole and Achenbaum perform a great service by introducing it, albeit indirectly. Historically, the aged were largely given a pass when it comes to behaviorism's strictures. They were not expected to work, and it was presumed that they would become ill and frail. Those who had worked had "earned" Social Security benefits (Ball, 2000), but even those who had not worked or whose Social Security credits were minimal were considered deserving, as seen in the Family Assistance Plan → SSI episode. As long as that image of the old prevailed, there was no call for application of the new behaviorism's code of conduct.

To a considerable although unknown degree, those politics built on a nega-tive stereotype of the old (Binstock, 1983) are shifting. Increasingly, policy re-formers are up against a world in which "a new population is encountering an old ideology" (Hudson, 1999). Though a reasonably faithful picture of the el-derly population 50 or 75 years ago, the negative stereotype of poverty, illness, and isolation no longer represents the elderly population's economic reality. The political question then becomes whether policy benefits for some or all of the old population, reflecting their heightened economic status, should be re-duced. Should those who can and wish to work and those who have saved enough to either work or retire be asked to rely increasingly on their own ac-cumulated resources? Should policies be modified to further encourage such individual reliance? Such suggestions reintroduce individualizing and privatizing responsibility for well-being in old age.

How far programmatic shifts and cuts might extend down the elderly well-being chain is obviously pure conjecture. The overall possibility does, however, raise a concern among advocates for the aging that the old-age constituency could be bifurcated, and efforts are clearly under way to bring this about. Some proposals to partially privatize Social Security would create a basic first tier for all; a second tier consisting of mandated private investments would grow ever larger. In the case of Medicare, efforts that can be understood to segment the old are already law. Beginning with Medicare+Choice (now Medicare Advantage) managed care options in 1996 and continuing with the privately administered Part D drug benefit under the Medicare Modernization Act in 2006, there are separate benefit, delivery, and financing streams already in place. As to the political ramifications, Bernstein and Stevens (1999) report that many elders now enrolled in Medicare managed care plans do not actually believe that they are participating in a government-sponsored program.

Again, it is interesting to place the Achenbaum/Cole "repotting" ideas into this shifting political landscape. Their recommendations are in the direction of breaking down age-based distinctions, which they find "lagging" behind both new realities and new opportunities. And in this, they may be correct. Certainly their disability/aging distinction is very much on the mark, though by definition it centers on questions of functional deficits. But their education points can resonate across the life cycle as well. Whether for reasons of vocation, education, or curiosity, educational opportunities can and should be opened across the age spectrum.

These suggestions could be problematic around the core "heavy-lifting" areas of aging policy—Social Security, Medicare, Medicaid. In the American welfare state, there is no reason to think that breaking down or even softening age-based categories will generate more support for the young, the middle-aged, or the old. Thus, for example, the idea of cutting spending for the old in order to increase benefits for the young is a political nonstarter. Never having had a social insurance program for the young, we nonetheless took the worst of our public assistance programs—AFDC for the young—and further reduced its scope. In a behaviorist era, a cut in benefits for the old would result in tax cuts or perhaps deficit reduction, but it would not result in added programming for the young.

As for the middle-aged, there was talk in the latter years of the Clinton administration that we should extend Medicare benefits to individuals 55 or older, thereby providing health insurance for older workers who were unemployed or otherwise forced to retire. Marilyn Moon (2005, p. 206) captures the dramatic shift in politics that has happened since: "Today, however, discussions of moving away from age-based policy would mean not expansion but rather elimination of Medicare." As for Medicaid, Colleen Grogan (2005) finds three political incarnations of the old since 1965: elderly people as too deserving for Medicaid's means-tested, stigmatizing benefit; elderly people as too well-off relative to other needy groups and therefore undeserving of Medicaid as a targeted program for the poor; and elderly people as deserving of Medicaid's social entitlement. The last stage is expansionary only in that it finds advocates acknowledging that, in the absence of public long-term-care insurance, "universalism within targeting" is the only road left open.

In short, the new politics of aging suggest that maintenance of age-based benefits may be the least bad strategy for those committed to public benefits for the old and, ironically, the young. While our only social insurance programs are heavily, although not exclusively, weighted toward the old (Social Security has survivor and dependent benefits; Medicare has benefits for the disabled and those with end-stage renal disease), a precedent-setting move to cut them would in all likelihood make expansion of social insurance benefits to other populations more rather than less remote. As difficult and as self-serving to the old as this perspective may seem, the young have nothing to gain by our cutting benefits to the old under the current political regime. The inability of President George W. Bush to rally younger people (as well as older ones) around his proposal to partially privatize Social Security suggests that this understanding may be resonating more widely than conventional generational wisdom would hold.

Conclusion

The boxes that Cole and Achenbaum would have us break out of are much associated with the Rileys' (1994) notion of structural lag, one of the truly innovative paradigms of social gerontology. There can be little question that the education, work, leisure sequencing is more permeable than may have once been the case. There is also a powerful normative case to be made that a deep-seated structural lag around politics and policies exists as well. Old age is no longer a reliable and near-unique proxy for need. The passage of time has seen heightened heterogeneity among the old and increasing similarities between older and younger populations. Questions of cross-age horizontal equity abound: individuals (of different ages) in similar circumstances receiving highly unequal benefits.

These emergent realities acknowledged, the raw politics of today do not lend themselves to or suggest a quick leveling of the inequities. Undoing aging benefits will not necessarily lead to larger or more equal population-based allocations. In structural lag terms, the unfortunate irony created by today's politics is that it may be *fortunate* that policies are lagging. The behaviorist strictures that have been relatively easy to impose on politically powerless welfare recipients could be extended to older people as well. Indeed, many will argue that they should be ("why aren't healthy 68-year olds working rather than receiving Social Security?"). Yet, if notions of reciprocity and reward for service are to be socially acknowledged, where will one draw the line? The philosophy that would erode old-age benefits is not one that will extend them to younger populations.

With much of the discussion above addressed to old-age benefits, we are left with a final thought on applying these concerns to Achenbaum and Cole's recommendations about education and disability. Politically speaking, I see little reason to believe new social benefits are about to accrue to the young; nor do I see much reason to believe that the educational benefits the young have long enjoyed will move meaningfully up the age range. Indeed, the behaviorist revolution recently overtook federal adult education policy, as the Adult Education Act, passed as part of Lyndon Johnson's Great Society in 1964, was repealed and replaced by the Workforce Investment Act of 1998 (PL 105-220).

The disability picture, however, is more encouraging, with Medicaid and SSI having long served low-income individuals of all ages. In the case of SSI, younger persons with disabilities have displaced the older poor as principal beneficiaries. In the case of Medicaid, as functional means-testing has been more stringently applied, disability has also made age less relevant (although there were never formal age gradients in the program). The most interesting age-relevant test relating to disability has occurred under the Older Americans Act and in the state agencies on aging that it spawned. Twenty-one of these traditional "aging agencies" are now also administering Medicaid home- and community-based service waivers for both the elderly and disabled populations (National Association of State Units on Aging, 2004). The worlds of aging services and those for adults with disabilities are clearly coming together, and as a result there is no question that state-level policy initiatives are reducing policy-related structural lag. Finally, the emergence of consumer-directed services—potentially for the old as well as for persons with disabilities—represents an especially potent step toward lessening "lag" in the worlds of chronic illness and disability (Mahoney et al., 2002).

Achenbaum and Cole are not predicting any near-term moves in support of their agenda, much as they might like to see them. In policy analytical terms, it may be unfortunate that they are not, because a strong normative case can be made to significantly reduce age-based segmentations. On the political front, however, it may be better to let sleeping agendas lie.

REFERENCES

Ball, R. 2000. *Insuring the Essentials.* New York: Century Foundation Press.
Bernstein, J., and Stevens, R. A. 1999. Public opinion, knowledge, and Medicare reform. *Health Affairs* 18:180–93.
Binstock, R. H. 1983. The aged as scapegoat. *Gerontologist* 23:136–43.
Burke, V., and Burke, V. 1974. *Nixon's Good Deed.* New York: Columbia University Press.
Campbell, A. L. 2003. *How Policies Make Citizens: Senior Political Action and the American Welfare State.* Princeton, NJ: Princeton University Press.
Campbell, A. L. 2004. The political consequences of program design: The case of Medicare. Department of Political Science, MIT. Unpublished manuscript.
Congressional Budget Office. 2004. *Federal Spending for Children and the Elderly.* www.cbo.gov/showdoc.cfm?index=2300&sequence=0.
Diamond, P., and P. Orszag. 2003. *Saving Social Security: A Balanced Approach.* Washington, DC: Brookings Institution Press.
Dychtwald, K., Erickson, T., and Morison, B. 2004. It's time to retire retirement. *Harvard Business Review,* March.
Esping-Andersen, G. 1985. *The Three Worlds of Welfare Capitalism.* Princeton, NJ: Princeton University Press.
Grogan, C. 2005. Politics of aging within Medicaid. In R. B. Hudson, ed., *The New Politics of Old Age Policy.* Baltimore: Johns Hopkins University Press.
Heidenheimer, A. J., Heclo, H., and Adams, C. T. 1983. *Comparative Public Policy.* New York: St. Martin's.
Holstein, M. 2005. A normative defense of universal age-based public policy. In R. B. Hudson, ed., *The New Politics of Old Age Policy.* Baltimore: Johns Hopkins University Press.
Hudson, R. 1991. Reflections on the "DIP" Decade. *Aging Today,* August–September.
Hudson, R. B. 1999. Conflict in today's aging policy: New population encounters old ideology. *Social Service Review* 73:358–79.
Kaim-Caudle, P. 1973. *Comparative Social Policy and Social Security.* London: Martin Robertson.

Kohli, M., Rein, M., Guillemard, A.-M., and Gunsteren, H. V., eds. 1991. *Time for Retirement.* New York: Cambridge University Press.

Lowi, T. J. 1990. Risks and rights in the history of American government. *Daedalus* 119:17–40.

Mahoney, K. J., Desmond, S. M., Simon-Rusinowitz, L., and Squillace, M. R. 2002. Consumer preferences for a cash option versus traditional services. *Journal of Disability Policy Studies* 13(2):74–86.

Marmor, T. R., Mashaw, J., and Harvey, P. 1990. *America's Misunderstood Welfare State.* New York: Basic Books.

Marshall, T. H. 1964. *Class, Citizenship, and Social Development.* Chicago: University of Chicago Press.

Mead, L. M. 1986. *Beyond Entitlement: The Social Obligations of Citizenship.* New York: Free Press.

Moon, M. 2005. Sustaining Medicare as an age-related program. In R. B. Hudson, ed., *The New Politics of Old Age Policy.* Baltimore: Johns Hopkins University Press.

Munnell, A. 2004. *Population Aging: It's Not Just the Baby Boom.* Chestnut Hill, MA: Boston College Center for Retirement Research.

Myles, J. 1984. *Old Age in the Welfare State.* Boston: Little, Brown.

Myles, J. 2005. What justice requires: Normative foundations for U.S. pension reform. In R. B. Hudson, ed., *The New Politics of Old Age Policy.* Baltimore: Johns Hopkins University Press.

National Association of State Units on Aging. 2004. *Forty Years of Leadership: The Dynamic Role of State Units on Aging.* Washington, DC: NASUA.

Nyce, S., and Schieber, S. 2004. Demographics matter: The economic reality of an aging society. *Public Policy and Aging Report* 14(3):17–21.

O'Rand, A. 2005. When old age begins: Implications for health, work, and retirement. In R. B. Hudson, ed., *The New Politics of Old Age Policy.* Baltimore: Johns Hopkins University Press.

Orloff, A. S. 1988. The Political Origins of America's Belated Welfare State. In M. Weir, A. S. Orloff, and T. Skocpol, eds., *The Politics of Social Policy in the United States.* Princeton, NJ: Princeton University Press.

Pear, R., and Hernandez, R. 2004. Campaign politics seen as bottleneck for welfare law. *New York Times,* July 6, pp. A1, A14.

Quinn, J. F., and Burkhauser, R. V. 1990. Work and retirement. In R. H. Binstock and L. K. George, eds., *Handbook of Aging and the Social Sciences,* 3rd ed. San Diego: Academic Press.

Riley, M. W., and Riley, J. W. 1994. Structural Lag: Past and Future. In M. W. Riley, R. L. Kahn, and A. Foner, eds., *Age and Structural Lag.* New York: John Wiley.

Rimlinger, G. 1971. *Welfare Policy and Industrialization in Europe, America, and Russia.* New York: John Wiley.

Skocpol, T. 1992. *Protecting Soldiers and Mothers.* Cambridge, MA: Harvard University Press.

Starobin, P. 1998. The daddy state. *National Journal,* March 28, pp. 678–83.

Thomson, D. 1989. The Welfare state and generation conflict: Winners and losers. In P. Johnson, C. Conrad, and D. Thomson, eds., *Workers and Pensioners.* New York: St. Martin's.

CHAPTER TWELVE

Is Responsibility across Generations Politically Feasible?

Robert H. Binstock, Ph.D.

In responding to the question "What changes will be needed in social policy and who will determine them?" W. Andrew Achenbaum and Thomas R. Cole (Chapter 10) make policy recommendations in three areas. In the arena of education, they suggest that lifelong learning should be more available, emphasizing that older workers should be "repotted" through training that equips them for jobs in the technologically oriented contemporary economy. In the realm of disability policy, they call for greater investment in vocational rehabilitation for disabled persons of all ages, as well as increased public funding for both treatment and rehabilitation for mentally ill persons. With respect to Social Security, they would like policy changed so that individuals can (1) borrow against their retirement accounts to pay for workforce repotting and other forms of lifelong learning and (2) receive Social Security credits for caring for children and for disabled family members of all ages.

These are commendable and constructive policy suggestions. However, with the baby boom cohort poised to join the ranks of old age, the primary policy goal (in my view) is to achieve continuity in American society's governmental responsibilities for older Americans that were constructed and strengthened from the 1930s through the 1970s. The top priorities are to sustain and improve existing old-age benefit programs without radical reforms that abandon present and future cohorts of older Americans to the risks of the market without adequate social protection. A key question is, What is the political feasibility of achieving these top-priority goals?

This chapter opens with a brief discussion that emphasizes the great importance of Social Security and Medicare for older persons, particularly those who are not wealthy, and outlines the economic challenges ahead if these programs are to be sustained. Then it examines changes in the political context of these programs over the years that make their preservation difficult. The chapter concludes with a suggestion for a politically feasible approach for assuring social protection for older people in the future. (Although providing support for long-term care through Medicaid and other measures is also a top priority, the appropriate mix of public and private responsibilities for long-term care is such a complex issue that it cannot be added into this discussion without exceeding the scope of a single chapter.)

The Impact and Future of Old Age Benefit Programs

From the enactment of Social Security in 1935 through the mid-1970s, American society incrementally constructed an old-age welfare state. The result is that through Social Security, Medicare, Medicaid, and a variety of other policies, we now spend more than one-third of our federal budget, more than $800 billion dollars, on programs benefiting older people (Congressional Budget Office, 2004a). These programs have substantially improved the status of older persons in American society over the years.

Social Security, for example, has helped reduce the percentage of older people in poverty from about 30 percent in 1965 (Clark, 1990) to less than 9 percent today (U.S. Census Bureau, 2005c). Moreover, payments from Social Security and means-tested old-age welfare, Supplemental Security Income (SSI), are essential sources of income for older persons who are not economically well off. For the lowest-income quintile of persons age 65 and older, Social Security and SSI account for 91.3 percent of income; for the second-lowest quintile, the two programs account for 82.2 percent of income (Federal Interagency Forum on Aging Related Statistics, 2004).

Similarly, Medicare and Medicaid have made access to health care possible over the years for tens of millions of older persons who would not have had it

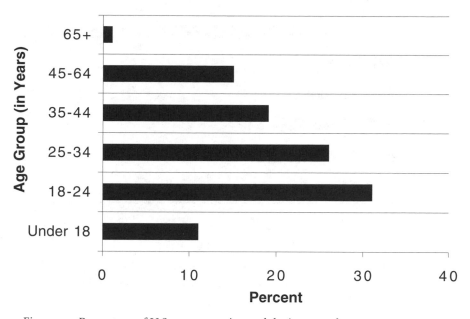

Figure 12.1. Percentage of U.S. persons uninsured during 2005, by age group
Source: U.S. Census Bureau, 2005b

otherwise. Because of these programs, older persons are the only age group of Americans that does not include millions of uninsured persons. As Figure 12.1 shows, less than 1 percent of people age 65 and older lack health insurance, compared with rates of 12 to 30 percent for all other age groupings.

To be sure, Social Security and Medicare have not solved problems of income adequacy and health care coverage for all aged Americans. Even those older persons who have made it up to the poverty line (or threshold) are in difficult economic straits. Consider that the federally established poverty line for an elderly couple in 2005 was $11,817 (U.S. Census Bureau, 2005c). Using the government's budgetary assumptions in constructing poverty lines, such a couple would have $38 a week, each, for food. In addition, the couple would have $325 a month for shelter and $325 a month for everything else: clothing; utilities; furniture; transportation; haircuts; toilet paper, soap, and other household supplies; and, notably, out-of-pocket expenses for health care including prescription drugs, copayments and deductibles, dental expenses, eye exams, and other health care expenses. This is the budget of a couple that has officially

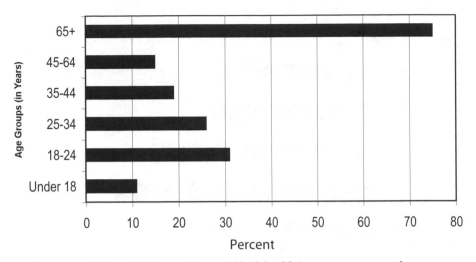

Figure 12.2. Without Medicare, who would lack health insurance coverage, by age group? *Source:* Binstock, based on estimates concerning Medicaid eligibility, employment-based insurance, steep premium prices, and exclusion of preexisting conditions

made it *out* of poverty, compared with the 3.5 million persons age 65 and older who are *below* the poverty line. As part of the broader picture, about two-fifths (38%) of older Americans have incomes that are less than 200 percent of the poverty threshold (U.S. Census Bureau, 2005a). Similarly, there are serious gaps in Medicare's coverage, such as long-term care and extended, financially catastrophic hospital stays. In addition, the prescription drug coverage provided for in the Medicare Modernization Act of 2003 is inadequate for most older patients (Moon, 2006).

However the situation would be much worse if Social Security retirement benefits were lower than they are at present and Medicare were unavailable or provided less coverage than it does. Retirement benefits currently account for 100 percent of income for one-fifth of Social Security recipients and more than 90 percent of income for another 13 percent of recipients (Social Security Administration, 2004). If Medicare did not exist, perhaps 75 percent of older persons would be completely without health insurance (see Figure 12.2).

Although Social Security and Medicare do not solve all of the income adequacy and health care access problems for older Americans, the ongoing levels of assistance and coverage they provide are critical for millions of aged persons at present and in the future. Yet projections regarding the future of these programs, especially for the years when the 76 million baby boomers will be aged, make clear that these levels will be difficult to maintain.

The Social Security Board of Trustees projects that in 2040 the program will be able to pay only 74 percent of scheduled annual benefits and will remain in actuarial deficit for decades to come (Social Security and Medicare Boards of Trustees, 2006). Social Security outlays, 4.4 percent of gross domestic product (GDP) in 2003, are projected to grow to 6.1 percent of GDP in 2030 (Congressional Budget Office, 2004b). Under a "middle-costs" scenario, Medicare is estimated to grow from 2.4 percent of GDP today to 8.3 percent in 2050. Projections such as these are likely to be inaccurate to some extent (Aaron, 2002). Yet they do indicate that major economic and political challenges lie ahead in sustaining these programs for the baby boom cohort (see Steuerle and Van de Water, 2002).

The Changing Political Contexts of Old-Age Policies

If the present political context of policies on aging were the same as it generally was when the old age welfare state was constructed, sustaining and improving Social Security and Medicare would not be as politically difficult as it is today. But the politics of old-age policies have gone through several changes in the last several decades.

The Era of Compassionate Ageism

From the New Deal until the late 1970s, public policy issues concerning older Americans were framed by an underlying *ageism* (see Palmore, 1990), the attribution of the same characteristics, status, and just deserts to a heterogeneous group that has been artificially homogenized as "the aged." Before the late 1970s, the predominant stereotypes of older Americans were compassionate. Elderly persons tended to be seen as poor, frail, socially dependent, objects of discrimination, and above all "deserving" (see Kalish, 1979). For more than 40 years—dating from the Social Security Act of 1935—American society accepted the oversimplified notion that all older persons were essentially the same and that all were worthy of governmental assistance. The lowest levels of economic status, health, and functional capacities that could be found among aged individuals became familiar as common denominators (Neugarten, 1970).

The American polity implemented this compassionate construct by adopting and financing major age-categorical benefit programs and, in addition, tax and price subsidies for which eligibility was not determined by need. Through the New Deal's Social Security, the Great Society's Medicare and Older Americans Act (an omnibus social service program), special tax exemptions and credits for being age 65 or older, and a variety of other measures enacted during President Nixon's New Federalism, elderly people were exempted from the screenings that are applied to welfare applicants to determine whether they are worthy of public help.

During the 1960s and 1970s, just about every issue or need that advocates for elderly people could identify as affecting older persons became a governmental responsibility: nutrition, legal, supportive, and leisure services; housing; home repair; energy assistance; transportation; employment assistance; job protection; public insurance for private pensions; special mental health programs; a separate National Institute on Aging; and on, and on, and on. By the late 1970s, if not earlier, American society had learned the catechism of compassionate ageism and had expressed it through a great many policies; a committee of the U.S. House of Representatives, using loose criteria, was able to count 134 programs benefiting aging people, overseen by 49 committees and subcommittees of Congress (U.S. House of Representatives, 1977).

"Greedy Geezers" and the Construct of "Intergenerational Equity"

Starting in 1978, the long-standing compassionate stereotypes of older persons began to undergo an extraordinary reversal. Older people came to be portrayed as one of the more flourishing and powerful groups in American society, and yet they were attacked as a burdensome responsibility. Throughout the 1980s and into the 1990s, the new stereotypes, readily observed in popular culture, depicted aged persons as prosperous, hedonistic, politically powerful, and selfish. For example, "Grays on the Go," a 1980 cover story in *Time,* was filled with pictures of senior surfers, senior swingers, and senior softball players. Elderly people were portrayed as America's new elite—healthy, wealthy, powerful, and "staging history's biggest retirement party" (Gibbs, 1988).

A dominant theme in such accounts of older Americans was that their selfishness was ruining the nation. The *New Republic* highlighted this motif with a drawing on the cover caricaturing aged persons, accompanied by the caption "greedy geezers." The table of contents "teaser" for the story that followed announced that "the real me generation isn't the yuppies, it's America's growing ranks of prosperous elderly" (Fairlie, 1988). This theme was echoed widely, and the epithet "greedy geezers" became familiar journalistic accounts of federal budget politics (e.g., Salholz, 1990). In the early 1990s, *Fortune* magazine declaimed that "The Tyranny of America's Old" is "one of the most crucial issues facing U.S. society" (Smith, 1992). These themes concerning seniors persist in public discourse, as evidenced by a story entitled "Meet the Greedy Grandparents" (Chapman, 2003) that commented on legislation in 2003 that provided some prescription drug coverage under Medicare.

Why the Reversal of Stereotypes?

The immediate precipitating factor for this reversal of stereotypes may have been the serious cash flow problem in the Social Security system that emerged within the larger context of a depressed economy during President Carter's administration (see Estes, 1983; Light, 1985). A high rate of unemployment substantially reduced the payroll tax base for Social Security revenue, while a high rate of inflation produced corresponding sharp increases in benefits through the program's cost-of-living adjustments.

Two additional elements contributed importantly. One was the tremendous growth in the amount and proportion of federal dollars·expended on benefits to aging citizens, which at that time had come to be more than one-quarter of our annual budget and comparable in size to expenditures on national defense. Journalists (e.g., Samuelson, 1978) and academicians (e.g., Hudson, 1978) began to notice and publicize this phenomenon in the late 1970s. By 1982, an economist in the Office of Management and Budget had pointed up the comparison with the defense budget by reframing the classical trade-off metaphor of political economy from "guns vs. butter" to "guns vs. canes" (Torrey, 1982). Another element in the reversal of the stereotypes of old age was dramatic improvements in the aggregate status of older Americans, in large measure due to the impact of federal benefit programs. The success of such programs had improved the economic status of aged persons to the point where journalists and social commentators could—with only superficial accuracy (see Quinn, 1987)—describe older people, on average, as more prosperous than the general population.

Intergenerational Equity: The Contemporary Dimension

In this unsympathetic climate of opinion, aged people emerged as a scapegoat for an impressive list of American problems, and the concept of so-called

intergenerational equity—really, intergenerational *inequity*—became prominent in public dialogue. At first, these issues of equity were propounded in a
contemporary dimension.

Demographers and advocates for children blamed the political power of elderly Americans for the plight of youngsters who have inadequate nutrition,
health care, and education and insufficiently supportive family environments
(e.g., Preston, 1984). One children's advocate even proposed that parents receive
an "extra vote" for each of their children, in order to combat older voters in an
intergenerational conflict (Carballo, 1981). Former secretary of commerce Peter Peterson (1987) suggested that a prerequisite for the United States to regain
its stature as a first-class power in the world economy was a sharp reduction in
programs benefiting older Americans. Widespread concerns about spiraling
U.S. health care costs were redirected, in part, from health care providers, sup-
pliers, administrators, and insurers—the parties that were responsible for
setting the prices of care—to the elderly persons for whom health care is provided. A number of academicians and public figures—including politicians—
expressed concern that health care expenditures on older persons would soon
absorb an unlimited amount of our national resources and crowd out health
care for others as well as various other worthy social causes (see Binstock and
Post, 1991). Some of them even proposed that old-age-based health care rationing was necessary, desirable, and just (e.g., Callahan, 1987).

By the end of the 1980s, the themes of intergenerational equity and conflict
had been adopted by the media and academics as routine perspectives for describing many social policy issues (see Cook et al., 1994) and had also gained
currency in elite sectors of American society and on Capitol Hill. For instance,
the president of the prestigious American Association of Universities asserted,
"The shape of the domestic federal budget inescapably pits programs for the
retired against every other social purpose dependent on federal funds" (Rosenzweig, 1990).

Indeed, the construct of intergenerational inequity had gained such a strong
foothold in the thinking of policy elites that they took it for granted as they analyzed American domestic policy issues. For example, in 1989 a distinguished
"executive panel" of American leaders convened by the Ford Foundation designated older persons as the only group of citizens that should be responsible
for financing a broad range of social programs for persons of all ages. In a report entitled *The Common Good: Social Welfare and the American Future*, the
panel recommended a series of policies, costing a total of $29 billion (Ford

Foundation, 1989). How did the panel propose that this $29 billion be financed? Solely by taxation of Social Security benefits. In fact, every financing alternative considered in the report assumed that elderly people should be the exclusive financiers of the panel's package of recommendations for improving social welfare in our nation. Apparently the Ford panel felt that the reasons for this assumption were self-evident; it did not even bother to justify its selections of these financing options, as opposed to others (also see, e.g., Beatty, 1990).

In this political climate, some of the long-standing structural features of old-age programs began undergoing significant revisions. A number of policy changes were made to reflect the diverse economic situations of elderly individuals (although the redistributive aspect of Social Security's benefit formulas had been quietly recognizing such diversity for many years). Some of the changes took benefits away from "greedy geezers." Others directed benefits toward poor older persons.

The Social Security Reform Act of 1983 began this trend by making Social Security benefits subject to taxation for the first time, at higher income levels. The Tax Reform Act of 1986, limited to just some older people the extra personal exemption that had been available to all persons 65 years and older when filing their federal income tax returns, and it provided new tax credits to very-low-income older persons on a sliding scale. The Older Americans Act programs of supportive and social services, for which all persons age 60 and older are eligible, became gradually targeted by Congress to low-income and minority elderly individuals. The Qualified Medicare Beneficiary and the Specified Low-Income Medicare Beneficiary programs, established by the Medicare Catastrophic Coverage Act (MCCA) of 1988, required Medicaid to pay Part B premiums, deductibles, and copayments for low-income older persons. The Omnibus Budget Reconciliation Act of 1993 continued this trend by adding to taxation of Social Security benefits.

The MCCA also introduced the notion that old-age benefits could be directly financed solely by program beneficiaries with no support from a payroll tax or general revenues. A portion of the bill (later repealed) provided that coverage for catastrophic hospital expenses be financed by surtaxes on the income of Medicare participants, calibrated on a sliding scale in relation to income.

These policy changes clearly established the principle that the diverse economic circumstances of older people can be addressed through politically feasible legislative reforms. Consequently, they set the stage for the legitimacy of complicated provisions of this kind that might be embodied in policy options to address both the still dire circumstance of many present older persons and the aging of the baby boom.

The Aging of the Baby Boom: Older People versus Society

The construct of intergenerational equity also had a future dimension, focusing on impending changes in the age structure of American society that would be brought about by the aging of the baby boom cohort, 76 million persons born between 1946 and 1964. One aspect of this issue was highlighted by the "generational accounting" analyses of economist Laurence Kotlikoff (1992) which, though controversial (see Haveman, 1994), received considerable attention. He suggested that future generations of older people will do less well than contemporary older people in terms of the taxes they pay for income security purposes and the subsequent lifetime payments they will receive through public programs.

But the more prominent aspect was concern about the consequences for society of sustaining the old-age welfare state in the twenty-first century when the baby boom becomes eligible for old-age benefit programs. This dimension was initially highlighted by the efforts of Americans for Generational Equity (AGE). Formed as an interest group in 1985, with backing from the corporate sector as well as a handful of congressmen who led it, AGE recruited some of the prominent "scapegoaters" of older people to its board and as its spokespersons. According to its annual reports, most of AGE's funding came from insurance companies, health care corporations, banks, and other private-sector businesses and organizations that are in financial competition with Medicare and Social Security (Quadagno, 1989).

Central to AGE's credo were the propositions that tomorrow's elderly baby boomers will be locked in an intergenerational conflict with younger age cohorts regarding the distribution of public resources. The organization disseminated this viewpoint from its Washington office through press releases, media interviews, a quarterly publication, a book (Longman, 1987), and periodic conferences with such titles as "Children at Risk: Who Will Support an Aging Society?" and "Medicare and the Baby Boom Generation." Although AGE faded from the scene at the end of the decade, its message concerning dire economic and social consequences of an aging society was taken up shortly thereafter by the Concord Coalition (1993), an organization founded by former senators Paul Tsongas and Warren Rudman.

The Era of Neoconservatism

Even as attention to the projected future costs and societal consequences of the aging of the baby boom characterized the politics of aging in the late 1980s and the 1990s, the broader political arena began to turn much more conservative than it had been since the New Deal. Bill Clinton, supported by the somewhat centrist Democratic Leadership Council, adopted the theme of "end big government as we know it." His most notable step in that direction was to sign the Republican-inspired Personal Responsibility and Work Opportunity Reconciliation Act (1996), commonly known as Welfare Reform.

Before the Republicans gained control of Congress in 1995, the U.S. old age welfare state was widely assumed to be a permanent feature of American society, especially the entitlement programs, Social Security and Medicare. Changes in these programs might take place, but their general contours would remain the same and their revenues and expenditures would probably continue to grow.

However, the escalation of conservatism as the Republicans took control of Congress in 1995, combined with growing concerns about the impact of an aging baby boom on future entitlement obligations, began to undermine that assumption. Another ingredient in the mix was the bipartisan belief at the time that growing budget deficits had to be brought under control, Social Security and Medicare being the two largest expenditure items.

Conservatism and Medicare

Toward this end, Congress submitted to President Clinton a budget bill for fiscal year 1996 that included a $452 billion reduction in projected Medicare and Medicaid spending over seven years. Although the president was willing to approve smaller reductions in Medicare and Medicaid spending, he vetoed the bill, citing the size of the reduction and some structural changes proposed for the programs among his reasons for doing so.

Meanwhile, Congress and the administration were shifting some measure of Medicare's financial risk to the private sector by encouraging the proliferation of Medicare managed care organizations (MCOs). In 1990, 3 percent of Medicare beneficiaries were enrolled in MCOs; by the end of 1997, the proportion had climbed to 14 percent (Medicare Payment Advisory Commission, 1998). In contrast to the traditional fee-for-service (FFS) reimbursement system under

Medicare, MCOs limit the federal government's financial risk in that Medicare makes a fixed per capita payment to these organizations for each Medicare participant they enroll; in turn, the MCOs are responsible for providing all needed services that are covered by Medicare.

The strategy of shifting financial risk from the government to the private sector was amplified by the Balanced Budget Act of 1997 (BBA97), which established the Medicare+Choice program. Through this program, beneficiaries could choose from a panoply of private-sector options for receiving their health care. The strategy proved to be less than a success, however. The percentage of Medicare enrollees opting for MCOs and other private-sector options reached a peak of 16 percent in 1999 before dropping to 11 percent in 2003 (Pear, 2003).

BBA97 also created the Bipartisan Commission on the Future of Medicare. A majority of the commission members wanted to complete the transition from the FFS system by proposing that each Medicare enrollee be given a voucher by the government to shop for insurance in the private sector. Two members who were sympathetic to the voucher proposal also demanded that adequate outpatient prescription drug coverage under Medicare be included in return for their votes supporting vouchers. Failing to win this concession, they did not join the majority, and the commission was unable to make an official recommendations when it concluded its work in 1998 (Pear, 1999; Vladeck, 1999). Yet these dynamics of the commission set the stage for further efforts to cover prescription drugs and to privatize Medicare.

During the 2000 presidential election campaign, both candidates pledged to secure Medicare prescription drug coverage. Then, when congressional Republicans took control of both houses in 2003, they joined President Bush in viewing legislation to cover drugs as an opportunity to curry favor with older voters, perhaps displacing Democrats as the traditional champions of Medicare. However, by the time a final bill was enacted—formally named the Medicare Prescription Drug, Improvement, and Modernization of Medicare Act (MMA) of 2003—it also contained many features to lure Medicare participants into private-sector health plans and to subsidize private Medicare plans to make them more attractive to both providers and potential enrollees (Freudenheim, 2004). According to the actuary of the Centers for Medicare and Medicaid Services, an estimated increase of $46 billion in Medicare payments would be provided to the private plans over the 10 years following the legislation (Pear, 2004). Ultimately, of course, a strategic goal of expanding Medicare enrollments in private plans is to shift the financial risk of paying doctors, hospitals, and other health care providers from the government to the private sector and to program beneficiaries.

Conservatism and Social Security

Privatizing Social Security has been on the agenda of conservatives and libertarian think tanks since the 1970s (Williamson, 1997) but did not reach the mainstream political agenda until the late 1990s. A key event was a 1997 report of an Advisory Council on Social Security that addressed long-term financing issues facing the Old-Age and Survivors Insurance (OASI) program. It presented three plans for partially privatizing OASI as a means of improving the long-range financial status of the traditional program and/or providing retired workers with a greater probability of sufficient income in retirement (Advisory Council on Social Security, 1997). Each called for investing tens to hundreds of billions of additional dollars in the private sector.

These and subsequent proposals for partial privatization, from Democratic and Republican members of Congress as well as other sources, transformed the politics of Social Security reform. The rapidity with which this notion gained political acceptability was underscored in the spring of 1998 when the Senate passed a resolution calling for private investment accounts to be part of any Social Security reform package (Stevenson, 1998b). By that summer, the president was seriously considering some form of equity investment as part of Social Security reform (Stevenson, 1998a).

George Bush picked up this theme during his 2000 election campaign, and in his first year in office he appointed a special commission on Social Security reform that included only members who were in favor of privatization ideas. Events related to 9/11 pushed these ideas and the commission's report into the background, but key members of the Bush administration continued to make clear that they intended to eventually move forward on the agenda of privatizing Social Security.

Sure enough, when President Bush began his second term in 2005, he launched a vigorous campaign to privatize Social Security. He personally undertook a speaking agenda, described by the White House as "60 stops in 60 days," to decry the status of the Social Security program. He repeatedly asserted that the program was imminently headed for disaster—that it soon would be "flat bust" (see, e.g., Bumiller, 2005) and that it was "headed toward bankruptcy" (see Bush, 2005). He blatantly ignored the fact that the shortfall estimated to be around 26 percent was not projected to begin until the 2040s—more than three decades hence. To undermine confidence in Social Security financing, President Bush even undertook a "photo-op" trip to an office building in Parkersburg, West Virginia, home of the U.S. Federal Bureau of Public Debt. There he ceremonially opened a file cabinet holding the U.S. Treasury bonds that have accrued as reserves in the Social Security Trust Funds and declared these U.S. bonds to be worthless; he described them as "just IOUs" and asserted that "there is no trust fund" (Vieth and Simon, 2005).

Political Obstacles to Contemporary Action

Although the economic and political challenges of sustaining (and perhaps improving) the old-age welfare state for the elderly years of baby boomers appear substantial, a number of politicians, policy analysts, commissions, committees, and organizations have generated proposals for dealing with them. An excellent example is Peter Diamond and Peter Orszag's chapter in this volume (Chapter 15). Yet U.S. political leaders seem reluctant to take action to meet these challenges other than through periodic minor measures to encourage Medicare enrollees to enroll in managed care.

What might happen if action is postponed until most baby boomers have reached the ranks of old age? Most analyses of this issue conclude that the economic costs will be far greater if Congress keeps waiting to deal with these challenges (e.g., see Congressional Budget Office, 2003; Social Security and Medicare Boards of Trustees, 2006). Various commentators have generated apocalyptic scenarios of the consequences of delaying action. Some have argued, for example, that it will be essential for Medicare to deny reimbursement for life-saving care of older people (e.g., Callahan, 1987). Others have suggested that aged baby boomers, in their self-interested pursuit of governmental benefits, will pose a fundamental threat to democracy and that class warfare will take place between the young and the old (e.g., Thurow, 1996). Although such apocalyptic visions are likely to be far off the mark, our society may find it difficult economically and politically to ensure adequate levels of income, medical care, and other supports for many older people if action is postponed until baby boomers have all joined the ranks of old age. Even now, there are some perennial political forces that tend to make such policy changes difficult.

The Aging of the Baby Boom Is Not an Immediate Crisis

Sustaining the old-age welfare state for aged baby boomers is not an immediate crisis. But elections are always imminent as crises for most politicians. Except for the rare individual who aspires to be a statesman—according to either contemporary or historical perspectives—today's politicians would lose little, if anything, by failing to deal with the policy challenges posed by an aged baby boom several decades hence. Most of them will be long gone from public life when the chickens come home to roost. In contrast, if they support policy changes that prove to be rather immediately unpopular, they could well incur substantial retribution from voters and other vested interests that have a substantial stake in the status quo.

Who Gains If Action Is Postponed?

The list of parties with vested interests in the status quo of the old-age welfare state is substantial. In addition to older people themselves, it includes the insurance industry, health care providers, long-term-care providers, the "retirement living" industry, "elder law" attorneys, financial counselors, pension funds, organized labor, and the aging services network, to name some—and even AARP (formerly the American Association of Retired Persons), which operates old-age affinity businesses for its 35 million members, yielding, together with dues, annual revenue of $878 million in 2004 (AARP, 2005).

What about the vested interest of today's older voters in the old-age welfare state? After all, a ubiquitous journalistic cliché for warning politicians is that "Social Security is the third rail of American politics—touch it and you're dead!"

Empirically, this cliché has not held up because there are many fundamental reasons why older people do not vote in a cohesive fashion, including the fact that they are as heterogeneous in their political attachments as the rest of the electorate (see Binstock and Quadagno, 2001). Even when old-age policy issues are prominent in presidential election campaigns (the arena most salient to old-age policies), the votes of older persons distribute among the major-party candidates in roughly the same proportions as do those of younger age groups (see Connelly, 2000).

Nonetheless, older voters do have an indirect latent group power that affects political elites, a power that does not necessarily require a behavioral reality of electoral cohesion. Members of Congress are characteristically concerned with how the next legislative vote they cast might become a defining issue—negative or positive—in their next electoral campaigns (see Arnold, 1992). Politicians at all levels know that older persons vote at a higher rate than other age groups and that they are a steadily increasing percentage of voters (Binstock, 2000). So politicians look for opportunities to curry favor with older voters, as exemplified by the efforts of President Bush and congressional Republicans to enact a Medicare prescription drug bill in 2003 (Toner, 2003). At the same time, they are wary of being cast as villains with respect to old-age policies. With the aging of the baby boom still a distant and abstract crisis, members of Congress are reluctant to make major changes in Social Security and Medicare to sustain the programs for the future.

What Might Enhance Action on Policies for the Aging of the Baby Boom?

Because of the political factors sketched out above, as well as for other reasons, there are no indications that political leaders are moving to take action on policies to sustain Social Security and Medicare for the baby boomers and beyond. What might make near-term adoption of such policies more politically feasible?

Advance Planning, Distant Startup, and Gradualism

Today's politicians might espouse and support a policy option that, though enacted now, calls for changes that would begin to take place in the near to medium-term future—and perhaps be implemented gradually from that point on. Such a policy would be unlikely to offend older or younger voters, and many of the various business and professional interests that are vested in the policy status quo would have sufficient time to adapt.

The Social Security Reform Act of 1983 provides an excellent illustration of this approach. Among other things, it enacted a change in the "normal retirement age" for full Social Security benefits, from age 65 to age 67. Yet the change was not scheduled to begin until 20 years later, in 2003, and to take an additional 24 years to be fully implemented in 2027. This policy change elicited little outrage, unrest, or opposition, either from voters or from vested interests (such as employers, whose successors would have to pay more months and years of payroll taxes for whatever employees they might have in the future).

In contrast, the portion of the Medicare Catastrophic Coverage Act of 1998 that required older persons to begin paying immediately out of their own pockets for insurance for extended hospital stays, at a rather steep rate, was repealed almost immediately following vociferous outcries from a minority of older persons (see Himmelfarb, 1995).

The change in Social Security's normal retirement age is a felicitous political model. It combined advanced planning with a far distant and gradually implemented policy change to deal with the aging of the baby boom. Consequently, it engendered little opposition from old-age advocacy groups or any other parties.

Unfortunately, from a policymaking point of view, the years when the baby boom will reach old age are not now far distant. Yet there is still some time left for the use of advance planning and gradualism to moderate political opposition.

Whatever policy options one has in mind, for example, they will probably involve measures for increasing dedicated revenue. Following the 1983 model of advance planning, an increase in the payroll tax, and/or the institution of a sales tax, or even a value-added tax, could be scheduled to begin some 5 to 10 or so years from now at minuscule rates. Then the tax (or taxes) could be scheduled to increase gradually over a number of years. Similarly, on the expenditure-reduction side, upward changes in the age of eligibility for benefits, for instance, could also be phased in gradually after a startup some years hence.

An approach of this kind, however, may not be sufficient in itself to enable a policy option to receive serious attention and possibly be adopted. Although the establishment of small new and gradually increased revenue sources, for example, would be unlikely to incur much of an outcry from voters, for whom the proposed changes would seem distant and relatively negligible, conservative politicians would be unhappy with the principle of "raising taxes." Employers would certainly oppose, say, an increase in their share of a payroll tax (although there is no inherent reason why the increase could not be confined to the employee share). Business and consumer groups could be expected to register opposition (although the distance and gradualism of implementation for such policies would be moderating factors). So, even if policy options to deal with the aging of the baby boom incorporated features of advance planning, distant start-up, and gradualism—more would be needed.

Crisis as a Context for Getting Attention

At various times in American history, relatively radical social legislation has been politically feasible because the economic and social contexts of the time generated a sufficient sense of public crisis to overcome our endemic fragmentation of power and the many vested interests in the status quo. Certainly, the New Deal (though hardly comprised of a single, integrated policy option) was the product of such a sense of crisis. One might also argue that the Great Society programs came out of a sense of crisis, whether that sense had its roots in the national reaction to the assassination of President Kennedy or in President Johnson's capacity to generate a sense of crisis concerning the plight of the poor and the social unrest in our inner cities—or both.

Perhaps near-term attention to sustaining Social Security and Medicare would be feasible if the aging of the baby boom were more successfully marketed as a crisis. Although many policy analysts and elite commentators keep writing and speaking about the aging of the baby boom as a looming crisis in American society (e.g., see Peterson, 1999), there is little sign, if any, that the general public or even the media are engaged with this set of issues from a crisislike perspective. This is understandable in the nature of the case—issues involving a far distant period portrayed by a lot of boring demographic and program expenditure projections.

Anthony Downs (1972) argued that there is an "issue-attention cycle" in American politics, rooted both in the nature of certain domestic problems and in the way major communications media interact with the public. With respect to the aging of the baby boom, we are in what he terms the "preproblem" stage of the cycle when the problem exists "but has not yet captured much public attention, even though some experts or interest groups may already be alarmed by it" (p. 39). What does it take to move from the "preproblem" stage to a "critical problem" stage? Downs suggests that "a problem must be dramatic and exciting to maintain public interest because news is 'consumed' by much of the American public (and by publics everywhere) largely as a form of entertainment" (p. 42).

How could the aging of the baby boom be made more dramatic and more successful in the competition for news coverage? I am far from being an expert in communications and marketing, but I will sketch out one approach at the risk of seeming unsophisticated in this realm of affairs.

The fundamental strategy would be to undertake a media campaign that portrays the aging of the baby boom as *a crisis for baby boomers, their families, and society—rather than a Social Security crisis and a Medicare crisis.* The central focus would be on *people rather than programs.* The key would be to convey the costs of policy inaction in terms of what it would mean tomorrow for older people, the nature of family obligations and lifestyles, and the fabric of familiar social institutions that are integral to daily life.

Such a campaign—perhaps undertaken by a president or some other political figure who can readily command media attention, or by some well-funded organizational entity—should be strategically targeted to the 76 million baby boomers and be strong enough to compete with anti-aging marketing campaigns that tell this audience how to avoid growing old (Mehlman et al., 2004). Its initial goal should be to convey to baby boomers (perhaps in a congratulatory fashion) that they will live for many, many years as older Americans. (If old-age-related marketing to baby boomers seems far-fetched, we should be mindful that AARP has been already engaged in doing so for some time. Witness the special issue of its magazine that pictured Susan Sarandon on the cover and featured a survey of the sex habits of Americans age 45 and older [Jacoby, 1999] and a recent cover story in *AARP—The Magazine* on the political attitudes of baby boomers [Keating, 2004].) Perhaps a complementary aspect of this first "congratulatory" phase would be to effectively inform baby boomers about the benefits of the old-age welfare state.

The next element would be to develop and convey scenarios that depict what life will be like for aged baby boomers if nothing is done to reconfigure the old-age welfare state and thereby sustain government supports at a level that is reasonably comparable to what older Americans experienced in the last three decades of the twentieth century. What will the budgets of elderly couples and aged widows be like in terms of how much they have to spend on food, shelter, clothing, utilities, transportation, medical care, and long-term care? For those who are less than wealthy, what limits might exist on their access to medical care and high-cost, high-tech medical interventions, particularly at advanced old ages? Will many older persons have to be financially supported by their children? Will American society witness, due to the necessity of family economics, the return of three- and perhaps four-generation households? Such questions could be countless.

The generation and promulgation of scenarios that answer these questions might be enough to help baby boomers and their families feel that a sufficient "crisis" looms in societal support for the basic needs of tomorrow's older people to warrant policy action in the near-term future. If an issue as abstract, unfamiliar, and seemingly distant in consequences as global warming can reach the policy agenda, then near-term policies to meet the challenges of population aging surely could if the not-too-distant consequences are conveyed in terms of daily lives rather than projected program deficits.

If the scenery for the play of daily life in our aging society can be effectively painted for the American public, what else is needed to mobilize popular support for dealing with an aging society? As implied above, the daily issues confronting older people are not now, and will not be then, hermetically sealed from the rest of society. Perhaps the way to gain widespread political support is to paint policy options for an aging society as *family policies* (see Harrington, 1999). If they prove to be effective, in many ways that is what—in effect—they will be.

Conclusion

When most of the baby boomers will have reached the ranks of old age, 20 or 25 years from now, our economy may not be prosperous. If we postpone until then the challenges of dealing with the aging of the baby boom, confronting them may be economically and politically overwhelming. Moreover, the circumstances of daily life for older people might well resemble the difficult economic and health care situations that earlier cohorts of older persons experienced before the construction of the old-age welfare state. Perhaps some of the apocalyptic visions of intergenerational conflict—class warfare between the young and the old—will become reality.

Although the adoption of forward-looking policies may seem politically difficult at the moment, my view is that it can be done in the near future. We need to take advantage of the fact that we still (but not for long) have time to employ the strategy of a semidistant startup for new measures, with gradual implementation. We need to convey a sense of crisis, in a futuristic dimension, by focusing on the crises that will be entailed for people, not programs. And we need political leadership that can frame the issues of the baby boom's old age in terms that enable us to understand that all of us—not just those of us who will be old at the time—will be affected. In short, if we can be brought to understand that "the beneficiaries 'R' us," we may have the political will to take action.

Acknowledgments

Portions of this chapter are adapted from "The Contemporary Politics of Old Age Policies," in *The New Politics of Old Age Policy,* edited by Robert B. Hudson. © 2005 The Johns Hopkins University Press.

REFERENCES

Aaron, H. J. 2002. Budget estimates: What we know, what we can't know, and why it matters. In S. H. Altman and D. I. Shactman, eds., *Policies for an Aging Society,* pp. 63–80. Baltimore: Johns Hopkins University Press.

AARP. 2005. *Annual Report 2004* and *Consolidated Financial Statements as of December 31, 2004.* Retrieved from www.aarp.org/about_aarp/aarp/_overview/a2003-06-24-annualreport-03.html (page discontinued).

Advisory Council on Social Security. 1997. *Report of the 1994–1996 Advisory Council on Social Security.* Vol. 1, *Findings and Recommendations.* Washington, DC: U.S. Government Printing Office.

Arnold, R. D. 1992. *The Logic of Congressional Action.* New Haven, CT: Yale University Press.

Beatty, J. 1990. A post–cold war budget. *Atlantic Monthly* 256(2):74–82.

Binstock, R. 2000. Older people and voting participation: Past and future. *Gerontologist* 40:18–31.

Binstock, R. H., and Post, S. G., eds. 1991. *Too Old for Health Care? Controversies in Medicine, Law, Economics, and Ethics.* Baltimore: Johns Hopkins University Press.

Binstock, R. H., and Quadagno, J. 2001. Aging and politics. In R. H. Binstock and L. K. George, eds., *Handbook of Aging and the Social Sciences,* 5th ed., pp. 333–51. San Diego: Academic Press.

Bumiller, E. 2005. Bush presses his argument for Social Security change. *New York Times,* January 12, p. A18.

Bush, G. W. 2005. Transcript: President Bush's state of the union address. *New York Times,* February 3.

Callahan, D. 1987. *Setting Limits: Medical Goals in an Aging Society.* New York: Simon & Schuster.

Carballo, M. 1981. Extra votes for parents? *Boston Globe,* December 17, p. 35.

Chapman, S. 2003. *Meet the greedy grandparents.* Slate, December 10. Retrieved from http://slate.msn.com/id/2092302/%20.

Clark, R. L. 1990. Income maintenance policies in the United States. In R. H. Binstock and L. K. George, eds., *Handbook of Aging and the Social Sciences,* 3rd ed., pp. 382–97. San Diego: Academic Press.

Concord Coalition. 1993. *The Zero Deficit Plan: A Plan for Eliminating the Federal Budget Deficit by the Year 2000.* Washington, DC: Concord Coalition.

Congressional Budget Office. 2003. *The Long-Term Budget Outlook.* Washington, DC: Congressional Budget Office. December.

Congressional Budget Office. 2004a. *The Budget and Economic Outlook: Fiscal Years 2005 to 2014.* Washington, DC: Congressional Budget Office. January.

Congressional Budget Office. 2004b. *The Outlook for Social Security.* Washington, DC: Congressional Budget Office. June.

Connelly, M. 2000. Who voted: A portrait of American politics, 1976–2000. *New York Times,* November 12, wk p. 4.

Cook, F. L., Marshall, V. M., Marshall, J. E., and Kaufman, J. E. 1994. The salience of intergenerational equity in Canada and the United States. In T. R. Marmor, T. M. Smeeding, and V. L. Greene, eds., *Economic Security and Intergenerational Justice: A Look at North America,* pp. 91–129. Washington, DC: Urban Institute Press.

Downs, A. 1972. Up and down with ecology: The "issue-attention cycle." *Public Interest* 28(summer):38–50.

Estes, C. L. 1983. Social Security: The social construction of a crisis. *Milbank Memorial Fund Quarterly/Health and Society* 61:445–61.

Fairlie, H. 1988. Talkin' bout my generation. *New Republic,* March 28, 19–22.

Federal Interagency Forum on Aging Related Statistics. 2004. *Older Americans 2000: Key Indicators of Well-Being.* Retrieved from www.agingstats.gov/tables%202001/tables-economics.html#Indicator%208.

Ford Foundation, Project on Social Welfare and the American Future, Executive Panel. 1989. *The Common Good: Social Welfare and the American Future.* New York: Ford Foundation.

Freudenheim, M. 2004. Using new Medicare billions, H.M.O.'s again court elderly. *New York Times,* March 9, p. A1.

Gibbs, N. R. 1988. Grays on the go. *Time,* February 22, pp. 66–75.

Harrington, M. 1999. *Care and Equality: Inventing a New Family Politics.* New York: Knopf.

Haveman, R. 1994. Should generational accounts replace public budgets and deficits? *Journal of Economic Perspectives* 8(winter):95–111.

Himmelfarb, R. 1995. *Catastrophic Politics: The Rise and Fall of the Medicare Catastrophic Coverage Act of 1988.* University Park: Pennsylvania State University Press.

Hudson, R. B. 1978. The "graying" of the federal budget and its consequences for old age policy. *Gerontologist* 18:428–40.

Jacoby, S. 1999. Great sex: What's age got to do with it? *Modern Maturity,* September–October.

Kalish, R. A. 1979. The new ageism and the failure models: A polemic. *Gerontologist* 19:398–407.

Keating, P. 2004. Wake-up call. *AARP—The Magazine,* September–October.

Kotlikoff, L. J. 1992. *Generational Accounting: Knowing Who Pays, and When, for What We Spend.* New York: Free Press.

Light, P. C. 1985. *Artful Work: The Politics of Social Security Reform.* New York: Random House.

Longman, P. 1987. *Born to Pay: The New Politics of Aging in America.* Boston: Houghton Mifflin.

Medicare Payment Advisory Commission. 1998. *Report to the Congress: Medicare Pay-*

ment Policy. Vol. 1, *Recommendations.* Washington, DC: U.S. Government Printing Office.

Mehlman, M. J., Binstock, R. H., Juengst, E. T., Ponsaran, R. S., and Whitehouse, P. J. 2004. Anti-aging medicine: Can consumers be better protected? *Gerontologist* 44:304–10.

Moon, M. 2006. *Medicare: A Policy Primer.* Washington, DC: Urban Institute Press.

Neugarten, B. L. 1970. The old and the young in modern societies. *American Behavioral Scientist* 14:13–24.

Palmore, E. B. 1990. *Ageism: Negative and Positive.* New York: Springer.

Pear, R. 1999. Medicare panel, sharply divided, submits no plan. *New York Times,* March 17, p. A1.

Pear, R. 2003. Fewer people on Medicare are dropped by H.M.O.'s. *New York Times,* September 9, p. A21.

Pear, R. 2004. Medicare actuary gives wanted data to Congress. *New York Times,* March 20, p. A8.

Personal Responsibility and Work Opportunity Reconciliation Act. 1996. Public Law No. 104-93.

Peterson, P. G. 1987. The morning after. *Atlantic Monthly,* October, pp. 43–49.

Peterson, P. G. 1999. *Gray Dawn: How the Coming Age Wave Will Transform America—and the World.* New York: Times Books.

Preston, S. H. 1984. Children and the elderly in the U.S. *Scientific American,* December, pp. 44–49.

Quadagno, J. 1989. Generational equity and the politics of the welfare state. *Politics and Society* 17:353–76.

Quinn, J. 1987. The economic status of the elderly: Beware the mean. *Review of Income and Wealth* 33(1):63–82.

Rosenzweig, R. M. 1990. Address to the president's opening session, 43rd Annual Meeting of the Gerontological Society of America, Boston, MA, November 16.

Salholz, E. 1990. Blaming the voters: Hapless budgeteers single out "greedy geezers." *Newsweek,* October 29, p. 36.

Samuelson, R. J. 1978. Aging America: Who will shoulder the growing burden? *National Journal* 10:1712–17.

Smith, L. 1992. The tyranny of America's old. *Fortune* 125(1):68–72.

Social Security Administration. 2004. *Income of the Aged Chartbook.* Retrieved from www.ssa.gov/policy/docs/chartbooks/income_aged/2001/iac01.pdf.

Social Security and Medicare Boards of Trustees. 2006. *Status of the Social Security and Medicare Programs: A Summary of the 2006 Annual Reports.* Retrieved from www.socialsecurity.gov/OACT/TRSUM/trsummary.hmtl (page discontinued; last accessed May 2, 2006).

Steuerle, E., and Van de Water, P. N. 2002. Long-run budget projections and their implications for funding elderly entitlements. In S. H. Altman and D. I. Shactman, eds., *Policies for an Aging Society,* pp. 81–108. Baltimore: Johns Hopkins University Press.

Stevenson, R. W. 1998a. Clinton may use Wall Street to ease Social Security ills. *New York Times,* July 28, p. A9.

Stevenson, R. W. 1998b. Privatization of Social Security is gaining ground. *New York Times,* April 6, p. A1.

Thurow, L. C. 1996. The birth of a revolutionary class. *New York Times Magazine,* May 19, pp. 46–47.

Toner, R. 2003. G.O.P. steals thunder. *New York Times,* June 28, p. A1.

Torrey, B. B. 1982. Guns vs. canes: The fiscal implications of an aging population. *American Economics Association Papers and Proceedings* 72:309–13.

U.S. Census Bureau. 2005a. *Annual Demographic Survey.* Retrieved from http://pubdb3 .census.gov/macro/032005/pov/toc.html (page discontinued).

U.S. Census Bureau. 2005b. People with or without health insurance coverage by selected characteristics: 2004 and 2005. Table 8. Retrieved from www.census.gov/ prod/2006pubs/p60–231.pdf (accessed December 4, 2006).

U.S. Census Bureau. 2005c. *Poverty Thresholds: Preliminary Estimates of Weighted Average Poverty Thresholds for 2005.* Retrieved from www.census.gov/hhes/www/poverty/ threshld/05prelim.html.

U.S. House of Representatives. 1977. *Federal Responsibility to the Elderly: Executive Programs and Legislative Jurisdiction.* Report of the Select Committee on Aging. Washington, DC: U.S. Government Printing Office.

Vieth, W., and Simon, R. 2005. President casts doubt on trust fund: Promoting his private account plan, Bush calls the Social Security bonds held for future beneficiaries "just IOUs" sitting in a filing cabinet. *Los Angeles Times,* April 6. Retrieved from http://pqasb.pqarchiver.com/latimes/advancedsearch.html.

Vladeck, B. C. 1999. Plenty of nothing—a report from the Medicare commission. *New England Journal of Medicine* 340:1503–6.

Williamson, J. B. 1997. A critique of the case for privatizing Social Security. *Gerontologist* 37:561–71.

IV / Health and Wealth

Whose Responsibility?

CHAPTER THIRTEEN

Social Security Reform and Responsibility across the Generations

Framing the Debate

John B. Williamson, Ph.D.

Recent projections by the Board of Trustees (2006), the group charged with overseeing the Social Security program, suggest that if no changes in policy are made and current trends continue, the Social Security trust funds will be depleted by 2040. Their prediction does not mean 2040 is the exact year in which the depletion would occur, since projections are made each year and it is common for them to fluctuate. Furthermore, it does not mean that in 2040 there would be no money to pay Social Security benefits, because billions of dollars in contributions would flow into the system in that year and in every year thereafter. In the unlikely event that no legislative changes are made between now and then and the trust funds are depleted, it will be necessary to either increase payroll taxes starting in that year or to reduce pension benefits substantially. The current estimate is that a balance of revenues and pension benefits could be achieved through either a 26 percent reduction in the pension benefits starting in 2040 (increasing to 30% by 2080) or an increase of the payroll tax by 5.1 percentage points (split evenly between employers and employees) starting in the same year (increasing to 6.3 percentage points by 2080). It is more likely that the gap would be filled by a combination of a benefit reduction of about half this size paired with a payroll tax increase of about half this size. However, even these changes would not keep the Social Security Trust Funds in balance indefinitely into the future. Over subsequent decades, it would likely be necessary to gradually phase in some combination of additional benefit cuts and payroll tax increases. All reputable Social Security analysts and commentators agree that by about 2040 the Social Security program will be facing a serious funding problem unless steps are taken between now and then to deal with the situation.

Is Social Security facing a funding "crisis," or is it facing a funding shortfall calling for modest reforms? The answer experts give to this question tends to reflect their political ideology, particularly with respect to social welfare issues. Both those on the right and those on the left believe they are being objective, and both believe people with opposing views are allowing their ideological beliefs to distort their perception about the seriousness of future funding problems and about the viability of various proposed solutions to the problem. This debate is part of the ideological contest between those on the right, who are seeking to reduce projected future increases in public spending on Social Security, and those on the left, who want to reform Social Security in such a way as to maintain its traditional structure and objectives.

The goals of this chapter are (1) to review the history of the debate over the so-called Social Security crisis, (2) to situate this debate within the more general contest between the right and the left over how to frame discourse about Social Security reform, and (3) to present policy alternatives linked to two of the most important frames (or interpretative packages) used in the debate over Social Security reform. In my discussion of policy proposals reflecting the generational-equity frame, I will focus on proposals suggested by a commission (President's Commission, 2001) set up by President George W. Bush. In my discussion of proposals reflecting the generational-interdependence frame, I will focus on proposals made in a recent book by Peter Diamond and Peter Orszag titled *Saving Social Security* (2004).

The Origins of the Debate over the Social Security "Crisis"

The so-called Social Security crisis has a long history. People on the right have been using this term since the late 1970s to describe both short-term and long-term projected shortfalls in Social Security funding. It was used in the debate leading up to the 1977 Social Security reforms and then again in the debate leading up to the 1983 Social Security reforms (Kingson, 1984; Williamson and Watts-Roy, 1999). Over the past 20 years the expression has continued to be employed, particularly in op-eds, and in the popular press more generally. However, it is of note that this expression has been used almost exclusively by those on the right. People on the left describe the same long-term projections in different terms. They have used such expressions as "projected funding shortfall" to label the same evidence with respect to the Social Security deficit currently projected to emerge in about 2042 if no policy changes are made between now and then other than those already legislated. The disagreement has been more over how to label these projected deficits than over their actual size.

What is going on? My interpretation is that Social Security commentators on the right prefer to use strong language in an effort to hype the seriousness of the problem so as to generate political support for their agenda, which is to introduce major structural reforms in Social Security designed to reduce its role as a source of retirement income in favor of some form of partial privatization. Given the pervasive popularity of Social Security as it is currently structured, the general public must first be convinced that the program really is in a state of crisis if they are to take seriously the rhetoric from the right calling for radical reforms. Social Security commentators on the left, in contrast, have responded by using language suggesting that the projected financing problems can easily be dealt with using a series of modest reforms that will retain the basic integrity of the current structure of the program.

During the early years of this debate, much of the effort from the right was aimed at convincing the general public that Social Security benefits to current retirees should be reduced or at least not allowed to grow in accordance with existing projections (Ferrara, 1982; Longman, 1982). One reason given was that when the baby boom generation retires, the program will go bankrupt (or in a slightly less polemic version of the argument, that it will be necessary to radically reduce benefits or radically increase payroll taxes) because of the projected spending bulge associated with the retirement of these boomers (Chakravarty and Weisman, 1988; Fairlie, 1988; Longman, 1985, 1987). The taxing power of the U.S. government, which could and would be used to prevent Social Security from going "bankrupt," was not mentioned; instead the analogy was frequently made to a family that exhausts its savings account by poor money management over the years. Eventually efforts by commentators on the right met with considerable, but not complete, success. They managed to convince a huge fraction of the population that the Social Security system was at high risk of going bankrupt. The critics of Social Security were successful in their efforts to undermine confidence in Social Security, but they were much less successful in their efforts to undermine support for the program (Reno and Friedland, 1997). This latter objective has long been and remains the ultimate goal for many of the most conservative analysts and commentators (Butler and Germanis, 1983).

During the past 15 years, there have been some shifts in the arguments made from the right in connection with the "Social Security funding crisis." There has been much more emphasis on the need to give workers ownership rights in connection with their Social Security pensions (Borden, 1995; Ferrara and Tanner, 1998). The objective has been to respond to the Social Security funding "crisis" by redefining the goals of the Social Security program. The traditional social insurance goals have been de-emphasized and arguments have been made suggesting that the program needs to be restructured so that it is much more of a retirement savings program (Bipartisan Commission, 1995). Instead of thinking of Social Security contributions as the analog to payments made in connection with a heath insurance policy, workers are urged to think of Social Security as a retirement savings account along the lines of a 401(k) plan. They are not encouraged to think about the program in terms such as shared risk or solidarity between generations. Instead they are prompted to envision the returns they are getting on their "contributions" relative to returns they would receive if those same contributions were made to their 401(k) accounts. In addition, they are often being asked to compare Social Security, a program that provides survivor benefits, provides disability benefits, and protects pension benefits from the effects of inflation after retirement, with a 401(k)-like scheme that does not include any of these major added benefits and protections.

Framing the Debate over Social Security Reform

During the 1980s, the "fiscal crisis" framing of the debate over Social Security reform evolved into what came to be referred to as the "generational equity" perspective on Social Security reform (Ferrara, 1985; Longman, 1985). The use of the generational-equity frame persists today, but its use has fallen off somewhat since the late 1990s (Williamson, McNamara, and Howling, 2003). This framing of the debate over Social Security reform proved to be useful as a vehicle linking the idea of a fiscal crisis to the idea that at least partially privatizing Social Security would be a sensible response to that crisis. In the following two sections I analyze the ideological contest between this "generational equity" frame on the right and an alternative "generational interdependence" frame that evolved as a response to the generational-equity frame from its critics on the left.

For the most part, what has come to be referred to as the generational-equity debate has taken place in the mass media, particularly the print media. The media provide a series of arenas, such as editorials and political cartoons, in which opposing camps put forth their perspective on the debate (Gurevitch and Levy, 1985). Because the mass media often report social issues as "crises," they are prone to interpret evidence of a projected funding shortfall in Social Security as a crisis. By framing programs such as Social Security and Medicare as being in crisis, advocates of the generational-equity perspective are attempting to create pressure for immediate and fundamental structure changes to these programs.

The Generational-Equity Framing of the Debate

At the heart of the generational-equity interpretative package is the idea that each generation should provide for itself (Beard and Williamson, 2004). Proponents of this perspective offer a way to view old-age policy that often leads to proposals to cut back on entitlement programs for elderly people and to place more emphasis on privatized alternatives such as the partial privatization of the Social Security program. Beginning in the mid-1980s, advocates of what has come to be referred to as the generational-equity perspective argued that there was a conflict of interest between elderly people, on the one hand, and the working-age population and/or their children, on the other. These advocates included a number of analysts linked to conservative think tanks such as the Olin Foundation and the Cato Institute and journalists associated with conservative magazines such as the *National Review* and conservative newspapers such as the *Wall Street Journal* (Williamson, McNamara, and Howling, 2003). This network also came to include some organizations formed specifically to advocate on behalf of public policies linked to the generational-equity perspective. Of particular note in this context was Americans for Generational Equity, founded by Senator David Durenburger and funded by several conservative foundations and large corporations (Binstock, 1999; Quadagno, 1989).

The writing of the well-respected demographer Samuel Preston (1984) was extensively cited as a source of scientific support for the generational-equity perspective. He presented evidence that the economic status of elderly people had been improving while that of children had been deteriorating in recent decades. His interpretation of these data was that, at least in part, the improving economic status of elderly people had been achieved at the expense of a decline in the economic status of children. From the generational-equity perspective, because of overly generous spending on elderly people in connection with Social Security, Medicare, and other programs for older Americans, young adults and children were being shortchanged.

The generational-equity frame combines the ideas of fairness and affordability (Marmor, Cook, and Scher, 1999). Proponents make five central arguments that go a long way in defining the perspective. First, they argue that whereas a few decades ago elderly people were often poor, today most are financially secure (Chakravarty and Weisman, 1988; Longman, 1987). While the assertion is true as far as it goes, it ignores or at least de-emphasizes the heterogeneity in the economic status among subgroups of the elderly population (Crown, 2001).

A second major claim made by advocates of the generational-equity frame is that affluent elderly people are getting more than their fair share of societal resources at the expense of young adults and children (Fairlie, 1988). According to this argument, the increase in federal spending on elderly people has contributed to an increase in the poverty rate for children. Critics of this perspective argue that there are many factors that have been contributing to the increase in poverty rates among children, factors that are quite independent of trends in the economic status of elderly people; one example is trends with respect to the prevalence of single parent households (Moody 1998).

Advocates of the generational-equity frame make a third argument, that a range of policies that are unfair to working-age adults and children have thrived due in large part to the political influence of old-age interest groups such as AARP (Fairlie, 1988; Longman, 1989). The claim that elderly people use their political power to promote unfair policies is loosely rooted in fact, since elderly people do form a larger percentage of the electorate today than do young adults and families with children (Binstock, 2000).

A fourth claim made by advocates of the generational-equity frame is that current old-age policies are unsustainable because of the nation's changing demographic structure. As the population ages, they argue, these policies will become unaffordable (Concord Coalition, 1993). Critics of this perspective agree that the dependency ratio of elderly people has increased, but they go on to point out that the dependency ratio for children has decreased (Marmor et al., 1999).

Finally, the fifth argument advocates of generational equity often make is that it is unfair to expect each generation to support the one that precedes it (Borden, 1995; Gokhale, Page, and Sturrock, 1999). If today's working-age adults cannot count on the same level of Social Security and Medicare benefits when they retire as their parents' generation receives today, the pay-as-you-go system is unfair. This argument is often used to support proposals calling for the introduction of privatized individual accounts as part of the Social Security system. The claim that old-age policies are unsustainable and unfair does not take into account the possibility that some relatively modest policy changes could prevent projected financing problems (Baker and Weisbrot, 1999).

The generational-equity frame has appeals to many Americans because it resonates so well with several of the most strongly and widely held values in American culture, such as individualism, autonomy, and self-reliance. Advocates of generational equity are generally not opposed to redistribution within families or voluntary redistribution in the context of charitable giving, but they oppose "mandatory" redistribution through government programs. Social Security by this argument infringes on individual freedoms and undermines incentives for citizens to consume less during their working years and to set aside the funds they will need to remain economically independent during their retirement years.

The Generational-Interdependence Framing of the Debate

Central to the generational-interdependence interpretative package is the idea that it is a mistake to privilege generational equity over other important forms of equity (Williamson and Watts-Roy, 1999). The generational-interdependence frame emerged largely as a liberal response to the conservative generational-equity frame. In addition to taking issue with a number of the claims made by advocates of the generational-equity frame, the generational-interdependence frame makes three distinctive claims.

The first is that the gains of one generation are not necessarily made at the expense of another (Kingson, Hirshorn, and Cornman, 1986). Robert Kuttner (1982), for example, mentions the ways in which the existence of Social Security benefits the children of elderly parents by making it possible for the elderly parents to maintain their independent households. Similarly, Joseph White

(2001) points to the relief Social Security provides to workers who, because of it, need not be concerned about their parents falling into poverty. Even with Social Security structured as it is today, some adult children find it necessary to take in their elderly parents. This practice would become even more common if we as a nation opted for a much diminished version of Social Security. Not only do those who are not elderly benefit from many programs often viewed as programs for elderly people, such as Social Security and caregiving services, but also many programs typically viewed as programs for those under age 62 benefit elderly people (for example, unemployment insurance and Medicaid).

The second claim is that there is a two-way flow of services and support between generations. The flow of financial resources in many families is primarily in the direction of the adult children until the elderly parents reach extreme old age. Many elderly people provide substantial caregiving services for their grandchildren or disabled adult children (Smith and Beltran, 2000).

The third distinctive claim is that elderly people are much more heterogeneous than implied by the opposing generational-equity frame. Some elderly people are affluent, but many are poor or nearly poor. It is also pointed out that the generational-equity frame focuses on one form of equity to the neglect of other important forms of equity, such as those based on gender, class, and race. In short, economically vulnerable groups tend to be neglected by the generational-equity frame; the generational-interdependence frame represents an effort to address this limitation (Adams and Dominick, 1995; Binstock, 1983; Kingson and Williamson, 1993).

Linking Ideological Frames and Policy Prescriptions

I have described the ways in which the contest between proponents of the generational-equity frame and proponents of the generational-interdependence frame shaped the debate over Social Security reform, particularly between the early 1980s and the mid-1990s. During the past decade or so the debate over generational equity has largely morphed into a debate between proponents and critics of the proposed partial privatization of Social Security. In the following two sections I present and briefly analyze two alternative sets of policy prescriptions for the reform of Social Security, one from each of these two perspectives. The conservative policy prescriptions are often defended using arguments linked to the generational-equity frame, whereas the progressive policy prescriptions are frequently defended using arguments linked to the generational-interdependence frame.

Given the sharp differences between these two competing conceptual frameworks, it should not be surprising to find that the policy prescriptions that emerge from proponents of these different perspectives differ dramatically. From the right the call is to restructure the Social Security program so as to gradually redefine it as primarily a retirement savings plan. As one example reflecting this perspective I will consider two of the major proposals made by the President's Commission to Strengthen Social Security as outlined in its 2001 report. In the other camp are those on the progressive left who favor efforts to retain Social Security as a broad-based social insurance program. They generally do not favor the creation of funded individual accounts, and they are reluctant to introduce changes that are likely to increase the burden on low-wage workers relative to higher-wage workers. As one example of this progressive perspective, I will consider a set of proposals made in a Diamond and Orszag's recent book (2004).

Conservative Policy Prescriptions: Social Security as Retirement Savings

Commentators and analysts associated with the conservative Cato Institute began to call for the privatization of Social Security during the early 1980s (Ferrara, 1982, 1985). Until the mid-1990s, the call to privatize Social Security did not get much attention; it was viewed as a political nonstarter associated with the radical right. But there was a dramatic shift in attitudes on this issue by the mid-1990s (Kingson and Williamson, 2001). By then, proposals calling for partially privatizing Social Security had been presented and vetted by two mainstream commissions: the Bipartisan Commission on Entitlement and Tax Reform (1995) and the Advisory Council on Social Security (1997). Both of these reports got a great deal of coverage in the media. More recently, the President's Commission to Strengthen Social Security (President's Commission, 2001) in its final report (hereafter called *Commission Report*) outlines additional alternatives for the partial privatization of Social Security. I will focus on the most recent set of proposals outlined in this report.

The first proposal would allow workers to redirect 2 percentage points (out of 6.2) of their payroll tax into personal accounts. When the worker retired, the Social Security pension based on the regular (or defined benefit) portion of the scheme would be lower owing to the diversion of a portion of the payroll tax into the new personal account. This plan calls for the addition of about $1.1 trillion in additional funding from general revenues between 2016 and 2043 to finance the transition. Even after 2043, the plan would still continue to run a deficit that would have to be made up in some way, but the deficit would be lower than that projected for the current scheme.

The second proposal would allow workers the option to redirect 4 percentage points of their payroll tax into personal accounts, but there would also be a cap of $1,000 per year on the amount that could be so diverted. At retirement the defined benefit portion of Social Security would be greatly reduced as a result of the diversion of this substantial fraction of the worker's payroll tax into the personal account. After 2009 there would be a shift from wage indexing to price indexing of the covered income used to compute the defined benefit portion of the benefit. This would add up to a huge benefit cut. A guaranteed minimum income would be added to help protect low-wage workers who would otherwise end up with very low pensions. If the worker's combined income from the defined benefit component and the personal accounts component were to fall below 120 percent of the poverty line, the difference would be made up by the government out of general revenues. The proposal calls for an infusion of about $900 billion between 2015 and 2029 from general revenues to help finance the transition.

The third proposal would allow workers to redirect 2.5 percentage points of their payroll tax into personal accounts, subject to a cap of $1,000 per year, but they would also need to add another 1 percent of their wages to these personal accounts. Again the defined benefit portion of the eventual pension would be reduced by an amount that reflects the extent of the diversion of payroll contributions into personal accounts. These pensions would also be further reduced by the proposed shift from wage indexing to price indexing of the pre-retirement wages used to compute the pension benefit. The proposal would increase the incentives for those who delay retirement (a reform that would end up affecting few workers) and increase penalties for those electing early retirement (a reform that would affect a lot of people). There would be a guaranteed minimum pension this time set at 100 percent of the poverty line. This proposal would require the infusion of approximately $400 billion in new money from general revenues between 2015 and 2028 to help pay for the transition. After this transition period there would still be a gap between benefits and revenues, but the gap would be less than that under current law.

In the comments that follow, I focus on proposals 2 and 3, since proposal 1 is at best a partial proposal. While both proposals 2 and 3 have their flaws, they also include a number of innovations. One innovation is to make participation in the personal accounts voluntary. Based on the British experience, this would help protect low-wage workers, many of whom would opt for the defined benefit option (Williamson, 2002). However, there is a catch. Both proposals 2 and 3 call for indexing changes that would result in substantial benefit cuts, changes that would impact all workers, not just those who elect the personal-account option.

The introduction of a rather generous minimum pension for proposal 2 (and a slightly less generous minimum pension for proposal 3) is another important innovation. The proposed minimum pension, modest as it is, would go a long way toward protecting many of the most vulnerable. However, here too there is a catch; this minimum pension would only become available after 30 years of participation, thus excluding many of the most vulnerable. Another concern I have is that in any final legislation, the minimum pension would be cut substantially and possibly eliminated entirely. There is a real risk that the groups that would be most dependent upon and affected by this provision would not be well represented when the final deal is cut behind closed doors. Another reason for concern is that the need for huge sums to pay for the transition costs associated with these reforms is likely to produce intense pressure to cut any benefits without a strong constituency. In addition, it is generally easier to cut proposed new benefits than it is to cut benefits that people have been receiving (or promised) for years.

Proposal 3 calls for splitting pension assets in the event of divorce. This innovative provision would benefit women who have been married for many years to high-wage spouses. However, it would not be of much help to women in low-wage households or those not legally married to their partners.

The *Commission Report* (President's Commission, 2001) does not give adequate attention to the issue of market risk or the consequences of being subjected to a sharp drop in financial markets during the months or years just before retirement. While a legitimate case can be made that the ups and down of the stock market tend to average out over a period of decades, risk is a big issue particularly for low-wage workers because they often end up so close to the poverty line that even a modest drop in benefits may push them into poverty. In addition, low-wage workers are much more dependent on Social Security for their retirement income than are the affluent, the ones who are the most enthusiastic about the introduction of personal accounts (Williamson, 1997).

Each of the three plans calls for a large infusion of funding from general revenues for a period of about 15 to 25 years to pay for the cost of the transition. This is extra funding that would be needed to meet Social Security obligations to the currently retired and disabled while diverted payroll taxes were being used to build up individual accounts. From the British experience, it is safe to assume that in the long run partial privatization would reduce the burden on the government (Liu, 1999), but in the short-term (15 to 25 years depending on the plan) the burden on the government would increase substantially.

Under both proposals 2 and 3, the shift from wage indexing to price indexing of preretirement earnings would bring about a major cut in Social Security benefits. When the extent of these cuts is made explicit, it is probably going to create major political problems for those attempting to build support for these privatization proposals.

Progressive Policy Prescriptions: Social Security as Social Insurance

The primary policy prescription that can be derived from the generational-interdependence framing of the debate over Social Security policy is that the emphasis should be on maintaining the program pretty much as it is. There is a recognition from this perspective that some changes will be necessary to bring the program into long-term financial balance, but the goal seems to be to keep the resulting program as close as possible to what we have today. Analysts from this perspective implicitly or explicitly emphasize that Social Security is a social insurance program, not a retirement savings program. While a social insurance program can be expected to provide income replacement for older workers, the emphasis is different. Such a program does not take as its primary objective obtaining the highest possible long-run return on payroll tax contributions made in the worker's name, and it is not structured so that pension benefits are strictly proportional to contribution.

Social insurance schemes have been created to cover a number of risks to income in modern societies, including disability, work injury, and the loss of income associated with old age and retirement. These schemes start with the assumption that in a modern market economy the risks and the benefits are unequally distributed and that some collective protection is needed for those who do not fare well. Social insurance is based in part on the assumption that workers who take the risks associated with a competitive economy need a certain level of collectively provided economic security (Dionne, 1999).

Given that there is a projected deficit for the Social Security program starting in 2042, even those who want to maintain Social Security much as it is recognize that some reforms are called for. One simple alternative would be to gradually raise the payroll tax. Were that done, it would be possible to meet the anticipated burden without any other changes in the program. The payroll tax may eventually have to increase by at least 3 percent for both the employer and for the employee by 2080 (Board of Trustees, 2006), but the total burden would still be lower than it is today in some European nations, such as Sweden. There are some analysts who support this alternative (Thompson, 2000), but most of those who represent the progressive social insurance framing of this debate reject this solution. Many believe that a call for a tax increase of this magnitude would not be politically viable. They also believe that it is unfair to put the entire burden on people in the labor force. While there may be disagreements with respect to how much of the burden should be borne by the retired as opposed to those who are still at work, there is general agreement among those in this camp that some sort of burden sharing is called for. One way to do this is to make a number of modest policy changes that produce a balance between benefit cuts and payroll tax increases.

A good example of a balanced set of policy changes is presented in *Saving Social Security*, by Peter Diamond and Peter Orszag.[1] Their proposals are structured to deal with three sources of the projected long-term deficit in Social Security: (1) increasing life expectancy, (2) increasing inequality in earnings, and (3) the legacy debt, the part of the projected debt that can be attributed to the generous benefits paid to early participants relative to the contributions they made before retirement. Their proposed reforms combine both tax increases and benefit cuts. President Bush's Commission to Strengthen Social Security proposed that we deal with the projected increase in life expectancy primarily by cutting benefits. Diamond and Orszag (2004), in contrast, offer an alternative that balances benefit cuts and payroll tax increases. Their alternative calls for an annual recomputation of the life tables and of the projected increases in the cost of the Social Security program due to any increase in life expectancy at the age at which a worker becomes eligible for a full (as opposed to a reduced) Social Security pension. Half of the projected increase in the cost of Social Security due to the increase in life expectancy would be dealt with by reducing the size of the worker's initial monthly retirement pension, based on his or her earnings history at retirement. The other half of the projected increase in the cost due to the change in life expectancy would be dealt with by a modest increase in the payroll tax.[2] This matched pair of reforms produces a relatively even split between the tax increase and benefit reduction over the long run.

The last major changes in Social Security policy were made in 1983. At that time, approximately 10 percent of all earnings were untaxed because they fell above the taxable maximum, the earnings level above which earnings are no longer taxed. By 2002, owing to the increase in income inequality (increases in earnings for those at the top of the income distribution relative to those at the lower end), approximately 15 percent of earnings were above this taxable maximum. One consequence of this shift is that the system is less progressive today than it was 20 years ago. Another is that today Social Security is projected to replace less of preretirement income in the decades ahead than it replaces today. This shift in the fraction of all earnings that are above the taxable maximum ($87,900 for 2004) is also part of the reason for the projected long-term deficit. The Diamond and Orszag proposal for dealing with this source of the deficit is to gradually increase the level of the taxable maximum until the percentage of earnings above the taxable maximum gets back up to 13 percent. I would suggest at a minimum moving it all the way back to 10 percent, but their desire to keep a balance between the extent to which benefits are cut and revenues are increased leads them to prefer the 13 percent figure, which turns out to be about the average level over the past 20 years.

The benefit cut Diamond and Orszag propose to balance the preceding tax increase is to make the payout formula used to compute Social Security pensions more progressive by gradually decreasing the size of the benefit for relatively high-wage workers, who currently get only a 15-cent increase in pension benefit for each additional dollar of AIME (average indexed monthly earnings), the income figure Social Security uses to compute the worker's PIA.[3] Their proposal is to gradually decrease it to 10 cents for each additional dollar of AIME for this group of high-wage workers. This same reform was proposed in connection with one of the three plans outlined by the President's Commission to Strengthen Social Security. Given the support for the idea in the *Commission Report* (President's Commission, 2001), it is likely that bipartisan support could be found for this proposal.

The third source of the projected Social Security deficit that Diamond and Orszag deal with is the legacy cost, the current and future costs due to benefits to early Social Security recipients that were in many cases far in excess of what could be justified on the basis of contributions to the program made before retirement. They estimate that between 3 and 4 percentage points of the 12.4 percent payroll tax is due to the need to finance this legacy debt. They propose three reforms to deal with this source of the projected deficit.

One is to require that all workers participate in the Social Security system, including those state and local government workers not currently enrolled in Social Security. Because many state and local pension schemes are more generous than Social Security, it would be politically easier to make these changes gradually, for new hires only. This proposal makes sense and it should be done. It is likely that there will be bipartisan support for this idea.

A second reform proposal designed to deal with the legacy debt is to add a new 3 percent tax on all earnings above the maximum taxable earnings specified under current law ($87,900 for 2004). Over time it is likely that this tax would have to be increased somewhat to keep up with the legacy debt. It is of note that this proposed tax would be about equal to the current Hospital Insurance component of Medicare, which is already financed on the basis of all earnings including those above the maximum taxable earnings limit. This proposal would be a good idea, but it is likely to run into strong political opposition from an influential segment of the population, those with high incomes. It might be more feasible politically to increase the taxable maximum to the level needed to bring in the same amount of revenue. In my view a new tax on the affluent is going to be harder to sell than increasing the taxable maximum more than is called for on the basis of inflation adjustments alone.

The third reform they propose is a "universal legacy charge." It calls for a reduction in pension benefits and an increase in the payroll tax. The benefit reduction for newly eligible beneficiaries calls for an additional 0.31 percent reduction each year starting in 2023. Thus, in 2024 the reduction would be 0.62 percent (relative to current law). The corresponding revenue increase (that would balance the 75-year actuarial effect of the benefit reductions just outlined) would take the form of a payroll tax increase sufficient to increase revenues by 85 percent of the amount saved from the reduction in pension benefits each year. This tax rate increase would be 0.26 percent (85% of the .31% benefit reduction each year) each year starting in 2023. Diamond and Orszag suggest that this set of benefit and revenue adjustments be reviewed and appropriate modifications made in each after 75 years. If history is any guide, such adjustments would most likely be made much sooner. This is a proposal that I would support, and I believe that it would make sense as part of a balanced program, but I fear that the prospect of the steady increase in the payroll tax called for is likely to generate a substantial amount of political opposition. The proposal to hold off starting the process of increasing the payroll tax until 2032 would help politically, particularly with older workers. Something along these lines might be politically feasible, but it might be a hard battle.

What I have outlined is a summary of the three major components of the Social Security reform plan outlined by Diamond and Orszag (2004). It is also of note that they go on to offer an alternative for one or more of the proposals that they have made. The alternative is to use the estate tax as an additional source of funding for Social Security. The Tax Relief Reconciliation Act of 2001 calls for reductions in the estate tax over the years and for the complete elimination of this tax as of 2010. However, without further legislation, that estate tax would return to its 2001 level the following year, an outcome that few expect will be politically acceptable. What Diamond and Orszag propose is that the estate tax be retained in the form it will have in 2009, that is, the tax would be at the level of 45 percent on the 0.5 percent of estates that are above $3.5 million. This source of revenue would then be used exclusively to help fund Social Security. A related proposal is to close existing loopholes in the estate tax. They also consider transforming the estate tax into an inheritance tax. The difference is that were it made into an inheritance tax, then the person who inherits the estate would pay the tax rather than the estate, but again the revenues would be earmarked to help fund Social Security. The idea of financing old-age pensions using an estate tax is not a new one. It is reported to have been suggested by Thomas Paine in 1797 (Diamond and Orszag, 2004).

Would it make sense to dedicate that portion of the estate tax that remains in 2009 to helping shore up Social Security? It would represent a shift from Social Security's long history of being financed entirely on the basis of a dedicated payroll tax. Many people would view it as a radical shift and would oppose it. However, the source of the funding might mute the opposition for two reasons: (1) it would not come from general tax revenues, and thus the number of people paying this tax would be limited, and (2) it would not be a new tax; rather it would be a tax the very rich are already paying. However, if this money is diverted into the Social Security system, how is the reduction in general government revenues to be made up? I would guess that the major alternative would be to increase income taxes. In the likely event that such a link would be made, political support might be undercut. While it would put the tax entirely on a relatively small segment of the population, the very wealthy (or, more precisely, their estates), this also happens to be a politically influential segment of the population, so the opposition could be fierce. How about the idea of transforming the estate tax into an inheritance tax? The major problem is again potential political opposition. At issue would be the view that it is a new tax, and it is always hard to get political support for a new tax.

A distinctive aspect of the set of proposals made by Diamond and Orszag is the way in which they divide the projected shortfall into three different sources and then provide a balanced set of benefit cuts and payroll tax increases to deal with each of these sources. The way in which they provide a balance between benefit cuts and payroll tax increase for each of the three sources of the projected deficit is going to make the package attractive to many policy analysts.

One of the most innovative aspects of their analysis is the inclusion of a set of reforms to deal with the legacy cost. I think many analysts are going to take an interest in the "universal legacy charge" they propose as part of the legacy cost problem.

While Diamond and Orszag's careful balancing of pension benefit cuts with payroll tax increases is a major strength that is going to contribute to the political viability of their proposals, this balance does not come without a cost. I would like to see the cap on the level of earnings subject to the Social Security payroll tax removed, as it already has been for the Hospital Insurance component of Medicare. I would also like to see earnings based on the exercise of stock options taxed as wage income when part of the employee's compensation package. But such reforms would violate the balance between payroll tax increases and benefit cuts that Diamond and Orszag (2004) so carefully crafted.

Conclusion

Is Social Security facing a substantial funding shortfall unless some modest tax increases and benefit cuts are made over the next few decades, or will it be facing a funding "crisis" unless fundamental structural changes are made—and soon? Many on the right who, for a variety of reasons, favor a radical restructuring of the program often use the crisis framing of the debate in an effort to build support for their proposals. Strong language is employed in an effort to undermine confidence in and support for what is arguably the nation's most popular social program. In contrast, many on the left who prefer to reform Social Security in such a way as minimize structural changes tend to use different language when describing the projected funding shortfall. Those on the right tend to use an interpretative package that emphasizes arguments linking Social

Security policy to such themes and values as individualism, self-reliance, personal freedom, and ownership. This is often referred to as the generational-equity perspective. Those on the left often use an alternative interpretative package that emphasizes a different set of themes, such as social insurance, shared risk, generational interdependence, and societal obligation to protect vulnerable groups from the sometimes harsh consequences of a market economy. This is often referred to as the generational-interdependence perspective. The debate between the right and the left over the future of Social Security is a symbolic contest being waged largely in the popular media, using carefully chosen metaphors and catch phrases designed to sell each interpretative package to as wide an audience as possible.

The generational-equity perspective has been used to build the case for a number of Social Security reform packages, the most widely discussed being those that have included a funded individual-account pillar (component). In this chapter I have presented and commented on one of the most recent sets of proposals, those outlined in the *Commission Report* prepared by the President's Commission to Strengthen Social Security (2001). The various proposals outlined in the *Commission Report* include a number of innovative ideas that subsequent commissions would do well to consider and others that are likely to prove seriously problematic. The proposed individual accounts would likely benefit some if not many affluent workers, but at a cost. These same proposals would not do an adequate a job of providing protection for those economically vulnerable groups that are most dependent upon Social Security pensions for their retirement income.

The generational-interdependence perspective has been used to build the case for a number of more progressive Social Security reform packages that give much more attention to the social insurance function of the program. Here I have presented and commented on the policy suggestions suggested in a recent book by Diamond and Orszag (2004) to illustrate the different policies that have been proposed from this alternative progressive perspective. In this case, the focus has not been on one major policy, such as the introduction of individual accounts; rather it has been on the creation of a basket of more modest reforms that leave the current structure of Social Security very much intact. These reforms have been carefully constructed so as to balance the burden of dealing with the projected deficit between future retirees and future workers, a balance between provisions that lead to modest benefit cuts and modest payroll tax increases without the introduction of funded individual accounts.

It is easy to take issue with one or another of the many policy changes that Diamond and Orszag proposed, but in so doing it is important not to miss a much more important point. Their major contribution has been to show how the long-term Social Security funding gap can be closed in such a way that the burden is evenly divided between individuals in the labor force and individuals who are retired. Furthermore, they show us how to achieve this goal without calling for the partial privatization of Social Security.

NOTES

1. Unless specified otherwise, the material presented here is drawn from chapter 5 of Diamond and Orszag 2004.
2. The payroll tax would be increased by the amount necessary to equal 85 percent of the decrease in the PIA (primary insurance amount), the pension benefit a worker is eligible for if she or he takes the pension at the age of eligibility for the full retirement benefit. See Diamond and Orszag (2004) for an explanation of why the 85 percent figure is used.
3. See note 2 for a definition of PIA.

REFERENCES

Adams, P., and Dominick, G. L. 1995. The old, the young, and the welfare state. *Generations* 19:38–42.
Advisory Council on Social Security. 1997. *Report of the 1994–1996 Advisory Council on Social Security.* Vol. 1, *Findings and Recommendations.* Washington, DC: U.S. Government Printing Office.
Baker, D., and Weisbrot, M. 1999. *Social Security: The Phony Crisis.* Chicago: University of Chicago Press.
Beard, R. L., and Williamson, J. B. 2004. Generational equity and generational interdependence: Framing the debate over health and Social Security policy in the United States. *Indian Journal of Gerontology* 18:348–62.
Binstock, R. H. 1983. The aged as scapegoat. *Gerontologist* 23:136–43.
Binstock, R. H. 1999. Scapegoating the old: Intergenerational equity and age-based health care rationing. In J. B. Williamson, D. M. Watts-Roy, and E. R. Kingson, eds., *The Generational Equity Debate,* pp. 185–203. New York: Columbia University Press.
Binstock, R. H. 2000. Older people and voting participation: Past and future. *Gerontologist* 40:18–31.
Bipartisan Commission on Entitlement and Tax Reform. 1995. *Bipartisan Commission on Entitlement and Tax Reform: Final Report.* Washington, DC: U.S. Government Printing Office.

Board of Trustees, Federal Old Age and Survivors Insurance and Disability Insurance Trust Funds. 2006. *The 2006 Annual Report of the Trustees of the Federal Old-Age and Survivors Insurance and Disability Insurance Trust Funds.* Retrieved from www.ssa .gov/OACT/TR/TR06/.

Borden, K. 1995. *Dismantling the Pyramid: The Why and How of Privatizing Social Security.* The Cato Project on Social Security Privatization SSP No. 1. Washington, DC: Cato Institute.

Butler, S., and Germanis, P. 1983. Achieving Social Security reform: A Leninist strategy. *Cato Journal* 3:547–56.

Chakravarty, S. N., and Weisman, K. 1988. Consuming our children. *Forbes,* November 14, pp. 222–32.

Concord Coalition. 1993. *The Zero Deficit Plan.* Washington, DC: Concord Coalition.

Crown, W. 2001. Economic status of the elderly. In R. H. Binstock and L. K. George, eds., *Handbook of Aging and the Social Sciences,* 5th ed., pp. 352–68. San Diego: Academic Press.

Diamond, P., and Orszag, P. 2004. *Saving Social Security: A Balanced Approach.* Washington, DC: Brookings Institution Press.

Dionne, E. J. 1999. *Why Social Insurance?* Social Security Brief No. 6. Washington, DC: National Academy of Social Insurance.

Fairlie, H. 1988. Talkin' bout my generation. *New Republic,* March 28, pp. 19–22.

Ferrara, P. J. 1982. *Social Security: Averting the Crisis.* Washington, DC: Cato Institute.

Ferrara, P. J. 1985. Social Security and the super IRA: A populist proposal. In P. Ferrara, ed., *Social Security: Prospects for Real Reform,* pp. 193–220. Washington, DC: Cato Institute.

Ferrara, P. J., and Tanner, M. 1998. *A New Deal for Social Security.* Washington, DC: Cato Institute.

Gokhale, J., Page, B. R., and Sturrock, J. R. 1999. Generational accounts for the United States: An update. In A. J. Auerbach, L. R. Laurence, and W. Leibfritz, eds., *Generational Accounting around the World,* pp. 489–517. Chicago: University of Chicago Press.

Gurevitch, M., and Levy, M. R. 1985. *Mass Communications Review Yearbook.* Vol. 5. Beverly Hills, CA: Sage.

Kingson, E. R. 1984. Financing Social Security: Agenda-setting and the enactment of the 1983 amendments to the Social Security Act. *Policy Studies Journal* 11:131–55.

Kingson, E. R., Hirshorn, B. A., and Cornman, J. M. 1986. *Ties That Bind.* Washington, DC: Seven Locks Press.

Kingson, E. R., and Williamson, J. B. 1993. The generational equity debate: A progressive framing of a conservative issue. *Journal of Aging and Social Policy* 5:31–53.

Kingson, E. R., and Williamson, J. B. 2001. Economic security policies. In R. H. Binstock and L. K. George, eds., *Handbook of Aging and the Social Sciences,* 5th ed., pp. 369–86. San Diego: Academic Press.

Kuttner, R. 1982. The Social Security hysteria. *New Republic,* December 27, pp. 17–21.

Liu, L. 1999. Retirement income security in the United Kingdom. *Social Security Bulletin* 62(1):23–46.

Longman, P. 1982. Taking America to the cleaners. *Washington Monthly* 14 (November): 25–30.

Longman, P. 1985. Justice between generations. *Atlantic Monthly,* June, pp. 73–81.

Longman, P. 1987. *Born to Pay: The New Politics of Aging in America.* Boston: Houghton Mifflin.

Longman, P. 1989. Elderly, affluent—and selfish. *New York Times,* October 10, p. 27.

Marmor, T. R., Cook, F. L., and Scher, S. 1999. Social Security and the politics of generational conflict. In J. B. Williamson, D. M. Watts-Roy, and E. R. Kingson, eds., *The Generational Equity Debate,* pp. 185–203. New York: Columbia University Press.

Moody, H. R. 1998. *Aging: Concepts and Controversies.* 2nd ed. Thousand Oaks, CA: Pine Forge Press.

President's Commission to Strengthen Social Security. 2001. *Strengthening Social Security and Creating Personal Wealth for all Americans: Report of the President's Commission.* Retrieved from www.csss.gov.

Preston, S. H. 1984. Children and the elderly: Divergent paths for America's dependents. *Demography* 21:81–86.

Quadagno, J. S. 1989. Generational equity and the politics of the welfare state. *Politics and Society* 17:353–76.

Reno, V. P., and Friedland, R. B. 1997. Strong support but low confidence: What explains the contradiction? In E. R. Kingson and J. H. Schulz, eds., *Social Security in the Twenty-first Century,* pp. 178–94. New York: Oxford University Press.

Smith, C. J., and Beltran, A. 2000. Grandparents raising grandchildren: Challenges faced by these growing numbers of families and effective policy solutions. *Journal of Aging and Social Policy* 12:7–17.

Thompson, L. H. 2000. *Sharing the Pain of Social Security and Medicare Reform.* Retirement Project Brief No. 11. Washington, DC: Urban Institute.

White, J. 2001. *False Alarm: Why the Greatest Threat to Social Security and Medicare Is the Campaign to "Save" Them.* Baltimore: Johns Hopkins University Press.

Williamson, J. B. 1997. A critique of the case for privatizing Social Security. *Gerontologist* 37:561–71.

Williamson, J. B. 2002. Privatization of social security in the United Kingdom: Warning or exemplar? *Journal of Aging Studies* 16:415–30.

Williamson, J. B., McNamara, T. K., and Howling, S. A. 2003. Generational equity, generational interdependence, and the framing of the debate over Social Security reform. *Journal of Sociology and Social Welfare* 30:3–14.

Williamson, J. B., and Watts-Roy, D. M. 1999. Framing the generational equity debate. In J. B. Williamson, D. M. Watts-Roy, and E. R. Kingson, eds., *The Generational Equity Debate,* pp. 3–37. New York: Columbia University Press.

CHAPTER FOURTEEN

Setting the Agenda for Social Security Reform

Eric R. Kingson, Ph.D.

Peter Diamond and Peter Orszag's chapter (Chapter 15) and their book *Saving Social Security* (2005) make sense of many of the uncertainties, policy proposals, and value choices associated with Social Security reform. Acknowledging the existence of a serious long-term financing problem, Diamond and Orszag present a coherent and creative set of reforms that addresses projected shortfalls without undermining the basic structure of Social Security or the program's capacity to provide widespread protection against losses of income associated with retirement, survivorship, or long-term and severe disability.

Following a review of the projected Social Security shortfall, my comments are organized in two parts. First I discuss why I believe the Diamond-Orszag approach provides rationale and policy proposals that strengthen the argument of those seeking to reform Social Security—the Old-Age, Survivors and Disability Insurance program (OASDI)—without compromising its underlying values or basic protections. Second, I discuss the near-term feasibility of passing proposals such as the ones they advocate. Like Diamond and Orszag, I believe it is preferable to address Social Security's financing problems sooner rather than later. But, as I will explain, and as I am sure they are aware, the near-

term political environment is not conducive to the type of reform they propose.

Background on Projected Shortfalls

In the next 10 to 25 years, it is virtually certain that Social Security will not
face projected short-term shortfall as it did in the early 1980s. It will, however,
need to come to terms with a projected long-term shortfall. Even so, how and
when this problem is addressed will have much more to do with the outcome
of a fierce ideological battle currently under way than with the mathematics of
the projected shortfall.

The most commonly accepted estimates suggest that OASDI has sufficient
funds to meet all its obligations until 2040. However, after that, its projected
revenues are sufficient to pay about 74 cents of every dollar promised over the
remaining 75-year estimating period. The projections suggest that tax revenues
(payroll tax receipts and receipts from taxation of benefits) will be exceeded by
outlays in 2017 but that income from all sources, including interest on trust
fund investment in U.S. government obligations, is expected to exceed expenditures through about 2027. After that, timely payment of benefits would require drawing down the assets of the OASDI trust fund until its depletion in
2040. Of course, the size of the actual problem could be larger or smaller. The
Social Security Administration's more pessimistic high cost estimates project a
shortfall beginning in 2031 that is roughly 150 percent larger than its most commonly accepted estimates. The SSA's more optimistic low cost estimates project that the OASDI trust funds can meet all of Social Security's obligations
through 2080 (See Board of Trustees, 2006).

Theoretically, the long-term financing problem could be addressed by immediately raising the Social Security payroll tax on employers and employees
from 6.2 to 7.2 percent or by immediately reducing all future benefits by about
14 percent. While this suggestion provides a sense of the size of the problem,
no one seriously advocates either approach. Another way to look at the Social
Security shortfall is as a percentage of GDP. Over the 75-year estimating period,
Social Security represents, on an annual basis, a shortfall of roughly 0.7 percent
of GDP; during the last 25 years of this estimating period—2056 to 2080—the
shortfall is projected at an annual 1.7 percent of GDP. Diamond and Orszag
present yet another way of understanding the dimensions of the problem: "1.92
percent of taxable payroll . . . corresponds to $3.8 trillion in present discounted

value. In other words, if $3.8 trillion were set aside today, the principle plus interest (accruing at a Treasury bond interest rate) would be just enough to cover the projected shortfall over the next seventy-five years. . . . Expressing the actuarial imbalance in dollars facilitates comparisons with other government actions that would have long-run financial effects" (2005, p. 31).

The facts surrounding Social Security's estimated shortfall are not highly disputed, but the perceived implications of the projected long-run shortfall fuel a lively and often rancorous policy debate (see Aaron and Reischauer, 1998; Altman and Shactman, 2002; Peterson, 1996, 1999; Quadagno, 1989; Williamson and Watts-Roy, 1999). Conflicting approaches to reform reflect differing views of the extent to which individuals versus the national community should bear responsibility for preparing for people's retirement, disability, or survivorship.

Conservatives view the projected long-term shortfall as a unique opportunity to shrink the federal government's role and move the nation toward a more individualistic "ownership society." Liberals consider conservative declarations of a "Social Security crisis" as ideologically driven, disinguous, and factually inaccurate—a carefully crafted assault on this most successful legacy of the New Deal. Much is at stake, including fundamental notions about the responsibility Americans have for each other and that government has to assure basic protections, especially for those likely to be at greatest risk. The traditional view emphasizes providing widespread, sure, and adequate protection as Social Security's fundamental purpose. Hence, stabilizing financing while assuring adequate benefits that are not subject to erosion by inflation, business cycles, and market fluctuations is the central reform concern. Strong commitment exists for moderate redistribution as a means of assuring that those who have worked for many years at relatively low wages will have minimally adequate retirement incomes. In contrast, those seeking to shift Social Security toward a more private-savings model—more closely aligned with libertarian principles—see the projected financing problem as a window of opportunity for structural change. They draw on their strong belief in individual responsibility, limited taxation, and freedom of choice. They argue that Social Security is not sustainable in its present form and emphasize maximizing rates of return and shrinking the role of government. While safeguards may be built in for some of the most disadvantaged, their proposals tend to be most beneficial to persons with higher earnings. For instance, most women would not fare well under a privatized retirement income savings program, because women tend to have more intermittent work histories and lower earnings and tend to live longer (see Williamson and Rix, 2000).

How to Reform, Not Destroy, Social Security

Into this fray step Diamond and Orszag, providing reasoned analysis and reform proposals that put the Social Security financing problems in perspective. Their analysis shows in "bas relief" that Social Security's projected shortfall is relatively small compared to revenues lost from continuing recent tax cuts. As they point out, "the 2001 and 2003 tax cuts, if continued over the next 75 years, would reduce revenue by about $12 trillion in present value, or roughly three times Social Security's actuarial imbalance over the same period" (2005, p. 31).

No doubt the projected growth in the number of beneficiaries relative to covered workers, the impending retirement of baby boomers, declines in fertility, increased life expectancies, and the slow-downs in the growth of the economy and real wages all contribute to the projected problem. Though acknowledging such factors, Diamond and Orszag's novel perspective on the causes of the projected shortfall introduces ideas that lay the foundation for innovative reforms.

Creative and sensible, the Diamond-Orszag analysis reinforces the rationale for maintaining Social Security as a program based on social insurance principles. Rejecting the libertarian assumptions of those advocating privatization, Diamond and Orszag argue that true Social Security reform will require a set of changes balancing benefit reductions and revenue increases, while also improving protections for especially vulnerable beneficiaries. Their reform package illustrates that it is possible and desirable to do so.

Addressing the Legacy Debt

Social Security aficionados understand that declining rates of return for current generations of beneficiaries relative to past beneficiaries and for future generations relative to current beneficiaries are a result of social insurance principles, which give primacy to adequacy—as opposed to individual equity—goals (see Hohaus, 1960). Social Security maintains a compromise between these competing principles that is best exemplified in its benefit formula, which assures proportionately larger benefits for low-wage beneficiaries but generally larger benefit amounts for higher-income workers making larger payroll tax contributions into the system. Importantly, the concern for adequacy is also given expression through decisions made early in the life of the program to provide relatively generous benefits to people who made payroll tax contributions for only a few years. Thus, Ida Fuller, the first Social Security beneficiary, in 1940, paid less than $100 in payroll tax contributions and received benefits for 35 years until she died in 1975 at the age of 100. Should Ida have received such generous treatment? The answer is no for those believing that the program should be structured on more individualistic principles; they prefer that it function more like a private insurance system, where benefits are in direct proportion to contributions. But for those considering the provision of widespread and adequate protection against identifiable risks as the driving force of Social Security, the answer is clearly yes. In keeping with these traditional social insurance concerns and beliefs about social responsibility, especially for those at greatest risk, Ida and other early beneficiaries were essentially given credit for past work and past contribution to the nation when the program was adopted and in subsequent benefit liberalizations. To do otherwise would have meant that Social Security would not address the economic security of those cohorts who were at far more economic risk than today's or tomorrow's elders.

Diamond and Orszag take this discussion one step further. Regardless of whether one agrees or disagrees with these past decisions (most would agree), a legacy debt is passed forward to current and future generations because of the largely pay-as-you-go nature of Social Security. They estimate that "in an actuarially balanced system, roughly 3 to 4 percentage points of the 12.4 percent of taxable payroll tax would be devoted to financing the program's legacy debt" (2005, p. 89). The only question is how the cost of financing the debt will be distributed fairly across and within future cohorts.

Their analysis of the legacy debt provides a rationale for (1) extending Social Security coverage to all state and local workers, so that those currently outside the system carry their fair share of the debt (addresses 13% of the projected financing problem); (2) adding a modest tax (initially 3%) on earnings above the maximum taxable earnings base, so that higher-income workers bear a more equitable share of the legacy debt (addresses 29%); and (3) a phased-in "legacy charge" split between small annual payroll tax increases and benefit reductions, beginning in 2023 when changes in the ages of eligibility are essentially phased in and the proposed rate of payroll tax increases declines (addresses 51%).

Addressing Increased Inequality of Earnings

Similarly, and importantly, Diamond and Orszag properly link the financing shortfall to the increased inequality in earnings. As the earnings distribution has become more unequal over the past 20 to 25 years, the percentage of earnings subject to payroll taxation has declined, and hence projected revenues have declined as well. The Social Security system has also lost substantial revenues as the relative growth of fringe benefits has further eroded the portion of employee compensation subject to payroll taxation. Moreover, larger fringe benefit packages are usually associated with higher wages and more stable employment, thus further exacerbating inequality and the loss of Social Security revenues connected to increasing inequality.

Immediately after enactment of the Social Security Amendments of 1983, 90 percent of cash compensation was subject to the Social Security (OASDI) payroll tax; today, only 85 percent is. The proportion of workers with incomes above the ceiling remains about the same—roughly 6 percent—but the growth in earnings by high-income workers has outstripped that of the bottom 94 percent, placing greater burden on this larger group for maintaining the progressivity of the system. Diamond and Orszag's solutions call for a modest and gradual increase in the proportion of cash compensation that is subject to the payroll tax, thereby addressing about 13 percent of the projected Social Security shortfall.

Their discussion also links increased life expectancies to declines in the progressivity of Social Security. Highly educated and higher-income persons experience greater rates of increase in life expectancy than those with more limited education and earnings. As a result, the system is less progressive because the gap is growing in how long these differing groups collect benefits. To offset this growth in inequality and to maintain balance between benefit cuts and revenue increases, Diamond and Orszag gradually phase in a change in the benefit formula that would result in modest benefit reductions, mostly among future beneficiaries with the largest monthly benefits (addresses 9% of the projected deficit).

Although I understand that Diamond and Orszag wanted to present a plan that balanced benefit reductions with revenue increases, I would like to suggest that their analysis highlights why consideration should be given to, at a minimum, raising the maximum taxable ceiling to cover 90 percent of taxable compensation. Moreover, their analysis is not inconsistent with eliminating the taxable ceiling for employers, just as has been done for the Medicare portion of the FICA tax. Given the widening inequality in the distribution of earnings, it is reasonable—although admittedly not politically feasible at this time—to spread more of the financing burden to firms offering disproportionately high salaries by subjecting 100 percent of the employer's payroll to FICA taxation. This step would address about half of the projected shortfall. Under this proposal, the maximum taxable ceiling would still apply to the employee's earnings, eliminating the need to give excessively large benefits in the future to the highest-income workers.

Addressing Other Implications of Increasing Life Expectancies

Increases in life expectancies have contributed and will continue to contribute to the projected financing problem. Life expectancies at age 65 or older have increased significantly since 1940, about four years for men and five for women. While the 1983 amendments introduced a gradual increase in the age of eligibility for full benefit to age 67 for workers reaching age 62 in 2022, no adjustments have been made for anticipated increases after 2022.

Retirement age increases (in the age of eligibility for full benefits with parallel reductions in the monthly benefit for earlier retirees) are a rather blunt policy instrument, not sensitive, for example, to health conditions that are more likely to drive lower-income workers to accept reduced early retirement benefits. Instead of retirement age adjustments, Diamond and Orszag propose small, automatic, and yearly adjustments based on actuarial projections of life expectancies made each year, beginning in 2012. Equal savings would come from slight reductions in annual benefits (i.e., shaving the worker's primary insurance amount) and slight payroll tax increases. This automatic adjustment would reduce uncertainties related to unexpected changes in life expectancies. It is also less disturbing of the progressivity of Social Security than retirement age increases. However, it may be easier to explain to the public that Social Security's ages of eligibility are being raised because "people are living longer" than to explain benefit formula changes, beginning in 2012, to adjust for anticipated increases in life expectancies.

Other Laudable Features

As noted, Diamond and Orszag provide a coherent and fully defensible approach to reforming Social Security. They are not dogmatic in their advocacy of policy changes. I agree that their plan is "balanced," although I am quite sure that those seeking to move away from the traditional social insurance structure of Social Security would disagree. Diamond and Orszag recognize that a balanced plan could incorporate other alternatives without undermining Social Security (e.g., dedicated estate or inheritance tax revenues or retirement age increases).

I share their analysis of the shortcomings of introducing individual accounts through a carve-out of a portion of the payroll tax and benefit reductions. Like many others (Marmor and Mashaw, 2002; Williamson, 1997), they point out that partial privatization proposals would create additional financing pressures on Social Security and potentially undermine the surety of benefits, progressivity, and protections for those at greatest risk. Individual accounts would be cumbersome and expensive to administer.

Importantly, Diamond and Orszag's plan goes beyond addressing the projected 75-year deficit. They propose changes (e.g., adjustments related to increasing life expectancies) that substantially reduce the risk of shortfalls 80, 90, or 100 years hence. Significantly, their plan produces sufficient savings and new revenues to fund proposals that would further reinforce the adequacy goals of the system. Thus, they include several proposals for slight improvements in protections for widows and widowers, long-term workers with low lifetime earnings, young survivors, and persons disabled early in their careers.

Setting the Agenda for Reform

Too often, advocates of the traditional Social Security program fall into the trap of simply saying what is wrong with various privatization proposals. Not Diamond and Orszag. Their analysis and proposal illustrates that it is far preferable and easier to reform Social Security without undermining its goals than to do otherwise.

I agree that addressing Social Security reform sooner rather than later is far preferable. I also agree that the approach that the 1982 National Commission on Social Security Reform has come to exemplify is an ideal way to think about going about reforming today's Social Security program. "The need for a suitable compromise is one of the lessons from the success of the balanced 1983 reform of Social Security. . . . [A] successful reform must involve both benefit reductions and revenue increases" (Diamond and Orszag, 2005, p. 45). Unfortunately, much has changed since the early 1980s, making reforms such as what

Diamond and Orszag advocate more difficult to move into prominence on the nation's political agenda. The conditions are not conducive to political action that reflects their perspective. Here's why.

Power is highly dispersed and fragmented in the American political system, so that it is difficult to gain consensus for complex policy changes such as Social Security reform. Substantial policy change is difficult to achieve on a national level under the best of circumstances, given House and Senate legislative processes, interest group politics, and potential political differences within and between the legislative and executive branches (see Binstock, 2002; Ornstein, 2002). Many problems compete for attention. Kingdon (2003) suggests that policy change requires a coupling of problems, policy prescriptions, and politics. Timing is crucial. Not only must a problem come into focus as requiring attention, but also substantial agreement must exist about causes and potential solutions, and the political environment (e.g., the national mood, congressional and executive leadership, and interest group incentives) must be favorable (see Kingdon, 2003). Change happens often as a response to crises—real and perceived; sometimes elections and political realignments foster change; and sometimes change occurs because policy facilitates the bringing together of problems, policies, and politics.

The politics surrounding Social Security reform are quite different today than they were in 1982–83 and do not favor the type of consensus building necessary for the type of reform Diamond and Orszag and others (like myself) would advocate. The 1983 amendments were enacted in a political environment that facilitated negotiation and compromise among political parties more than the current environment does.

The Politics of Social Security in 1982–83

The Social Security politics of the early 1980s were certainly contentious. When President Ronald Reagan appointed the bipartisan National Commission on Social Security Reform, few expected its members to reach consensus (Kingson, 1984; Light, 1995). In 1981 many Republicans were arguing that the projected financing problems of Social Security were potentially much larger than others predicted. But most Republicans were reticent to advance proposals because they did not want to be positioned in an election year as advocating benefit reductions; after all, "Social Security was a 'Democratic issue.'" Some Democrats and liberal supporters of Social Security argued that there was not necessarily a problem, and in any event it was not necessarily as large as projected. The Reagan administration, in an otherwise successful first year in office, stumbled domestically in 1981 when it floated a proposal for large cuts to address projected shortfalls in OASDI, cuts that would have produced savings far in excess of what was needed to address the financing problems. When that proposal was announced, many viewed the Commission as simply a vehicle for keeping Social Security "out of politics" until after the 1982 midterm congressional elections (see Berkowitz, 2004; Kingson, 1984; Light, 1995).

Shortly after the November 1982 elections, the Commission met and reached agreement that helped lay the foundation for the 1983 amendments. The members of the Commission unanimously (1) rejected means-testing and voluntary approaches (e.g., individual accounts); (2) recommended that Congress "should not alter the fundamental structure of the Social Security program or undermine its fundamental principles" (National Commission on Social Security Reform, 1983); and (3) agreed on the existence and size of the financing problems. While failing to agree on a financing package, the members of the Commission reached consensus on a number of important proposals that were later included as part of the 1983 amendments. Democratic members acknowledged that some benefit reductions would be necessary, and Republicans agreed that revenue increases would be necessary as well (see Berkowitz, 2004; Kingson, 1984; Light, 1995).

Ultimately, President Reagan agreed early in 1983 to a compromise that balanced revenue increases (e.g., taxation of benefits, acceleration of preexisting payroll tax increases, changed tax treatment of the self-employed, and expansion of coverage to new federal employees) and benefit reductions (e.g., a six-month permanent delay in the COLA and a gradual increase in the age of eligibility for full benefits).

There are a number of reasons—all instructive for today's Social Security politics—why this relatively moderate set of reforms moved quickly through Congress with bipartisan support.

- Importantly, there really was an immediate short-term financing crisis. Without remedial legislation early in 1983, Social Security would not have had sufficient revenue to meet all promised benefits, a situation that would not be politically tenable for Democrats or Republicans.
- President Reagan had a strong incentive for reaching a compromise with the Democratic leadership before delivering his annual budget to

Congress in late January. Without the revenues being generated by the proposal agreement, the president's budget would show a substantial deficit.

- A political compromise that balanced benefit reductions and revenue increases was a necessary ingredient of bipartisan compromise. President Reagan and the Democratic Speaker of the House, Tip O'Neill, needed to reach agreement, and O'Neill, a strong supporter of the traditional Social Security program, would not—and could not politically—agree to large benefit cuts.

- Politicians need political cover to enact "dedistributive" policy reforms—changes that distribute pain to many constituencies (Light, 1995). Hence, reaching bipartisan agreement on a package that can be sold as distributing modest benefit reductions and revenue increases across many groups provides critical protection to members of both political parties.

Today's Politics of Social Security

Today's long-term financing problem is quite similar in cause and size to the problem confronting policymakers in the early 1980s. But the similarities in the politics of Social Security stop with this observation.

First and perhaps most important, Social Security is financially sound in the short run. There is no immediate crisis. Politicians are generally reluctant to expend political capital for a problem that is likely to be salient 20 or more years in the future, even one so important as Social Security's long-term financing. Social Security reform of the type proposed by Orszag and Diamond would require taking a stand on how to distribute pain to various constituents. Absent a short-term crisis, the political incentives do not point in such a direction.

Second, the politics of Social Security are more ideological today. Throughout the 1980s and 1990s, neoconservatives were successful in moving their critiques of Social Security and their proposals for structural reforms (e.g., partial privatization) from the periphery to the center of Social Security policy discussions (see Quadagno, 1989; Williamson and Watts-Roy, 1999). Beginning with the 2000 presidential campaign, President George W. Bush is on record as strongly favoring some type of reform that includes individual accounts.

Third, there are more institutional barriers to reform. Congressional politics are more polarized. Republican control of the presidency and both houses of Congress creates less incentive for compromise. Democrats—as the minority party—need to maintain distinctions on key issues such as Social Security. More congressional districts are considered "safe" for incumbents, meaning that incumbents need to be more concerned with primary challenges from within their parties than with the general election. This situation creates incentives to move away from the political center, because officeholders must place greater attention on maintaining the political support of party activists and primary voters, who tend to be more ideologically driven. Potential for compromise is further dampened by ideological and even personal contentiousness among members of Congress (see Binstock, 2002; Ornstein, 2002).

Conclusion

Barring major political realignment, the Diamond-Orszag proposal or similar proposals will not be enacted as a legislative package in the near future. But this reality takes nothing away from Peter Diamond and Peter Orszag's efforts and accomplishment. Neither do I think it comes as a surprise to them.

Their proposal is an admirable example of what Social Security reform should be. Well-reasoned, it illustrates the feasibility of addressing the Social Security financing problem while preserving its basic structure and protections. It carefully balances benefit reductions and revenue increases, while managing to strengthen protections for some at-risk groups. It connects to the values given eloquent expression years ago by Princeton economist J. Douglas Brown. Brown wrote of an implied covenant in Social Security, arising from a deeply embedded sense of mutual responsibility in civilization that underlies "the fundamental obligation of the government and citizens of one time and the government and citizens of another time to maintain a contributory social insurance system" (Brown, 1977, pp. 31–32). The Diamond-Orszag proposal also implicitly reflects an understanding of Social Security as an institution that gives expression to values supporting mutual aid and the obligation to care for our neighbors and ourselves. As the Social Security debate heats up, it will be important to not lose sight of this moral dimension of the program, which is one of the joining institutions of our society.

By introducing new ways of looking at and addressing the Social Security financing problem and by restating the case for a Social Security program based on social insurance principles, Diamond and Orszag provide backing for those seeking to block radical and counterproductive privatization proposals and strengthen the argument for productive reform in the future.

REFERENCES

Altman, S. H., and Shactman, D. I., eds. 2002. *Policies for an Aging Society.* Baltimore: Johns Hopkins University Press.

Aaron, H. J., and Reischauer, R. D. 1998. *Countdown to Reform: The Great Social Security Debate.* New York: Century Foundation Press.

Berkowitz, E. D. 2004. *Robert Ball and the Politics of Social Security.* Madison: University of Wisconsin Press.

Binstock, R. H. 2002. The Politics of Enacting Reform. In S. H. Altman and D. I. Shactman, eds., *Policies for an Aging Society.* Baltimore: Johns Hopkins University Press.

Board of Trustees, Federal Old Age and Survivors Insurance and Disability Insurance Trust Funds. 2006. *2006 Annual Report of the Trustees of the Federal Old-Age and Survivors Insurance and Disability Insurance Trust Funds.* Washington, DC: U.S. Government Printing Office.

Brown, J. D. 1977. *Essays on Social Security.* Princeton, NJ: Princeton University Press.

Diamond, P. A., and Orszag, P. R. 2005. *Saving Social Security: A Balanced Approach.* Rev. ed. Washington, DC: Brookings Institution Press.

Hohaus, R. A. 1960. Equity, Adequacy, and Related Factors in Old Age Security. In W. Haber and W. J. Cohen, eds., *Social Security Programs, Problems, and Policies.* Homewood, IL: Richard D. Irwin.

Kingdon, J. W. 2003. *Agendas, Alternatives, and Public Policies.* New York: Longman.

Kingson, E. R. 1984. Financing Social Security: Agenda-setting and the enactment of 1983 amendments to the Social Security Act. *Policy Studies Journal* 11(3):131–55.

Light, P. C. 1995. *Still Artful Work: The Continuing Politics of Social Security Reform.* New York: McGraw-Hill.

Marmor, T. R., and Mashaw, J. L. 2002. The case for universal social insurance. In S. H. Altman and D. I. Shactman, eds., *Policies for an Aging Society.* Baltimore: Johns Hopkins University Press.

National Commission on Social Security Reform. 1983. *Report of the National Commission on Social Security Reform.* Washington, DC: National Commission on Social Security Reform. January.

Ornstein, N. J. 2002. Enacting reform: What can we expect in the current political context? In S. H. Altman and D. I. Shactman, eds., *Policies for an Aging Society.* Baltimore: Johns Hopkins University Press.

Peterson, P. G. 1996. *Will America Grow Up before It Grows Old?* New York: Random House.

Peterson, P. G. 1999. How will America pay for the retirement of the baby boom generation? In J. B. Williamson, D. M. Watts-Roy, and E. R. Kingson, eds., *The Generational Equity Debate,* pp. 41–57. New York: Columbia University Press.

Quadagno, J. S. 1989. Generational equity and the politics of the welfare state. *Politics and Society* 17:353–76.

Williamson, J. B. 1997. A critique of the case for privatizing Social Security. *Gerontologist* 37:561–71.

Williamson, J. B., and Rix, S. E. 2000. Social Security reform: Implications for women. *Journal of Aging and Social Policy* 11(4):41–68.

Williamson, J. B., and Watts-Roy, D. M. 1999. Framing the generational equity debate. In J. B. Williamson, D. M. Watts-Roy, and E. R. Kingson, eds., *The Generational Equity Debate,* pp. 3–37. New York: Columbia University Press.

CHAPTER FIFTEEN

A Summary of *Saving Social Security: A Balanced Approach*

Peter A. Diamond, Ph.D., and Peter R. Orszag, Ph.D.

Social Security is one of the most successful U.S. government programs. It has helped millions of Americans avoid poverty in old age, on becoming disabled, or after the death of a family wage earner. As President Bush emphasized, "Social Security is one of the greatest achievements of the American government, and one of the deepest commitments to the American people."[1] Despite its successes, however, the program faces two principal problems.

First, Social Security faces a long-term deficit, even though it is currently running short-term cash surpluses. Addressing the long-term deficit would put both the program itself and the nation's budget on a sounder footing. Second, there is broad agreement that benefits should be increased for some particularly needy groups—such as those who have worked at low pay rates over long careers and widows and widowers with low benefits. The history of Social Security is one of steady adaptation to evolving issues, and it is time to adapt the program once again.

Restoring long-term balance to Social Security is necessary, but it is not necessary to destroy the program in order to save it. Social Security's projected financial difficulties are real. Addressing these difficulties sooner rather than later would make sensible reforms easier and more likely. The prospects are not so dire, however, as to require undercutting the basic structure of the system. In other words, our purpose is to save Social Security both from its financial problems and from some of its "reformers."

In this chapter we review the financial position of Social Security, present a plan for saving it, and explain why Social Security revenue should not be diverted into individual accounts. Our approach recognizes and preserves the value of Social Security in providing a basic level of benefits for workers and their families that cannot be decimated by stock market crashes or inflation and that lasts for the life of the beneficiary. It also eliminates the long-term deficit in Social Security without resorting to accounting gimmicks; thereby it puts the program and the federal budget on a sounder financial footing. Our plan combines revenue increases and benefit reductions, the same approach taken in the last major Social Security reform, that of the early 1980s, when Alan Greenspan chaired a bipartisan commission on Social Security. That commission facilitated a reform including adjustments to both benefits and taxes. Such a balanced approach was the basis for reaching a consensus between President Ronald Reagan and congressional Republicans, on one hand, and congressional Democrats, led by House Speaker Thomas P. O'Neill, on the other. We hope to move the discussion toward a basis for such a compromise.

Social Security's Long-Term Deficit

Social Security faces a long-term deficit, requiring some type of reform to put the system on a sounder financial footing. According to the most recent projection done by the Office of the Chief Actuary of Social Security, from its current balance of roughly $1.5 trillion, the trust fund is projected to first rise and then fall, reaching zero in 2042. At that time, revenue from payroll taxes and the income taxation of benefits would still be sufficient to cover about three-quarters of the projected expenditure. That fraction then declines slowly to slightly less than 70 percent in 2080. Thus, although some observers refer to the "bankruptcy" of Social Security, in fact, a substantial revenue flow would still be dedicated to Social Security even after the trust fund is exhausted. As such, concerns that there will be nothing from Social Security for future generations are misplaced. Even so, everyone agrees that a serious political problem arises when the trust fund reaches zero. At that point, the system cannot pay all promised benefits out of the existing revenue structure.

Some observers have argued that the problem will arrive much sooner than that, when the flow of revenue from taxes first falls short of annual expenditure in 2018. We see no basis for attaching any significance to such a date, however, and are unaware of any rigorous presentation of an argument for why that date represents a crisis.

Another description of the financial picture comes from considering an "actuarial balance" figure. This measure reflects the degree to which the current trust fund and projected revenues over some period are sufficient to finance projected costs. The period conventionally chosen is 75 years. When the projection shows insufficient resources to pay scheduled benefits over that period, the Office of the Chief Actuary calculates what level of additional resources would be sufficient to close the gap and leave the trust fund with a projected balance (considered a "precautionary balance") equal to projected expenditure for one additional year after the end of the period. This measure of the actuarial deficit, presented as a percentage of taxable payroll over the next 75 years, is the key traditional criterion for evaluating Social Security's finances.[2] In the 2004 trustees' report, the actuarial imbalance was 1.89 percent of taxable payroll. One interpretation of this number is that it indicates what payroll tax increase would be sufficient to finance benefits over the 75-year horizon (and leave a precautionary balance as defined above), provided the increase began immediately and remained in force for the full 75 years. Reporting the imbalance in this way is not meant to recommend that the payroll tax rate be raised by this amount; rather, it is a way of summarizing the magnitude of the financial difficulties at hand. People may disagree about whether a shortfall of 1.9 percent of taxable payroll is a large problem or a small one, but it is a straightforward way to present the problem.

One of the primary goals of a Social Security reform plan should be to achieve 75-year actuarial balance. But this should not be accomplished through the "magic asterisk" approach of simply assuming transfers from the rest of the budget (discussed in the next section). Nor should one adopt the deceptive approach of using the higher expected returns on stocks relative to bonds to eliminate the projected deficit.

Many factors have contributed to the change from projected balance at the time of the 1983 reform to the current imbalance. Because there are many ways to attribute the change to specific factors, any particular allocation is somewhat arbitrary. Rather than attempt an accounting of the contributions to the long-term deficit from all the different factors, we simply focus on three important contributing factors: improvements in life expectancy, increases in earnings inequality, and the burden of the legacy debt resulting from Social Security's early history. These factors interact with one another, further underscoring the arbitrary nature of such classifications. Nonetheless, each of these three factors, examined by itself, has an adverse effect on Social Security's financing and motivates a component of our reform plan.

Increasing Life Expectancy

Life expectancy at age 65 has increased greatly since the creation of Social Security. It has risen by four years for men and five years for women since 1940 and is expected to continue rising in the future. Increasing life expectancy contributes to Social Security's long-term deficit. Because Social Security pays a benefit that continues as long as the beneficiary is alive, any increase in life expectancy, counting from the age at which benefits commence, increases the cost of Social Security, unless there is an offsetting decrease in the monthly benefit level. The last major reform of the program, in 1983, increased the full benefit age gradually over two six-year periods (2000–2005 and 2017–22), in anticipation of increased life expectancy, which effectively reduced monthly benefits for those affected by the change. But the 1983 reform did not include any ongoing adjustment for life expectancy after 2022. So, as time goes on and life expectancy continues its steady increase, the projected cost of Social Security steadily rises.

Although demographers, actuaries, and other experts agree that mortality rates will continue to decline well into the future, there is heated debate in academic and actuarial circles about how rapid an improvement to expect. This is not an appropriate place to assess that dispute, but the debate underscores the fact that projections of mortality improvements are subject to considerable uncertainty. Indeed, this uncertainty is one of our motivations for proposing that Social Security be indexed to future mortality levels, so that rather than trying to make adjustments now based on today's mortality projections, such adjustments will be made automatically as time goes on and actual improvements in mortality become known. Such improvements have historically varied from year to year, and indeed even from decade to decade. Thus, one should expect to see significant deviations in the future from current mortality projections, even if those projections are accurate on average over long periods.

One might think that any adverse financial effect on Social Security from increased life expectancy would be substantially diminished by longer careers, as people choose to spend part of their longer expected lives continuing to work. That is not the case, however, for two reasons. First, it seems unlikely that longer life expectancy will be associated with significant increases in career lengths. Second, even if people did extend their careers, the effect on Social Security would be relatively modest because the system is roughly actuarially fair. Working longer (and claiming benefits later) does not have much effect on Social Security's financing because annual benefits are increased when the initial benefit claim is postponed. The bottom line is that increased life expectancy, whether or not it is accompanied by longer careers, imposes financial costs on Social Security.

The steady increases in life expectancy that have occurred since the 1983 reform of Social Security are not a total surprise. Indeed, the actuarial projections done at the time of the reform assumed steadily improving life expectancy. But the target in 1983 was to restore actuarial balance for the following 75 years, not forever. Now we are more than 20 years into that 75-year projection period, and with the 75-year projection period including an additional 20 years, financing difficulties are again on the horizon. (This is a reflection of what is called the "terminal" or "cliff" problem. Under Social Security's current structure, the years beyond the 75-year projection horizon have larger cash flow imbalances than earlier years. Extending the horizon, as a new projection is done, then worsens the projected balance.) Because ongoing increases in life expectancy contribute to the terminal year effect, and because that terminal year effect helps to explain the reemergence of a 75-year deficit since 1983, life expectancy increases are one cause of the long-term deficit in Social Security.

In thinking about how Social Security should be modified to deal with increases in life expectancy, it is helpful to examine how a worker would sensibly react to a change in life expectancy, both under conditions in which the worker relied only on his or her own resources and under different types of pension systems. On learning that she or he will live longer than previously expected, an individual worker could adjust in any of three ways to the resulting need to finance consumption over a longer life: by consuming less before retirement (that is, saving more), consuming less during retirement, or working longer. A sensible approach would likely involve all three.

Social Security benefits are higher for those who start them at a later age and are higher for each additional year of work that raises the worker's average indexed monthly earnings. The current system thus already allows for one response to increases in life expectancy: working longer to enjoy higher annual benefits.

The other two elements of individual adjustment can be thought of as corresponding to an increase in the payroll tax rate (consuming less and saving more before retirement) and a reduction in benefits for any given age at retirement (consuming less during retirement). Both responses involve reductions in consumption, one before retirement and the other after. Our approach includes both of these, given that Social Security already provides the opportunity for higher benefits from more work.

Automatic adjustment of benefits and taxes for ongoing increases in life expectancy would enhance the financial soundness of Social Security, but they still leave open a key question, namely, the extent to which the adjustment should be divided between taxes and benefits. Sweden's approach and a proposal from President Bush's commission allocate all of the adjustment for longer life expectancy to benefit cuts. We consider that an extreme approach and instead propose a balanced combination of benefit and tax adjustments.

Specifically, under our proposal, in each year the Office of the Chief Actuary would calculate the net cost to Social Security from the improvement in life expectancy observed in the past year for a typical worker at the full benefit age. This would be done by comparing the cost of benefits for different cohorts, using successive mortality tables.[3] Half of this "net cost of increased life expectancy" would be offset by a reduction in benefits, which would apply to all covered workers age 59 and younger (once a worker reaches age 60, the rules for his or her benefits would be finalized and would not change further in response to ongoing life expectancy changes). An accompanying payroll tax change would roughly balance the actuarial effects of the benefit reductions over a 75-year period.[4]

The first benefit adjustment would occur for those initially eligible to receive benefits in 2012, and the first adjustment to the payroll tax rate would also occur in 2012, with additional changes each year thereafter (as a result, benefits for those age 55 and older in 2004 would be unaffected). Each tax rate change would affect all earnings below the maximum taxable earnings base from then on. Because the already-legislated increases in the full benefit age are supposed to reflect improvements in life expectancy, the adjustment of benefits from this provision would be decreased to the extent that scheduled increases in the full benefit age already reduce benefits in the relevant years. To do otherwise would be to compensate twice for the same change in life expectancy.

It is worth emphasizing that our proposal would *not* change either the full benefit age or the earliest eligibility age. Indeed, we do not support any simple principle for adjusting Social Security based on an expectation of how much longer people should work in response to lower mortality rates. The reason is that the age at which it is sensible for a worker to retire depends on more than just life expectancy. It depends as well on how a worker's ability to work and interest in work and the availability of jobs vary as mortality decreases. It also depends on the extent to which, because of higher earnings, workers are more interested in retiring earlier. Furthermore, the diversity in the labor force and the appropriateness (in some cases the need) for some workers to take early retirement also underscore the importance of preserving early retirement options. Future declines in mortality will widen the variance in ages at death, which is also exacerbated by the income-related difference in the rate of decline in mortality rates. These factors, if anything, *increase* the importance of providing an option of early retirement for those with shorter life expectancy.

Implementing this proposal would reduce the 75-year actuarial deficit by 0.55 percent of taxable payroll, or slightly less than one-third of the currently projected deficit. Moreover, the change would attenuate the terminal-year effect of moving from one 75-year projection period to the next.

Increasing Inequality of Earnings

A second factor affecting Social Security's financing is earnings inequality. Here we examine two aspects of earnings inequality: the increase in the share of earnings that is untaxed because earnings are above the maximum taxable earnings base, and the widening difference in life expectancy between lower earners and higher earners.

These changes, by themselves, have made Social Security less progressive on a lifetime basis over the past 20 years. But many factors affect the overall progressivity of Social Security, and it is not our intent to address all of them. For example, the increased tendency of women to have substantial careers outside the home has diminished the relative importance of the spousal benefit. The spousal benefit has tended historically to reduce Social Security's progressivity, because it has accrued disproportionately to spouses in high-income families; the decline in the relative importance of the spousal benefit therefore makes Social Security more progressive as a whole (see, e.g., Smith, Toder, and Iams, 2001; Cohen, Steuerle, and Carasso, 2001). Although some of these other factors are also important, we focus on just the effect of earnings inequality, which we believe particularly warrants a policy response.

Over the past two decades, earnings have risen most rapidly at the top of the earnings distribution, that is, among those workers who already were receiving the highest earnings. Economists have explored a variety of explanations for this increase in earnings inequality. The leading explanation involves technological changes that have increased the wages earned by better-educated workers compared to less-well-educated workers, although social norms also seem to play an important role.

The increase in the share of earnings accruing to the top of the income distribution affects Social Security's financing because the Social Security payroll tax is imposed only up to a maximum taxable level ($87,900 in 2004). The increasing inequality of earnings in recent years implies that a much larger fraction of aggregate earnings is not subject to the payroll tax than in the past. In other words, when the earnings distribution changes so that more of total earnings goes to those earning more than the taxable maximum, the fraction of total earnings subject to Social Security tax decreases.

The fraction of aggregate earnings that was above the maximum taxable earnings base has risen substantially since the early 1980s, from 10 percent in 1983 to 15 percent in 2002. The increase in the fraction of earnings not subject to tax reflects the fact that earnings growth at the top of the income distribution has been much more rapid than the growth of average earnings. Surprisingly, the fraction of workers with earnings at or above the maximum taxable earnings base has remained roughly constant since the early 1980s. In each year since the early 1980s, about 6 percent of workers have had earnings at or above the taxable maximum. Thus the increase in earnings that escape the payroll tax does not reflect an increase in the fraction of workers with earnings above the maximum, but rather an increase in the average earnings of those workers relative to other workers. For example, in 1983 the average earnings of workers who earned more than the taxable maximum were five times the average earnings of all other workers; by 2001 the same relationship was more than seven to one.

To offset this effect, we would raise the maximum taxable earnings base so that the percentage of aggregate earnings covered is closer to that which prevailed in 1983. The large increase since 1983 in the share of earnings that is untaxed because those earnings are above the taxable maximum does not reflect a policy decision, but rather the outcome of changes in earnings patterns in the

economy over the past quarter century. One could argue that policymakers implicitly agreed in 1983 that only about 10 percent of earnings should escape taxation by virtue of being above the maximum. Thus one reasonable approach
would gradually increase the maximum until the 1983 share is restored. But this
would generate so much revenue as to result in a large imbalance between our
proposed revenue and benefits adjustments in this category. Therefore, to
achieve a closer balance between the two, we adopt instead the more moderate
approach of returning the share of earnings above the taxable maximum about
halfway to its 1983 level, that is, to 13 percent, which is approximately its average over the past two decades. We also phase in this reform over an extended
period to allow workers time to adjust to the change. In particular, each year
after the plan is adopted, the maximum taxable earnings base would increase
by 0.5 percentage points more than the percentage increase in average wages,
until 2063, when it is projected that 87 percent of covered earnings will be subject to payroll taxation.[5]

Increasing the maximum taxable earnings base would affect only the 6 percent of workers in each year with earnings at or above the current maximum.
Moreover, although it would raise their payroll tax payments, it would raise
their subsequent benefits as well (the increase in benefits associated with earnings in the relevant range would, however, only partly offset the increase in revenue, because of the progressivity of Social Security's benefit formula). Gradually returning the share of untaxed earnings to 13 percent would reduce the
75-year actuarial imbalance by 0.25 percent of payroll, or about one-eighth of
the existing deficit.

The second piece of our earnings inequality adjustment involves differential
trends in life expectancy. The trend to longer life expectancy and its impact on
Social Security are widely known. Somewhat less well known, but also bearing
implications for the program, is the fact that people with higher earnings and
more education tend to live longer than those with lower earnings and less education. Even less well known is that these mortality differences by earnings
and education have been expanding significantly over time.

This increasing gap in mortality rates by level of education has two implications for Social Security. First, to the extent that projected improvements in
life expectancy reflect disproportionate improvements for higher earners (a
reasonable supposition because higher earners tend to have more education
than lower earners), the adverse effect on Social Security's financing is larger
than if the projected improvement occurred equally across the earnings distri-

bution. The reason is that higher earners receive larger annual benefits in retirement; a disproportionate increase in their life expectancy therefore imposes a larger burden on Social Security than an equivalent increase in life expectancy for other beneficiaries. Second, when one thinks of the progressivity of Social Security on a lifetime basis, rather than an annual basis, the changing pattern of mortality tends to make Social Security less progressive than it would be without such a change, because it means that higher earners will collect benefits for an increasingly larger number of years, and thus enjoy larger lifetime benefits, relative to lower earners.

In response to the increase in earnings inequality and the growing spread in life expectancies between higher earners and lower earners, our plan would increase the progressivity of the Social Security benefit formula. A worker's monthly Social Security benefits are based on a primary insurance amount (PIA), which is itself computed by applying a three-tiered formula to the worker's Average Indexed Monthly Earnings (AIME), the measure of lifetime earnings used to compute Social Security benefits. In the highest tier of the PIA calculation, which is relevant only for relatively high earners, benefits are increased by 15 cents for every extra dollar in AIME. To respond to the effect of increasing differences in mortality rates, we would gradually reduce this 15 cents in benefits on each dollar in the top tier by 0.25 cent a year for newly eligible beneficiaries in 2012 and thereafter, until it reaches 10 cents in 2031. This benefit adjustment, which was also adopted by one of the three plans proposed in 2001 by the President's Commission to Strengthen Social Security, reduces the 75-year deficit by 0.18 percent of payroll.

This reduction would affect approximately the highest-earning 15 percent of all workers. If the change had been fully in effect in 2003, for example, it would have affected only those whose AIME exceeds $3,653, or almost $44,000 a year. Social Security data suggest that only about 15 percent of newly retired and disabled workers have consistently had earnings at or above this level over their lifetime. Furthermore, the change would have larger effects on higher earners than on those whose earnings just barely put them in the 15-cent tier. For example, reducing the 15-cent rate to 10 cents would ultimately reduce benefits by 1.6 percent for those with an AIME of $4,167 (and therefore career-average annual earnings of $50,000) but would reduce benefits by 8.7 percent for those with the maximum AIME of $7,250 (and therefore, career-average annual earnings of $87,000).

The Legacy Debt Burden

A third important influence on the future financing of Social Security reflects, somewhat ironically, the past. That is the fact that the benefits paid to almost all current and past cohorts of beneficiaries exceeded what could have been financed with the revenue they contributed. This history imposes a legacy debt on the Social Security system. That is, if earlier cohorts had received only the benefits that could be financed by their contributions plus interest, the trust fund's assets today would be much greater. Those assets would earn interest, which could be used to finance benefits. The legacy debt reflects the absence of those assets and thus directly relates to Social Security's funding level. In this section we use the legacy debt as an alternative lens through which to view Social Security's financing challenges.

The decision, made early in the history of Social Security, to provide the first generations of beneficiaries benefits disproportionate to their contributions represented sound policy. It was a humane response to the suffering imposed by World War I, the Great Depression, and World War II on Americans who came of age during those years, and it helped to reduce unacceptably high rates of poverty among them in old age. Moreover, the higher benefits not only helped the recipients themselves but also relieved part of the burden on their families and friends, and on the taxpayers of that era, who would otherwise have contributed more to their support. Thus the decision to grant generous Social Security benefits to workers who had contributed little or nothing to Social Security during their careers provided crucial assistance to more people than just those workers themselves.

But whatever the rationales for and positive effects of those decisions, all workers covered by Social Security now face the burden of financing them. To measure that burden and explore in detail how it accumulated, one can examine how much each cohort paid and is projected to pay in Social Security taxes (in present value) and how much that cohort received and is projected to receive in benefits (again in present value).

Figure 15.1 shows, for each cohort born from 1876 to 1949, the difference between what that cohort paid or will pay in taxes to Social Security, and what it received or is projected to receive in benefits, in present value. The dotted line in Figure 15.1 shows that the earliest cohorts received more from Social Security than they paid into it. Because the program as a whole was small in those

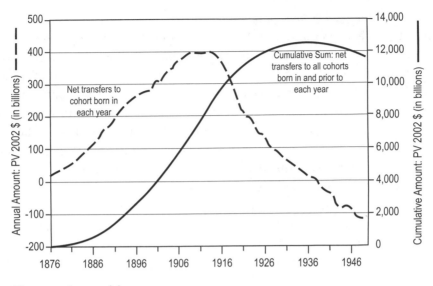

Figure 15.1. Legacy debt

early years, the total net transfer was not large, either for each cohort individually or for all the early cohorts cumulatively (depicted by the solid line). As the program grew, however, it continued to provide more generous benefits than could have been financed by previous contributions (plus a market rate of interest), and the cumulative transfer grew rapidly. Following the 1983 reforms, all cohorts starting with those born in 1936 are now scheduled to pay in more than they receive in present value, thereby reducing the legacy debt that is passed on to the future.

The effect of the early generosity is that the "rate of return" received on contributions by younger workers is lower than a market interest rate, and a "legacy cost" is borne because of this difference between the return on contributions under Social Security and the market interest rate.

Nothing anyone can do today can take back the benefits that were given to Social Security's early beneficiaries, and most Americans would be unwilling to reduce benefits for those now receiving them or soon to receive them. Those two facts largely determine the size of the legacy debt. For example, on one reasonable assumption, namely that benefits will not be reduced for anyone age 55 or older in 2004, the legacy debt amounts to approximately $11.6 trillion.

Because the size of the legacy debt is mostly already determined, the only remaining issue is how to finance it across different generations, and different people within generations, in the future. To be sure, the legacy debt does not have to be paid off immediately. Indeed, some of it need never be paid off, just as there is no need ever to pay off the entire public debt. But any ongoing legacy debt, like other outstanding public debt, incurs a cost for continuing to finance it, which, if not paid as it accrues, increases the debt. And just as a continuously rising public-debt-to-gross-domestic-product ratio would eventually become unsustainable (as holders of the debt come to doubt whether they will be repaid in full), so, too, the legacy debt cannot grow faster than taxable payroll indefinitely without disrupting the functioning of Social Security.

That workers today bear a cost of financing the legacy debt does not necessarily mean that Social Security is a bad deal for those workers. Many workers, no doubt, are pleased that their parents and grandparents received higher benefits than their contributions would have paid for. Just as in the past, some current workers benefit from the fact that Social Security reduces the need for them to support their parents directly. Also, Social Security provides today's workers with life insurance, disability insurance, and an inflation-indexed annuity, and it does so at a remarkably low administrative cost, far lower than the private financial market could match. Moreover, the mandatory nature of Social Security avoids the problem of adverse selection that can arise in private insurance markets. (Adverse selection stems from the fact that those who expect to benefit more from insurance are more likely to buy it; this raises the average cost of insurance to the insurer, leading to price increases and possibly a vicious cycle of ever-fewer participants and ever-higher prices.) Finally, Social Security's mandatory character also protects individuals and their families from myopically undersaving and underinsuring themselves. Thus, although younger workers will receive less in benefits from Social Security than they would have in the absence of the legacy debt, they still stand to inherit a system that will provide them with valuable benefits, some of which cannot be duplicated in the market.

We propose changing the way in which the program's legacy debt is financed, in three ways: through universal coverage under Social Security; through a legacy tax on earnings above the maximum taxable earnings base, with the tax rate beginning at 3 percent and gradually increasing over time; and through a universal legacy charge that would apply to workers and beneficiaries in the future.

Universal Coverage

About 4 million state and local government employees are not covered by Social Security.[6] It is unfair to workers who are covered by Social Security (including the great majority of state and local government workers) that many state and local government workers are not included in the program and so do not bear their fair share of the cost of the system's past generosity. On average, state and local government workers are well paid. It therefore seems appropriate that they, along with other higher earners, pay their fair share of Social Security's redistributive cost (the cost of relatively more generous benefits for low earners) as well as the cost of more generous benefits to earlier cohorts.

Pension systems for state and local government workers are generous, on average, compared with those available to privately employed workers. Such generosity can be maintained for current workers while revising the system's parameters for newly hired workers. Of course, state and local governments would need several years to design suitable changes in their systems, and so any requirement that newly hired workers be included in Social Security should only begin sometime after legislation is enacted requiring such inclusion. We propose a three-year time frame, which was the phase-in period adopted in 1983 for inclusion of newly hired federal workers in Social Security.

Moreover, inclusion in Social Security would result in a net benefit to some state and local government workers and their families. The clearest beneficiaries are some of those workers who leave state and local government employment before retirement to take jobs in the private sector that are covered by Social Security. Eligibility for Social Security disability benefits does not begin until a worker has held Social Security-covered employment for a given number of years. For example, a worker who has been in uncovered work for ten years would not have Social Security disability coverage for at least five years after beginning covered work. Because many employers do not provide such coverage, many of these workers would thus find themselves without any disability coverage. This gap in coverage can be a source of great financial hardship in the event of disability during the early years of a new job.

Coverage under Social Security would also help workers who leave state and local government jobs before their retirement benefits vest. Even those with vested benefits who leave early in their careers may benefit from being covered under Social Security, because the real value of their state or local government pension typically declines with any inflation that occurs before they reach retirement age; such a decline does not occur under Social Security. After retirement, many (but not all) state and local government plans do provide automatic adjustment of benefits for inflation, but in many cases these increases are capped at 3 percent, whereas Social Security has no such cap.

In addition, the retirement and survivor provisions of some state and local government pension plans do not offer all the protections to workers and their families provided by Social Security. For example, in the event of death before retirement, some systems offer only a lump sum that reflects the employee's past contributions plus a modest return, and some only refund the contributions, without any return. Instead, Social Security provides annuitized benefits to the deceased worker's young children and, on retirement, to his or her spouse. After retirement, workers in state and local government plans can choose between single life and joint life annuities, implying that some surviving spouses (those whose spouse chose the single life annuity) will no longer receive benefits once the worker dies. Thus, Social Security coverage offers elements of real value to state and local government workers, over and above what their current pension plan offers.

We therefore propose that all state and local government workers hired in and after 2008 be required by law to be included in Social Security.[7] This change would reduce the 75-year actuarial deficit by 0.19 percent of taxable payroll, or roughly 10 percent of the deficit itself.

A Legacy Tax on Earnings above the Maximum Taxable Earnings Base

Estimates suggest that, in an actuarially balanced system, roughly three to four percentage points of the 12.4 percent payroll tax would be devoted to financing the program's legacy debt (Geanakoplos, Mitchell, and Zeldes, 1998, p. 148). Yet those with earnings above the maximum taxable earnings base do not bear a share of this legacy cost proportional to their total earnings. Thus we propose a tax on earnings above the taxable maximum; the tax rate would begin at 3 percent (1.5 percent each on employer and employee) and gradually increase over time, along with the universal charge to be described next, reaching 4 percent in 2080. By itself, this change would reduce the 75-year actuarial deficit by an estimated 0.55 percent of taxable payroll, but there is a significant interaction between this provision and the proposed increase in the maximum earnings subject to taxation.

How onerous would this legacy tax be? It is worth noting that the 2.9 percent payroll tax for the Hospital Insurance component of Medicare already applies to all earnings. The tax we propose is approximately equal to this tax. Furthermore, the legacy tax would be smaller than the 4.6 percentage-point reduction in the top marginal income tax rate since the beginning of 2001. Both of these considerations suggest that the tax would not have substantial adverse effects on either the higher earners to whom it would apply or the economy as a whole.

A Universal Legacy Charge on Payroll Taxes and Benefits

The legacy debt arises from decisions that we as a society made decades ago, and it is fitting that future workers and beneficiaries should contribute a fair share toward financing that debt. The final element of our proposal therefore involves a universal legacy charge on both benefits and tax rates, which would apply to all workers and newly eligible beneficiaries from 2023 forward. We select this starting date because the increases in the full benefit age continue until 2022. After 2023, we smoothly increase the legacy charge, because the growth rate in taxable payroll declines thereafter, calling for an increasing offset to the legacy cost.

The benefit adjustment would reduce initial benefits by 0.31 percent a year for newly eligible beneficiaries in 2023 and later. The benefit reduction would increase for newly eligible beneficiaries in 2024 to 0.62 percent relative to current law, and so on.[8] This benefit reduction spreads part of the legacy cost over all retirees thereafter.

The revenue adjustment would raise the payroll tax rate by 85 percent of the benefit reduction percentage from this component of our plan. (The logic for this 85% factor is the same as that for the life expectancy component of the plan; that is, benefits for newly eligible beneficiaries equal 85% of total benefits over a 75-year horizon, whereas all earnings within that horizon are subject to the higher tax rate.) The result is that the tax rate would increase by 0.26 percentage point (0.13 each on employer and employee), or 85 percent of 0.31, each year starting in 2023. Between them, the tax and benefit universal legacy cost offsets would reduce the 75-year actuarial deficit by an estimated 0.97 percent of taxable payroll.

Taken together, these means of financing the legacy debt represent a balance between burdening near-term generations and burdening distant generations with the entire debt, between burdening workers and burdening future retirees, and between burdening lower-income workers and burdening higher-income workers. The phased-in nature of the universal legacy cost adjustment also helps the Social Security system to adjust to the reduced fertility rates that have occurred since the 1960s.

The Estate Tax as an Alternative Source of Revenue

Throughout its history, all Social Security tax revenue has been linked to benefits in some way, either through the payroll tax (with earnings subject to tax being the basis for benefits) or through the taxation of benefits. The third component of our proposal would set a precedent in that earnings above the taxable maximum would be subjected to partial taxation but would not affect the calculation of benefits.[9] An alternative deviation from the historical pattern could come from dedicating some other source of revenue to Social Security. Given that unified federal budget deficits are projected for the foreseeable future, however, any reform proposal should devote only dedicated revenue to Social Security rather than an unspecified source of general revenue. Moreover, any such dedicated revenue that makes use of existing revenue sources should be devoted only if such revenue would otherwise be eliminated through tax cuts; if the alternative to using an existing stream of revenue for Social Security is that the revenue would disappear, the dedication of such revenue to Social Security does not exacerbate the government's overall deficit. One possible source of dedicated revenue for Social Security is a reformed estate tax. Such revenue could substitute for one or more of the specific revenue proposals in our plan. The idea of using an estate tax to finance benefits for elderly persons and disabled workers is not new. Indeed, it is more than 200 years old, Thomas Paine having proposed it in 1797.[10]

The Center on Budget and Policy Priorities estimates that retaining the estate tax in its 2009 form (that is, with a $3.5 million per person exemption and a 45% top rate) rather than allowing it to be repealed altogether would result in only 0.5 percent of estates—the largest five of every 1,000—being subject to taxation in 2010. The total number of estates taxed at all in a given year would be approximately 10,000, and these estates would enjoy lower estate tax rates and a higher exemption than today. More important for our purposes, the revenue raised by retaining the estate tax in its 2009 form—rather than repealing it—would address about 20 percent of the 75-year actuarial deficit in Social Security. A reform that closed loopholes in the estate tax would add to its revenue potential at any given tax rate and could be used to replace one or more of our proposed reforms.

Our three-part proposal would restore 75-year actuarial balance to Social Security, as summarized in Table 15.1. These proposals were designed to achieve actuarial balance while also achieving "sustainable solvency" by ensuring a sta-

Table 15.1. Summary of Effects of Proposed Reforms

	Effect on Actuarial Balance	
Proposed Reform[a]	As Share of Taxable Payroll	As Share of Actuarial Deficit[b]
Adjustments for increasing life expectancy		
Adjust benefits	0.26	13
Adjust revenue	0.29	15
Subtotal	0.55	29
Adjustments for increased earnings inequality		
Increase taxable earnings base	0.25	13
Reduce benefits for higher earners	0.18	9
Subtotal	0.43	22
Adjustments for fairer sharing of legacy cost		
Make Social Security coverage universal	0.19	10
Impose legacy tax on earnings over taxable maximum	0.55	29
Impose legacy charge on benefits and revenue	0.97	51
Subtotal	1.71	89
Reforms to strengthen social insurance functions[c]		
Enhanced benefits for lifetime low earners	−0.14	−7
Increased benefits for widows	−0.08	−4
Hold-harmless provisions for disabled workers and young survivors	−0.21	−11
Completion of inflation protection of benefits[d]	0.0	0
Subtotal	−0.43	−22
Interactions of above reforms	−0.26	−14
Total effect	2.00	104
Alternative: reform existing estate tax[e]	0.60	31

Source: Authors' calculations.

[a]See text for details of specific proposed reforms.

[b]The 75-year deficit is currently estmated to be 1.9% of taxable payroll over that period. Numbers may not sum to totals because of rounding.

[c]These reforms and their separate impacts on actuarial balance are described in the chapter.

[d]Not included in the package of reforms officially scored by the Office of the Chief Actuary, but should have de minimis actuarial effect.

[e]This reform could be enacted in place of one of the other proposed reforms that affect primarily higher earners.

ble Social Security trust fund ratio at the end of the projection period, thereby addressing the terminal-year problem. Moreover, they also provide the revenues to finance the proposed benefit increases for needy groups.

Strengthening Social Security's Effectiveness as Social Insurance

Our plan for restoring long-term balance also provides financing for provisions that would buttress Social Security's protections for the most vulnerable beneficiaries. Our goal is to ensure that Social Security continues to provide an adequate base of inflation-protected income in time of need and to cushion family incomes against the possibility of disability, death of a family wage earner, or having one's career not turn out as well as expected. That is one of the reasons that our plan combines benefit reductions and revenue increases, rather than relying excessively on benefit reductions.

Even the relatively modest benefit reductions workers would experience under our plan, however, would be too much for Social Security's most vulnerable beneficiaries to bear. Three groups that would be particularly affected are workers with low lifetime earnings over a long career, widows and widowers with low benefits, and disabled workers and young survivors. We propose ways to mitigate or in some cases eliminate any adverse consequences for these groups from the benefit cuts needed to restore long-term balance. In addition, we propose augmenting the program's protection against unexpected inflation, to shelter all beneficiaries from its potentially serious effects.

Provisions for Workers with Low Lifetime Earnings

People with low lifetime earnings receive meager benefits under Social Security despite the progressive benefit formula. For example, a worker claiming retirement benefits at age 62 in 2003, who had steadily growing earnings ending at about $15,500 a year, would receive an annual benefit of under $7,000 (by "steadily growing," we mean that the worker's wage grew each year at the same rate as average wages in the economy). That is about 25 percent below the official poverty threshold for a single elderly person. A person who works 2,000 hours a year at the current minimum wage of $5.15 has annual earnings of $10,300. Such a worker who has had steadily increasing earnings over his or her career and claims Social Security benefits at age 62 in 2003 would receive an annual benefit of less than $6,000.

Low lifetime earnings can arise from a variety of causes. Some people labor at full-time, low-paying jobs over an entire career. Others are in and out of the formal workforce at different points in their lives, and therefore their average lifetime earnings (counting the years they are not in the paid workforce as zero earnings) are relatively low. Finally, some workers have relatively low lifetime earnings as counted by Social Security simply because most of their career is spent in jobs currently not covered by the program. In designing reforms to improve Social Security's protections against poverty, it is important to distinguish among these various reasons for having low lifetime earnings; in particular, we should avoid giving windfalls to workers whose lifetime earnings are understated by Social Security simply because they worked outside Social Security for some extended period.

In 1993, taking into account all sources of income, 9 percent of retired Social Security beneficiaries lived in poverty. Of these poor beneficiaries, 10 percent had worked for 41 or more years in employment covered by Social Security, and more than 40 percent had worked between 20 and 40 years. Many policymakers remain concerned, as do we, that workers who have had such substantial connections to the workforce throughout their careers nonetheless face poverty in retirement.

Before 1982, Social Security included a minimum benefit for low earners, which supplemented what they received under the regular benefit formula. This benefit, however, was not well-targeted to workers with low-paying employment over a career: it also provided significant benefits to workers with higher wages who had not worked many years in jobs covered by Social Security. That minimum benefit was eliminated for beneficiaries becoming entitled in 1982 and thereafter. A more targeted special minimum benefit, created in 1972, still exists but is phasing out because the value of regular Social Security benefits, which are indexed to wages, is increasing more rapidly than the special minimum benefit, which is indexed to prices. Indeed, under the intermediate cost assumptions of the 2000 Trustees' Report, the special minimum benefit will no longer be payable to any retired workers becoming eligible in 2013 or later (Olsen and Hoffmeyer, 2001–2).

In the light of the declining role of the special minimum benefit under current law, various reforms have proposed strengthening the minimum benefit within Social Security, including the reform plan proposed in 2001 by Representatives Jim Kolbe (R-AZ) and Charlie Stenholm (D-TX)[11] and the plans proposed by the President's Commission to Strengthen Social Security.[12]

Analysis undertaken by the Social Security Administration suggests that a minimum benefit would provide some support to a substantial fraction of workers, even though only a modest number of workers would receive the full minimum benefit. Researchers studied the effect of a minimum benefit that would provide 60 percent of income at the poverty level for workers with 20 years of covered earnings and 100 percent of the poverty level for workers with 40 or more years (Sandell, Iams, and Fanaras, 1999).[13] For workers reaching age 62 between 2008 and 2017, this minimum benefit would provide at least some benefit supplement to 21 percent of men and 49 percent of women. The full minimum benefit would be provided to only a small fraction of these beneficiaries: 3 percent of retired men and 6 percent of retired women. The effect is more pronounced among lower earners, where more than two-thirds of both men and women with average indexed monthly earnings of less than $1,200 (in 1998 dollars) would receive some benefit from the proposal. Roughly one-tenth of low-income retired workers would receive the full minimum benefit.

We propose a benefit enhancement for low earners that is quite similar to the Kolbe-Stenholm proposal and the approach adopted by the President's Commission to Strengthen Social Security. Our low-earner enhanced benefit would apply to workers with at least 20 years of covered earnings at retirement; for such workers with steadily rising earnings that amount to $10,300 in 2003, the benefit at age 62 would be increased to equal 60 percent of the poverty threshold in 2012. The benefit enhancement would increase with each additional year of covered earnings, so that benefits would equal 100 percent of the poverty threshold in 2012 for newly eligible workers with at least 35 years of covered and steadily rising earnings that amount to $10,300 in 2003.[14] For such workers, the benefit increase would amount to almost 12 percent.[15]

After 2012, the benefit enhancement would increase in line with retirement benefits for an average earner under our plan. Because the official poverty threshold increases in line with prices, whereas retirement benefits for the average worker tend to grow faster than prices under our plan, the minimum benefit would tend to increase relative to the official poverty threshold over time. As a result, Social Security would become increasingly effective at ensuring that people who have worked their entire careers will not live in poverty in old age. This proposal would cost 0.14 percent of payroll over the next 75 years.

Provisions for Widows and Widowers

A second area in which Social Security should be strengthened is its financial protection of widows and widowers. Widows typically suffer a 30 percent drop in living standards when their husbands die (Holden and Zick, 1998). This decline represents a challenge for many widows, pushing some into poverty. Indeed, whereas the poverty rate for elderly married couples is only about 5 percent, that for elderly widows is more than three times as high (Favreault, Sammartino, and Steuerle, 2002, table 6.1, p. 183).

Social Security's spousal and survivor benefits were designed decades ago, when work and family patterns were very different from what they are now. With increasing female labor force participation and evolving family structures, many have come to question this basic structure of benefits. A number of panels and commissions have reviewed this issue but failed to come up with an overall reform that attracted wide support. The reason is that all of the proposed reforms would have helped some groups but, because any improvements must be paid for, would have hurt others. The fact that most of the affected groups include both high-income and low-income individuals makes it almost impossible to do good for some without also harming many vulnerable beneficiaries. Rather than tackle the full array of issues involved in reforming Social Security's benefit structure for families, we propose only a partial adjustment in the area where the most agreement exists and where the need for reform may be the most urgent: improving survivor benefits.

Consider a retired husband and wife covered by Social Security. Should either die, the survivor will receive a benefit that is some fraction of the total benefits the couple was receiving while both were alive. In the current system, this "survivor replacement rate" varies with the couple's earnings history. In the case of a one-earner couple, the survivor receives two-thirds of what the couple was receiving, apart from any changes as a result of actuarial reductions and delayed retirement credits. In contrast, for married earners both of whom have identical earnings histories, the replacement is only one-half.

Several reforms have suggested raising the survivor benefit so that it equals at least three-quarters of the couple's combined benefits. The goal would be to increase the benefits of widows, who are generally recognized as making up the majority of survivors. One approach, proposed by Richard Burkhauser and Timothy Smeeding of Syracuse University (1994), would finance this increase

in the survivor replacement rate by reducing the spousal benefit. Such a reduction would have little or no effect on two-earner couples, because both
members qualify for their own retirement benefit and therefore rely little, if at
all, on the spousal benefit. But the reduction in the spousal benefit would have
significant effects on one-earner couples, who do rely heavily on that benefit.
In other words, the increase in the survivor benefit would benefit all couples,
but the method of financing that increase would place a large burden on one-
earner couples. The package as a whole thus would redistribute from single-
earner couples to two-earner couples. Such an approach would also reduce
benefits for many divorced spouses, a group with a high poverty rate. To avoid
increasing their poverty rate, benefits for divorced spouses could be made
larger than benefits for still-married spouses, but that seems unlikely to be politically acceptable and would have some adverse incentives. Another approach,
implicitly followed by the President's Commission to Strengthen Social Security, would finance the increase in the survivor replacement rate out of the program's general resources.

Our alternative proposal makes use of two approaches. For survivors with
low benefits, we rely on resources from the program as a whole. For survivors
with higher benefits, we take a different approach.

We propose that the survivor benefit for couples with modest benefits be
raised to 75 percent of the combined couple's benefit. To limit the cost of the
proposal and target its benefits toward reducing poverty, this enhancement
would be capped at what the survivor would receive as a worker with the average primary insurance amount for all retired workers (President Bush's Commission to Strengthen Social Security also would have imposed this limit). This
targeted proposal would cost 0.08 percent of payroll and would be financed by
the program as a whole.

For higher-income couples, we also endorse a survivor replacement rate of
75 percent, financed by reducing the couple's own combined benefits while
both are alive and using the funds to raise the benefit for the survivor (here and
below, we use the word *endorse* to indicate changes we would support but that
are not officially scored in our plan). In other words, for survivors who would
receive the average PIA or more, and therefore would have received a capped
benefit or would not be affected by the above proposal, we support a redistribution of the couple's expected benefits toward the survivor and away from the
time when both members of the couple are alive. For these couples, the goal

would be to produce no expected effect on the couple's combined lifetime benefits.[16] Such an approach would merely involve redistribution across time for the couple.[17]

A related issue involves Supplemental Security Income and Medicaid. Increasing survivor benefits or other Social Security benefits in very old age could disqualify some people from the SSI program by increasing their income above the threshold for eligibility in the program. In most states, access for elderly people to Medicaid is tied to SSI eligibility; disqualification from the SSI program could thus result in the loss of Medicaid benefits.[18] Reforms to the SSI eligibility rules are required to avoid this steep implicit tax on increased Social Security benefits.

Provisions for Disabled Workers and Young Survivors

Two groups of vulnerable beneficiaries deserving protection from the adverse effects of restoring long-term solvency to Social Security are disabled workers and the young survivors of deceased workers. Despite Social Security's protections, disabled workers and their families have higher poverty rates and are more financially vulnerable than the general population.[19] For example, those who become disabled at a young age typically have substantially less in assets than retired workers—and less than workers who become disabled later in their careers. But even workers who become disabled late in their careers tend to have less in assets than retired workers. Whether this differential reflects smaller accumulations of assets while working or the adverse financial effects of disability is unknown, but probably both are relevant.

Given the financial vulnerabilities of disabled workers despite Social Security's benefits, various reforms to the disability program seem worthy of further examination. An extensive study of these issues should be undertaken by a nonpartisan group, either appointed by Congress or formed by the National Academy of Social Insurance, perhaps on congressional request. In the absence of a more exhaustive study, we merely propose that, in the aggregate, disabled workers as a group be held harmless from the benefit reductions that would otherwise apply under our plan over the next 75 years. Our reform plan thus imposes no net reduction in benefits for the disabled beneficiary population as a whole relative to the scheduled benefit baseline over the next 75 years.

We do not propose simply maintaining the current benefit formula for disabled workers, however, for two reasons. First, it would add to the tensions already associated with application for disability benefits for those nearing or passing the earliest eligibility age for retirement benefits. The incentive to claim disability benefits arises because, unlike retirement benefits, disability benefits are not actuarially reduced at those ages. For example, consider a worker age 62. If such a worker claims retirement benefits, those benefits are reduced because the worker is claiming before the full benefit age. If the worker succeeds in qualifying for disability benefits, however, her or his benefits are not reduced. Under the current system, there is thus an incentive for workers to claim disability benefits rather than early retirement benefits. If retirement benefits were further reduced but disability benefits were not, this incentive would be strengthened, and concerns about gaming of the system would become more worrisome. To avoid exacerbating that tension and to better target disability benefits to the most needy disabled workers, we propose redistributing benefits toward workers who become disabled very young and therefore are deprived of the opportunity to enjoy the rising earnings that are typical of American workers.

A second reason not to simply maintain the current benefit formula for the disabled is that workers who become disabled at younger ages should not be locked into lower real benefits than workers who become disabled at older ages to the degree that occurs under the current system. Imagine disability benefits as replacing the retirement benefits that would have occurred had one not become disabled, as well as providing a bridge to retirement. Then one can see how the current rules leave those who became disabled at young ages far behind where they might have been if the disability had not occurred or had occurred later. In calculating the PIA for a retired worker, past earnings are indexed to the average wage up to the year when the worker turns 60. Then the PIA formula is applied to this indexed earnings level. After disability benefits start, however, benefits only keep pace with prices, as they do for retired workers after age 62. Thus, for a given cohort of workers, the continued growth of productivity in the economy raises retirement benefits for workers who are not disabled, but workers who have been disabled do not share in these productivity gains. From the perspective of social insurance, the result is an inadequate benefit for workers who become disabled at a young age.

Table 15.2 shows this effect for a 25-year-old average-earning worker in 2003 who continues to earn the average wage until becoming disabled. If this worker becomes permanently disabled at age 30, he or she will receive an inflation-adjusted benefit of less than $16,000 for the rest of his or her life (most dis-

Table 15.2. *Disability Benefits for Average-Earning Workers Age 25 in 2003, by Age at Disability*

Age at Disability	Year in which Worker Becomes Entitled to Disability Benefits	Real Benefit Level (2003 dollars)
30	2008	15,408
35	2013	16,326
40	2018	17,203
45	2023	18,089
50	2028	19,062
55	2033	20,104

Source: 2003 Annual Report, 2003, table V1.F11.
Note: Data are estimates based on retirement benefits for medium earners turning 62 in the indicated year and subsequently claiming benefits at the full benefit age.

ability beneficiaries do in fact remain permanently eligible for benefits once they have begun receiving them). Had the same worker become disabled at age 55 instead, he or she would have enjoyed 25 years of additional real wage growth and would therefore receive slightly more than $20,000 a year in benefits.

To allow workers who become disabled at younger ages to share partially in the benefits of aggregate productivity growth that occurs after their disability, we propose indexing disability benefits *after* they have been initially claimed to a combination of wage and price growth rather than to price increases alone. The determination of initial disability benefits would continue to rely on wage indexation, as under current law.

Specifically, to raise real benefit levels over time for workers who become disabled earlier in their careers, our plan includes a "super" cost-of-living adjustment (COLA) for disability benefits. The super-COLA would have the effect, relative to the current structure of disability benefits, of increasing benefits for those who become disabled at younger ages compared with those who become disabled at older ages. The size of the super-COLA is chosen so disabled workers as a whole would be held harmless from the benefit reductions in our plan over the next 75 years. In particular, the super-COLA would increase disability benefits by 0.9 percentage point a year more than the overall inflation rate. (Although the actuarial evaluation was based on using this figure each year, the actual super-COLA in each year would depend on wage and price growth. The expected value of the super-COLA given the Board of Trustees' 2003 projections for wages and prices is inflation plus 0.9 percentage point.)

This approach has several advantages relative to the alternative of not applying any benefit changes to disabled beneficiaries. First, it retains the close connection between disability benefits and retirement benefits; as under current law, disabled beneficiaries would transfer seamlessly to retired worker status at the full benefit age. Second, as noted above, making no changes whatsoever to disability benefits while reducing retired worker benefits would create even stronger incentives for workers to apply for disability rather than retirement benefits before the full benefit age. Our approach attenuates this problem by redistributing lifetime benefits within the disabled population toward workers who become eligible for disability benefits at younger ages, even while holding disabled workers as a whole harmless from our changes. It strikes us as implausible that younger workers would apply for disability benefits, and thereby forgo substantial future labor earnings, just to offset part or all of the reductions that would otherwise apply to their retirement benefits. Finally, the redistribution seems to us valuable even in the absence of other changes, because workers who become disabled at younger ages seem more needy and are locked into lower real annual benefits than workers who become disabled at later ages.

Two other implications of our approach should be noted. First, workers who become disabled in the near future would receive higher lifetime benefits than under current law, because they would experience little reduction in their initial benefit level and then would receive a super-COLA. Second, workers who become disabled at older ages in the distant future would receive lower lifetime benefits than under the scheduled benefit baseline. In other words, this approach holds the disabled worker beneficiary population as a whole harmless from the benefit reductions we would impose over the next 75 years, but it does not necessarily hold each cohort of disabled workers harmless.

We would apply the same system of super-COLAs to benefits for young survivors. Together with the super-COLAs for disabled workers, this change would cost 0.21 percent of payroll over the next 75 years. That is precisely the effect over the same period of the other provisions of our plan on benefits that apply to all disabled workers and young survivors.

The result is that our proposal to restore long-term balance to Social Security over the next 75 years does not rely on any net reduction in benefits for these vulnerable beneficiary groups. Rather, we hold both disabled workers and young survivors as a whole harmless from the benefit reductions that would otherwise apply over the next 75 years.

Closing Gaps in the Protection of Benefits against Inflation

Our fourth reform to strengthen the social insurance differs from the previous three: we endorse enhancing Social Security's protections against unexpected inflation, thus providing improved insurance to all beneficiaries. (Again, we "endorse" rather than "propose" this reform because this element of our plan was not officially scored by the Social Security actuaries; however, it should have de minimis actuarial effects.)

Social Security benefits were first indexed for inflation in 1972; legislation enacted in 1977 introduced some changes in the system of indexation. The result is that moderate inflation now has little effect on either real benefits or the fiscal position of Social Security; however, a gap remains in the indexing of Social Security, such that a return to high inflation would have adverse effects on some generations, while saving money for Social Security. We propose to fill this gap in a revenue-neutral way.

The gap in indexing results from the way in which benefits are adjusted for inflation after the determination of the AIME. For any year after the year a worker turns 62, benefits are increased by the inflation rate from the year that worker turns 62 until the current year. But the AIME is based on average indexed career earnings until the year a worker turns 60, and the key components of the benefit formula are indexed in the same way. Thus there is a two-year gap, between ages 60 and 62, in the protection against inflation.

If inflation happened to be particularly severe in some two-year period, workers age 60 at the start of that period would experience a significant decline in their inflation-adjusted benefits. For example, a repeat of the inflation rates of 1980 and 1981 (which resulted in Social Security cost-of-living adjustments of 14.3 percent and 11.2 percent, respectively) would reduce real benefits for that unfortunate cohort by more than 20 percent. Although inflation above the level used in the actuarial projection would reduce real costs for Social Security, there is no reason to subject workers to the risk of an unknown level of inflation during those two years. Thus we propose that the indexing of benefits for inflation start from the year in which a worker turns 60 rather than the year in which a worker turns 62.

By itself, such a change would increase benefits, and thus the actuarial imbalance. To preserve projected revenue neutrality, we combine this change in indexing with an across-the-board percentage reduction in benefits meant to leave all workers in the same position relative to expected inflation. The goal is neither to make nor to lose money for Social Security, and neither to increase nor to decrease lifetime projected benefits, but rather to remove an element of risk that arises from the lack of indexing during these years. This rule applies to disabled workers as well as retirees, because the gap is present in both cases.

Social Security reform should do more than merely restore long-term financial balance to the program. It should also improve Social Security's protection of some of the most vulnerable beneficiaries: low earners, widows and widowers, and disabled workers and survivors. Because restoring long-term financial solvency to the program is likely to require some benefit reductions, balancing those reductions with selective improvements in critical areas seems essential, to cushion the impact of these reductions on the most vulnerable. Our plan therefore not only achieves long-term solvency but also strengthens Social Security's social insurance protections for these beneficiaries.

Implications for Benefits and Revenue

In evaluating reform plans, it is important to be clear about the baseline against which the proposed benefits and revenues are compared. In presenting our proposals above, we compared all our proposed benefit changes against the scheduled benefit baseline, which reflects what would be paid in the future under the current benefit formula and current projections if all benefits are paid. The proposed tax changes were described relative to the current tax structure, even though that structure is insufficient to finance scheduled benefits. This combination seemed the most straightforward way to explain the proposed changes to ensure that they were properly understood.

Actuarial Effects

Figure 15.2 shows the projected path of the trust fund ratio under current law and under our reform plan (the trust fund ratio is the ratio of the assets of the Social Security trust fund to the program's expenditures in a given year). As the figure illustrates, our plan achieves a positive trust fund ratio throughout the next 75 years and leaves the trust fund ratio stable at the end of that period, under the 2003 intermediate cost projections used by the Office of the Chief Actuary.

Note that, under our plan, the trust fund ratio peaks somewhat higher and

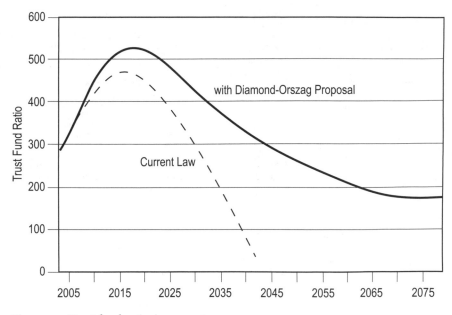

Figure 15.2. Trust fund ratio, in percentages

somewhat later than under current law and then begins a steady decline. This decline is relatively rapid at first, as the continued financing of benefits to baby boomer retirees draws the trust fund down. Over time, however, as the baby boomers die and our changes to both taxes and benefits are slowly phased in, the decline in the ratio slows. By the end of the projection period, the trust fund ratio is again beginning to rise.

Combined Effects

As we emphasized, our plan combines benefit reductions and tax changes to restore long-term solvency to Social Security. Table 15.3 shows the overall benefit reductions that our plan would impose on a worker with average earnings. For lower earners, the reductions in annual benefits would be smaller than shown because of the low-earner benefit enhancement. For higher earners the reductions would be larger than shown, because the income inequality adjustment to the top PIA factor would apply to them and not to lower earners.

As the table also shows, real benefits under our plan would continue to rise from one generation to the next, despite the reductions from baseline, because benefit increases due to ongoing productivity gains are projected to more than

Table 15.3. Benefit Reductions under Proposed Reform for Average Earners

Age at End of 2004	Change in Benefits from Scheduled Benefit Baseline	Inflation-Adjusted Benefit at Full Benefit Age Relative to 55-Year-Old[a]
55	0.0%	100
45	−0.6	110
35	−4.5	118
25	−8.6	125

Source: Authors' calculations.

[a]For a retired worker with scaled medium preretirement earnings pattern. This scaled earnings pattern allows wages to vary with the age of the worker but ensures that lifetime earnings are approximately equal to those of a worker with the average wage in every year of his or her career.

Table 15.4. Payroll Tax Rates under Proposed Reform
(Percentage of earnings)

Year	Employee Rate	Combined Employer-Employee Rate
2005	6.20	12.40
2015	6.22	12.45
2025	6.35	12.69
2035	6.59	13.18
2045	6.84	13.68
2055	7.09	14.18

Source: Authors' calculations.

offset our modest benefit reductions. An average-earning worker age 25 today would receive an annual benefit at the full benefit age that is roughly 25 percent more than a 55-year-old average-earning worker today. Because of the minimum benefit, low-earners have less of a benefit reduction (and some have an increase), while medium earners are having the effects just described. Also higher earners would experience larger benefit reductions than the average.

The combined revenue effects of our plan give rise to a gradual increase in the payroll tax. As Table 15.4 shows, the employee payroll tax rate under our plan slowly increases from 6.2 percent in 2005 to 7.1 percent in 2055. The combined employer-employee payroll tax increases from 12.4 percent today to 12.45 percent in 2015, 13.2 percent in 2035, and 14.2 percent in 2055.

By 2055, the tax rate is thus 14 percent higher than under the current tax structure ($14.18/12.40 = 1.14$). For an average worker becoming eligible for retirement benefits in that year, the PIA is also 14 percent lower than under the current benefit formula. This reflects the rough balance between benefit and revenue changes that we have pursued in our plan.

The overall results for benefit reductions and tax increases underscore that it is possible to restore long-term balance to Social Security while retaining the program's core social insurance role and spreading the legacy costs from the program's history fairly across generations. For the vast majority of workers, the provisions included in our plan would involve quite modest changes. The payroll tax rate would rise slowly in response to increasing life expectancy and to adjusting the ratio of legacy costs to taxable payroll; by 2035, the combined employer-employee payroll tax rate under our plan, at 13.2 percent, would be less than 1 percentage point higher than today's 12.4 percent. The benefit reductions would also be modest and gradual: today's average-earning 35-year-olds, for example, would experience less than a 5 percent reduction in annual benefits compared with the current benefit formula. To be sure, the required adjustments for higher earners would be larger, but so is their ability to absorb those adjustments.

Individual Accounts

Unlike many other proposals for Social Security reform, our plan does not call for the creation of individual accounts within Social Security. Individual accounts, which include tax-favored private-sector accounts such as 401(k)s and Keoghs, already provide an extremely useful supplement to Social Security, and they can be improved and expanded. But they are simply inappropriate for a social insurance system intended to provide for the basic tier of income during retirement, disability, and other times of need. Moreover, the trend in private pensions from defined benefit to defined contribution structures makes individual accounts less attractive, because the trend adds to the correlation of the risks already being borne by workers to the risks in individual accounts.

Furthermore, individual accounts could potentially reduce the actuarial deficit in Social Security only if they are linked to reductions in traditional benefits in some way, either explicitly or implicitly. They would not, by themselves, improve the ability of the Social Security system to finance its traditional benefits, and they might undermine that ability. In particular, if individual accounts were financed by diverting payroll tax revenue away from the Social Security trust fund, the immediate effect would be to *increase* the deficit within Social Security. In that case, individual accounts could help reduce the projected deficit only if they more than compensated for the diverted revenue either by directly returning sufficient funds to Social Security or by being linked in some less direct way to benefit reductions within the traditional system.

However, reducing traditional Social Security benefits to make room for individual accounts would be, in our opinion, a bad deal for society as a whole. The reason is that the benefits that would be financed from a system of individual accounts are likely to differ from the benefits that Social Security provides today in several important ways, including the following:

- Retirement benefits under Social Security provide an assured level of income that does not depend on what happens in financial markets.[20] Instead, benefits are related to the beneficiary's average lifetime earnings and when the beneficiary chooses to retire. With an individual account, by contrast, benefits during retirement depend on the value of the assets accumulated in the account, which likewise depends in part on lifetime earnings and retirement timing but also depends on how well one has invested and on how financial markets happened to perform during one's career. It is entirely appropriate and indeed beneficial in some settings for individuals to accept the risks of investing in financial markets; it does not, however, make sense to incur such risks as a way of providing for a base level of income during retirement, disability, or other times of need. This observation is particularly important for those workers who expect to rely heavily or exclusively on Social Security in retirement; recall that Social Security represents the *only* source of income for one-fifth of elderly beneficiaries.

- Retirement benefits under Social Security are protected from inflation and last as long as the beneficiary lives. A retirement system based on individual accounts could, in principle, achieve similar protection by requiring account holders, on retiring, to convert their account balances into a lifelong series of inflation-adjusted payments (that is, an inflation-indexed annuity), but many proposals for individual accounts do not include such a requirement. Furthermore, any such requirement might not be politically sustainable. Individual accounts have been promoted on the grounds that they would enhance "personal wealth" and "ownership" of one's retirement assets; this seems inconsistent with maintaining substantial restrictions on how account holders may access and use their accounts. The goal of "bequeathable wealth," an explicit selling point of some proposals, is in direct conflict with the financing of benefits that last as long as the beneficiary lives. One cannot use the same assets to both maximize benefits during one's own lifetime and leave something for one's heirs. Not all retirement income need be protected against inflation and last for the life of the beneficiary, but some base level of income during retirement, disability, or other times of need should be so protected. Again, this observation is particularly important for workers with little or no retirement savings other than Social Security.

- Social Security benefits come as a joint-life annuity, protecting surviving spouses. Just as annuitization might not be sustained for individual accounts, so too protection of spouses might be undercut.[21]

- The Social Security benefit formula is progressive: it replaces a larger share of previous earnings for lower earners than for higher earners. Most plans do not incorporate this type of progressivity in the individual accounts and some do not preserve comparable progressivity in remaining benefits. For the nation, the progressivity of Social Security helps reduce poverty and narrow income inequalities; for the individual, it can cushion the blow from a career that turns out to be less rewarding than one hoped. These protections would be strengthened under our plan, which includes provisions to improve Social Security benefits for the most vulnerable members of society.

- There is no political pressure to give earlier access to Social Security benefit. In contrast, there is likely to be considerable pressure for individual accounts to mimic 401(k)s and IRAs, which allow earlier access through loans and early withdrawals. This could undermine the preservation of funds for retirement.

- Social Security provides other benefits in addition to basic retirement income. Some of these, such as disability benefits, would be difficult to integrate into an individual account system. Under some individual account proposals, disabled workers would not have access to the accumulated assets in their accounts before they reach retirement age; thus the accounts would be of no help to them when needed most. Even with such access, workers who become disabled before retirement age will have had less time than other workers to accumulate a balance in their accounts. Thus, even though disabled workers are on average in worse financial condition than retirees, a movement to individual accounts is likely to treat them even worse than retirees.

- A system of individual accounts would require certain administrative costs to maintain those accounts, costs that the present structure of Social Security avoids. The higher these costs, the less generous the benefits that a given history of contributions can finance. Also, inevitably, some workers managing their own individual accounts will make poor investment choices that will leave them stranded in time of need, even if financial markets have performed well. Although some individual account proposals have rules that would limit administrative costs and restrict the opportunities for workers to make poor investment choices, other proposals leave scope for high administrative charges and misguided investment decisions. Thus, there is great uncertainty about the types of protective rules that may or may not accompany any individual account plan that is actually implemented.

To sum up, Social Security has certain core principles, including the following: to provide benefits to workers and their families in the form of a real annuity after the disability, retirement, or death of a family wage earner; to provide higher annual benefits relative to earnings for those with lower earnings; and to provide similar replacement rates on average to cohorts that are close in age. A system of individual accounts could well move away from all of these principles. Benefits might be provided as a lump sum that might be outlived, leaving the worker or a surviving spouse much less well off than under an annuity; any access to account balances before retirement could leave less for retirement; replacement rates, rather than being progressive, could be proportional to earnings within a cohort if its members held the same portfolios and faced the same charges; and these replacement rates could vary dramatically from one generation to the next as financial markets fluctuate. Finally, under the current system, the level of benefits becomes predictable as workers approach retirement age; under an individual account system, benefits could be far less predictable, depending on possible sudden changes in asset values and interest rates.

Financing of Individual Account Plans

In addition to providing less satisfactory benefits to workers, individual accounts that divert revenue away from Social Security make Social Security financing more difficult. If Social Security revenue were diverted into individual accounts without any corresponding reduction in benefits, Social Security's financial standing would clearly be worsened. To avoid this, individual accounts financed by such revenue diversion must be linked in some way to a reduction in traditional benefits sufficient to offset the cost of the diverted revenue. To examine the effects of individual account plans that are linked in this manner, we begin with an example of an account structure in which traditional benefits that would otherwise be paid to the individual account holder are reduced in such a way that traditional Social Security finances are unaffected over the account holder's lifetime. This holds the Social Security trust fund harmless over the lifetime of the average worker from the diversion of revenue, but not in each year.[22]

For our example, assume that a flow of revenue, such as payroll tax revenue, that otherwise would have flowed into the Social Security trust fund, goes instead into a system of individual accounts (it does not matter whether the revenue is an existing flow or a new, additional flow, as long as it is assumed that it would have gone to the trust fund were it not being diverted to the individual accounts). To ensure that the traditional Social Security system is held harmless from the diversion, a worker with an individual account in our example is considered to owe a "debt" to the Social Security trust fund. On retirement, the debt is repaid by reducing the worker's traditional Social Security benefits. For the trust fund to be held harmless over the lifetime of the worker, those reductions in benefits must exactly equal the amounts diverted from the Social Security trust fund to the individual accounts, plus the interest the trust fund would have earned on the diverted funds had they remained in the trust fund.

This example raises several issues: the timing of cash flows, the differences between benefits provided by the current Social Security structure and benefits provided by the combined individual accounts–Social Security system, the likelihood that revenue available to the individual accounts would otherwise have been available to Social Security, and possible differences in policy actions due to the presence of the individual accounts.

In our example, a reduction in traditional benefits is what holds Social Security harmless over the lifetime of a worker for the flow of revenue into the individual account rather than into the Social Security trust fund. For each worker, however, the bulk of the flow of revenue into the individual accounts would precede by many years the offsetting reductions in traditional benefits.

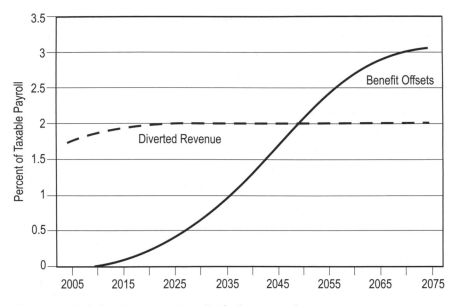

Figure 15.3. Cash flow from generic individual account plan

For example, the benefit offset for a worker age 25 would occur over a period of several decades that does not begin until about four decades hence. Revenue would thus be diverted from the trust fund over many years before the corresponding "debt" would be repaid.

Currently, roughly 85 cents of every dollar in noninterest Social Security revenue is used to pay benefits during the same year. If revenue were diverted into individual accounts, the reduced cash flow would drive the trust fund balance to exhaustion sooner than currently projected, requiring either some source of additional revenue to continue paying benefits or a reduction in current benefits to offset the reduced revenue flow.

To examine our example in more detail, we assume that 2 percent of payroll is diverted to individual accounts, with an offsetting reduction in traditional benefits for account holders on retirement, as stipulated above.[23] Figure 15.3 shows the cash-flow effects. Over an infinite horizon, the individual accounts have no effect on the trust fund in present value terms—the trust fund is eventually paid back in full for the diverted revenue; however, the aggregate cash flow from the individual accounts is negative over a period of more than 45 years, because the diverted revenue exceeds the benefit offsets until almost 2050.

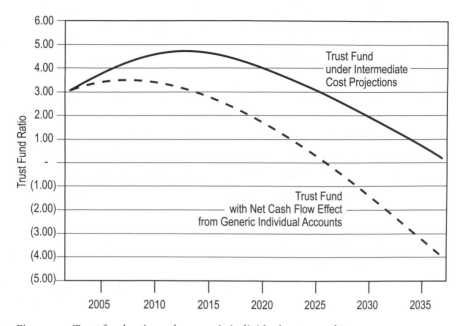

Figure 15.4. Trust fund ratio under generic individual account plan

While the present value of the impact on the trust fund of the accounts is zero on an infinite horizon basis, at each point of time the trust fund is lower than it would have been. Indeed, the loss of the trust fund relative to taxable earnings is steadily increasing throughout the projection period, as shown in Figure 15.4. The delay between the revenue flow and the corresponding benefit reductions thus poses a significant problem for the Social Security system. The net cash outflow shown in the figure causes the trust fund to be exhausted more than a decade earlier than in the absence of the accounts. To offset this negative cash flow, it would be necessary either to phase in benefit reductions more rapidly, to provide additional revenue to Social Security, or to allow Social Security to borrow from the rest of the budget. The problems with general revenue transfers and borrowing are discussed later in the chapter.

With these individual accounts, workers can make deposits and purchase financial assets such as stocks and bonds, in effect financing those deposits with decreases in their future traditional benefits. Because the benefit decreases, including interest, are calculated using a Treasury bond interest rate, workers would in effect be doing an "asset swap," substituting a mixed portfolio of stocks and bonds for an all-bond portfolio. It is important to remember, however, that in an efficient financial market, higher expected returns are earned only by taking on greater risks. Most investors do not like risk. To induce risk-averse investors to place money in riskier assets, those assets must offer higher expected average returns. Risk is one of the principal reasons that stocks tend to have a relatively higher expected average rate of return than other financial assets.

Because individuals are averse to risk, comparing average rates of return on assets with different risk characteristics is misleading; an asset with a higher average return but substantially more risk may not be preferable to a lower-yielding, lower-risk asset. The average return on the riskier asset will be higher, but so will be the risk; some who invest in the asset will receive low returns, whereas others investing at different times will receive high returns. To analyze the relative attractiveness of different assets, virtually all economists believe it is necessary to adjust for risk.

To do this, economists calculate for risky assets a rate of return that adjusts for the risk associated with the asset. If the measured rate of return on an asset is high only because it is riskier than other assets, its risk-adjusted rate of return will not be so high: the risk adjustment will partly or fully eliminate the difference between the measured rates of return. The risk-adjusted rate of return thus allows one to evaluate the measured rates of return of different assets on a comparable basis. Only to the extent that the risk-adjusted rate of return is higher on one asset than another would that asset necessarily be preferable as an investment.

To compute risk-adjusted rates of return for various assets, economists have developed a variety of tools for measuring and correcting for risk; however, the task remains difficult. For example, the cost of bearing risk depends on a wide variety of factors, which vary from individual to individual, including especially the other risks to which they are exposed. Here we focus merely on the relative returns of stocks and bonds, abstracting from the other dimensions of risk.

One critical question is whether the higher returns to stocks observed in the past can be explained solely by the greater riskiness of stocks than bonds. Some economists have concluded they cannot—that the rate of return on stocks is higher than can be explained by their greater riskiness alone. The complexities of risk adjustment make it difficult to reach a definitive conclusion.

On the one hand, for many workers covered by Social Security, who also hold significant portfolios of assets outside of Social Security to help finance their retirement, the diversification is of little or no value. A worker accumulating assets for retirement can hold stocks and bonds in existing retirement accounts as well as outside of such accounts. Adding the opportunity to substitute stocks for bonds within Social Security, as our generic example of an individual account system effectively shows, does not alter the overall composition of the package of assets the worker can choose unless the worker is holding few or no bonds outside Social Security. In other words, a worker with a diversified portfolio will generally hold both stocks and bonds, with the shares of each reflecting the worker's risk aversion. An opportunity to become more exposed to stocks through Social Security does not alter this worker's opportunities, if the worker already had the opportunity to sell some of her or his bonds and buy some more stocks. For someone already holding a diversified portfolio, the risk adjustment that is appropriate shows that stocks are worth no more than Treasury bonds.

On the other hand, for workers with so little financial wealth that they are holding no stocks at all, the opportunity our generic example offers is a new one. Such workers may experience a small gain from this opportunity, but the opportunity does involve taking on additional risk (see, for example, Geanakoplos, Mitchell, and Zeldes, 1998; and Diamond and Geanakoplos, 2003). Even for such workers, *some* risk adjustment is therefore appropriate, and the fact that Social Security is the primary tier of retirement income may affect the size of that adjustment. Furthermore, evidence from workers' actual 401(k) investment choices makes it clear that many workers without investing experience have trouble making sensible investment decisions in the absence of significant financial education or extremely restricted portfolio choices.[24] Ensuring that workers have adequate financial education to manage their individual accounts would be expensive, effectively adding to the administrative costs imposed under such a system.

It is worth noting that we do not object to individual accounts on grounds that the stock market is excessively risky. Indeed, if we were advising a large group of individuals saving for retirement, we would recommend a diversified portfolio, not one comprising only bonds. Our discussion of risk is intended primarily to help the reader interpret the presentations of proponents of individual accounts, some of whom regularly report the benefits that such accounts could finance without *any* adjustment for risk. Such presentations should be taken with a large grain of salt.[25]

Finally, if the judgment was made that diversification into equities does provide benefits even after adjusting for risk, such diversification could also be undertaken directly or indirectly through the Social Security trust fund, without the need for individual accounts.

The bottom line is that the swap of bonds for stocks inherent in our generic example of individual accounts would be of no value to many workers. For those with little financial wealth, the swap may be of some value, provided the opportunity is pursued with good investment choices and to a sufficiently limited extent, in keeping with the risk aversion appropriate for someone relying heavily on Social Security. Any potential advantages of such a swap, however, need to be considered along with the disadvantages associated with the potential changes in how benefits are provided. It is precisely those with limited financial wealth who are likely to gain the most from the annuitized benefits provided by the current system and from its progressivity. Thus, those who stand to gain from the change in asset holdings are also those most at risk of losing from other aspects of individual accounts.

Sources of Revenue

Our individual accounts analyzed above assumed that a given level of revenue is available either to traditional Social Security or to the system of individual accounts. Some analysts, however, argue that an increase in revenue is more feasible politically if it is devoted to a system of individual accounts than if it is devoted to the existing system. Edward Gramlich has been perhaps the most prominent advocate of this perspective.[26] Gramlich proposes a system of individual accounts financed by contributions beyond the existing payroll tax; the mandatory additional contributions would be tantamount to a payroll tax increase that is specifically directed to the individual accounts. This implicit tax increase would then be combined with a reduction in traditional benefits sufficient for the two together to restore actuarial balance to Social Security as a whole.

It may indeed be easier to legislate an implicit tax linked to individual accounts than an explicit payroll tax increase of the same size, although it is difficult to know for sure because strong backing is not currently in evidence for either approach. Our view is that the political system can provide adequate revenue without the crutch of individual accounts and that the shortcomings of such accounts make it worthwhile to seek a reform without them. That is, we think the American public is sufficiently supportive of Social Security that it would continue to reelect legislators who voted for a modest payroll tax increase to shore up the system. To us it does not seem necessary to link payroll tax increases to individual accounts, although we acknowledge that this is a political judgment with which others may differ.

Some individual account proposals have not identified a specific source of contributions to the accounts but instead have simply assumed that the ultimate source will be the rest of the federal budget. For example, general revenue could be directly deposited into individual accounts, or existing payroll revenue could be diverted into the accounts and the trust fund compensated with general revenue transfers. In light of the substantial deficits projected for the federal budget, however, any proposal for transfers that does not identify a specific funding source seems to us strikingly irresponsible. Many individual account proposals are particularly problematic in this regard, because they rely on massive assumed general revenue transfers.

More generally, after more than 70 years, the basic structure of Social Security is well settled: Americans have implicitly agreed to use Social Security to provide for a certain range of social insurance goals and not for other purposes. Any radical change in the program's structure would reopen largely settled questions about the broad approach through which the political process will meet this range of goals. In short, drastic changes in Social Security would alter the political environment from one of basic agreement to one of substantial flux and uncertainty. That is a risk anyone who benefits from the current structure, or is concerned about those who rely on the current structure for their well-being, should regard as worrisome (see Heclo, 1998). Indeed, the wide variety of rules proposed across the various individual account plans offered to date is itself evidence of how it is hard to predict what will come from such proposals if and when they are enacted, much less over time as political forces evolve.

Individual Account Proposals

The President's Commission to Strengthen Social Security proposed a system linking individual accounts to traditional benefit reductions similar to our generic example. Unlike our generic example, however, both model 2 and model 3 as proposed by the Commission would have *subsidized* the individual accounts by charging an interest rate on the liability accounts (that is, on the amounts diverted from the trust fund), which is projected to be lower than the return the trust fund earns on its reserves. Because the interest rate on the diverted funds would be lower than what the trust fund would have earned otherwise, these individual account proposals would worsen Social Security's financial status even on an infinite-horizon basis. Stated another way, the trust fund earns the interest rate paid on Treasury bonds on each dollar that is not diverted into an individual account; but on each dollar that is diverted into an individual account, under this proposal, the trust fund would earn only the interest rate charged on the liability account, which is lower. This amounts to a subsidy from the trust fund to the individuals who establish individual accounts. We see no reason why such a subsidy is warranted.[27]

Other methods of linking individual accounts and traditional benefit reductions have been proposed. For example, under so-called clawback provisions, withdrawals from an individual account on retirement would trigger proportional reductions in Social Security benefits or other transfers back to Social Security. Thus, the returns on individual accounts subject to a clawback, unlike those in our generic example, would affect not only the individual investor but also the financial position of Social Security. Alternatively, some plans would simply take revenue from the individual accounts without changing traditional benefits. Such a mechanism has been proposed by Representative Clay Shaw (R-FL), among others.[28]

Under the Shaw plan, a worker who retired or became disabled would receive 5 percent of his or her account balance in a lump-sum payment. The other 95 percent of the account balance would be transferred directly back to Social Security.[29] In the absence of countervailing measures, such a structure could create incentives for risky investments in the accounts, because the Social Security system would subsidize 95 percent of any losses and tax 95 percent of the gains.[30] In the Shaw plan, however, workers would be forced to invest in a specified portfolio comprising 60 percent stocks, held in broad market indexes, and 40 percent bonds, to avoid the potential gaming problems associated with this type of clawback. A plan with 95 percent of asset balances returned to Social Security is merely a gimmick to take advantage of the actuarial scoring rules.

Administrative Costs and the Structure of Individual Accounts

Our generic example did not examine the administrative costs of individual accounts. Individual accounts would unquestionably entail administrative costs not present under traditional Social Security. Thus, for the net returns available to finance benefits to be the same with individual accounts as with matching trust fund investments, the costs of the accounts must be implausibly low. How high those costs would be in reality would depend on a number of factors, including how centralized the system of accounts was and how limited the investment choices were; the level of service provided (for example, whether individuals enjoyed unlimited free telephone calls to account representatives, frequent account balance statements, and other services); the size of the accounts; and the rules and regulations governing them. The higher the administrative costs, the lower the ultimate benefit a worker would receive, all else equal, because more of the funds in the accounts would be consumed by these costs and less would be left over to pay retirement benefits. For example, if administrative costs amounted to 1 percent of assets each year over a typical worker's career, the level of retirement benefits that could be financed would be roughly 20 percent less than what could be financed without the administrative costs. If the costs were half as large, the reduction in benefits would also be roughly half as large.[31]

Conclusion

Proposals to establish a system of individual accounts within Social Security raise many issues. Diverting revenue into these accounts and away from the existing Social Security system would generate a cash-flow problem for Social Security, even if the system was eventually reimbursed for the diverted funds. Advocates of individual accounts tend to play down this cash-flow problem or simply assume it away. We, however, view the prospect of the Social Security trust fund being exhausted more than a decade sooner than otherwise as a serious political economy problem. Furthermore, the various alternatives for "solving" the problem—including transferring funds from the rest of the budget or reducing current benefits to match the reduced level of revenue—are unappealing. Indeed they leave Social Security at risk.

Furthermore, individual accounts would likely not generate any significant gains in overall economic efficiency. Finally, because individual accounts would likely fail to provide the social insurance protections the current system offers, it simply makes little sense to scale back that system to finance an alternative system of individual accounts in addition to the individual accounts (401(k), Keogh, IRA) that already exist on top of Social Security.

A Final Note

The long-term deficit projected in Social Security should neither serve as an excuse for undermining the program's social insurance structure, nor be "eliminated" with accounting or other gimmicks that promise to erase the deficit without any pain. Eventually the bill for those gimmicks will come due. The American public deserves a well-informed and honest debate over Social Security's future, not obfuscation. As our proposal shows, Social Security can be reformed without dismantling its important insurance protections and without resorting to accounting tricks. It can also be done without undercutting the functioning of Social Security itself or of the economy—indeed, reform can improve their functioning.

Our plan meets important criteria: It would restore actuarial balance while addressing the terminal-year problem. It would not directly increase the burden on the rest of the federal budget (or rely on gimmicks that take advantage of actuarial scoring rules). It would distribute the legacy cost fairly. It would preserve and improve the social insurance character of Social Security. And it would protect and improve the functioning of the economy by contributing to national saving.

Our plan comprises a moderate set of reforms that would restore long-term balance to Social Security by addressing three main sources of its long-term deficit: increases in life expectancy, increased income inequality, and the legacy debt from the system's history. The plan combines revenue increases and benefit reductions to achieve long-term solvency. Its design builds on the tradition set in 1983, when policymakers from both parties came together to embrace a balanced set of reforms.

A quarter century later, the debate over Social Security reform has loomed large in presidential and other elections, but we have failed to fix the program. Extreme positions held by some and denial of the problem by others have so far impeded progress. It is time that we once again pursued a balanced approach to reforming Social Security.

Acknowledgments

This chapter is an adapted extract from our book *Saving Social Security: A Balanced Approach,* Revised Edition. © 2005 Brookings Institution Press.

NOTES

1. President George W. Bush, announcing the formation of the President's Commission to Strengthen Social Security, in the Rose Garden at the White House, May 2, 2001, www.csss.gov/press/press050201.html.

2. The Office of the Chief Actuary has established a set of criteria that must be met for the system to be deemed in actuarial balance. If the system's short-run finances (current revenue plus the trust fund balance) are insufficient to pay scheduled benefits, the system is clearly not in balance. Over longer periods, however, the reliability of the projections declines. Actuarial balance based on long-run considerations therefore allows some small degree of shortfall; if the shortfall is modest enough, corrective action is not necessarily warranted and the system is deemed to be in balance.

3. Specifically, using the period mortality table for the most recent available period and the one available for the previous year, and using the interest rates projected the previous year, the Office of the Chief Actuary would determine the percentage reduction in the Primary Insurance Amount for that cohort that would keep unchanged the lifetime cost, at present value, of a dollar of benefits commencing at the full benefit age. With this approach, changes in benefit levels depend not on assumed changes in life expectancy, but on actual changes in mortality by age.

4. Because the 75-year cost of benefits to all newly eligible beneficiaries is roughly 85 percent of the 75-year cost of benefits in total, the percentage increase in the tax rate would be 85 percent of the percentage decrease in the Primary Insurance Amount. This does not result in precisely a 50–50 balance between changes in taxes and changes in benefits over the initial 75-year period. Rather, our thought was to produce a rolling 75-year balance from each annual change, recognizing that the initiation of this policy involves anticipation of many future changes. In addition, to avoid the administrative complexities associated with de minimis changes, the tax rate would change only when the accumulated computed change from this provision and later provisions since the last adjustment exceeded 0.05 percent of payroll.

5. Interestingly, model 3 of President Bush's Commission to Strengthen Social Security also implicitly proposed a similar change in the maximum taxable earnings base to increase revenue. Although the Commission was prohibited from recommending any tax increases, model 3 included revenue that matched what would be generated if the taxable maximum were increased. Specifically, the scoring of the general revenue transfers under model 3 assumed that the fraction of covered earnings subject to tax increased to 86 percent between 2005 and 2009 and was then maintained at that level thereafter. In what may be the only dissenting words in the report, the Commission noted that "some members . . . believed that a substantial portion of this [revenue transfer to Social Security under model 3] should come from an increase in the payroll tax base. . . . However, this suggestion was deemed inconsistent with the principles in the executive order establishing the Commission" (President's Commission, 2001, p. 131, note 41).

6. Much of the material in this section is drawn from Munnell, 2000.

7. With universal coverage, the Government Pension Offset and Windfall Elimination Provision under current Social Security law will eventually no longer be needed. These provisions were legislated so that those covered by Social Security for only part of their careers, or whose spouses were not fully covered by Social Security, did not receive unwarranted benefits from the program's progressive benefit formula. Some have argued instead for eliminating these provisions, but we think that in the absence of universal coverage they serve an important role in targeting higher benefits to those intended to receive them, although there is room for improvement. See our paper "Reforming the GPO and WEP in Social Security" (Diamond and Orszag, 2003).

8. The benefit reduction would be calculated as $1 - 0.9969^{t - 2022}$, where t is the year in which the worker becomes eligible for benefits.

9. One could instead allow full or partial inclusion of such earnings in benefit calculations. We chose not to pursue this approach because those with such high earnings are not likely to be crucially reliant on Social Security for benefits. Thus, a higher tax rate with partial benefit credits would not serve an important social insurance purpose beyond ensuring that high earners bear a fair share of the legacy cost.

10. Paine also wanted to use part of the revenue to give a grant to those turning 21 to help launch their careers. See Paine, 1925.

11. Under the Kolbe-Stenholm approach, workers with a 20-year history of covered earnings under Social Security would receive a benefit at the full benefit age of at least 60 percent of the poverty level. The minimum benefit would increase for workers with longer careers; for workers with at least 40 years of covered earnings, the minimum benefit at the full benefit age would equal 100 percent of the poverty level. The minimum benefit target would be indexed to prices over time under the Kolbe-Stenholm plan, as is the poverty level.

12. The Commission's model 2 proposed a new minimum benefit for low-wage workers with at least 20 years of covered earnings. This benefit would increase with years of additional covered earnings. For workers with at least 30 years of covered earnings, the benefit at the full benefit age was expected to reach 120 percent of the poverty threshold by 2018 and then stabilize at approximately that level. Model 3 also proposed a minimum benefit for workers with at least 20 years of covered earnings. This benefit, too, would increase with additional years of coverage; for workers with at least 30 years of covered earnings, the minimum benefit at the full benefit age would equal 100 percent of the poverty threshold in 2018 and exceed the threshold thereafter.

13. This minimum benefit was simulated assuming that Social Security had been modified to take 40 years into account in computing regular benefits, rather than 35 years as under current law. Because that assumption reduces regular benefits, the marginal effect of the minimum benefit is somewhat exaggerated relative to adding a minimum benefit to the scheduled benefit level. Our plan, however, would also involve some reduction in regular benefits relative to the scheduled benefit level; the results presented here may therefore still provide at least some insight into the marginal effect of a minimum benefit of this type under our plan.

14. For workers who become disabled or die before age 62, the years of coverage required to receive (or for their survivors to receive) the minimum benefit would be scaled to the length of the elapsed period from age 22 to the year of benefit eligibility.

15. As specified, this provision would create a "notch" between those becoming eligible in 2011 and before and those becoming eligible in 2012 and thereafter. The notch could be eliminated by phasing the provision in over time rather than having it take full effect all at once in 2012.

16. Specifically, each year the Office of the Chief Actuary would produce tables that would indicate, for any couple, the change in benefits on a break-even basis that would achieve the proposed survivor replacement rate. That is, when the second member of a couple claims benefits, the Office of the Chief Actuary would first determine what the benefits would be under current law (adjusted for any legislated changes in benefit levels). Then it would adjust the time profile of benefits to ensure a target survivor replacement rate of 75 percent. To do so, it would proportionately reduce the benefits of

both members of a couple while alive to finance the higher survivor benefit level after one spouse dies. There would also be a need for rules to cover the possible return of one of the retirees to work. We envision the use of a period mortality table for this calculation to avoid disputes about the mortality rate projection and to allocate slightly more benefits to later in life.

17. To the extent that the couple's expected mortality experience differed from the population's, there would also be some redistribution toward or away from the couple. Note that because the actuarial calculation is based on a 75-year horizon, and the benefit reductions for the couple would precede the benefit increases for the survivor, this proposal would improve the system's 75-year actuarial balance. However, we did not request that the implied increase be included in the official actuarial evaluation of our plan, because we prefer to restore actuarial balance without having this change contribute toward the actuarial balance.

18. For further details, see Kijakazi, 2001.

19. For data on the circumstances of people with disabilities, see Reno, Mashaw, and Gradison, 1997.

20. This is not to say that benefits as described by current law will never be changed; indeed, we are proposing to make changes to the benefit structure. But Social Security can be designed so that the need for legislation is infrequent. With advance planning, legislated changes can protect those nearing retirement and involve only moderate and gradual changes for others active in the labor market. In contrast, financial market changes can be large and sudden and affect those on the verge of retirement, and even those already retired if they continue to rely on a diversified portfolio of assets. For one recent study of how older workers have reacted to substantial financial market fluctuations, see Gardner and Orszag, 2003.

21. Social Security provides spouse and survivor benefits without reducing the worker benefit for a worker with a spouse. In contrast, individual account annuitization pricing would reduce worker annuities to finance spouse and survivor benefits. The current structure is controversial, with some analysts believing that the current structure is too generous to married workers relative to single workers and makes benefits too dependent on the division of earnings between husband and wife.

22. This design was applied in somewhat different form in the plans proposed by the President's Commission to Strengthen Social Security. A form of this approach was originally proposed by the General Accounting Office in response to requests from Representative John Porter (R-IL). See U.S. General Accounting Office, 1990. We ignore the complications arising from workers who die before starting retirement benefits.

23. More specifically, we assume that payroll is diverted into individual accounts for workers age 54 and younger at the beginning of 2002. We also base the projections on the 2001 intermediate cost assumptions of the Social Security trustees' report. These assumptions allow us to use a variety of calculations already undertaken by the Office of the Chief Actuary for model 1 of the President's Commission to Strengthen Social Security. To ensure that the Social Security trust fund is held harmless over a worker's lifetime, the benefit offset must reflect the diverted revenue accumulated at a 3 percent real interest rate, which is the real interest rate assumed to be earned by the trust fund. To compute the benefit offsets, we combine the figures calculated by the Office of the Chief Actuary for model 1, which assumed a 3.5 percent real interest rate for the benefit offsets, and for model 3, which assumed a 2.5 percent rate. The figures for model 3 are scaled

by 2.0/2.965, because the offset amounts under model 3 are based on a total 2.965 percent-of-payroll contribution rate (including 1% of payroll in add-on contributions).

24. For example, many workers seem to have difficulty understanding the value of diversification, recognizing the meaning of different points on a risk-return frontier, and avoiding risk-increasing attempts to time markets. Many of these problems could be avoided by allowing little or no discretion in portfolio choice, but that might not be politically sustainable.

25. Furthermore, we would not recommend that individuals with small retirement savings borrow to invest in stocks. That seems too risky. But carve-out accounts as proposed by President Bush's Commission to Strengthen Social Security would effectively allow for such borrowing. One of the major objectives of Social Security reform should be to put Social Security on a firm footing, to ensure that future retirees can more readily rely on a basic, assured stream of income. Carve-out accounts are inconsistent with this objective.

26. See the individual account plan proposed by Gramlich and Mark Twinney with the report of the 1994–1996 Advisory Council on Social Security. A description is available at www.ssa.gov/history/reports/adcouncil/report/gramlich.htm. See also Gramlich, 1998.

27. For a further description of the Commission's proposals, see Diamond and Orszag, 2002.

28. Martin Feldstein earlier proposed a similar mechanism. The Feldstein Social Security Plan is available at www.cbpp.org/12-16-98socsec.htm. Feldstein cites a memo from Stephen C. Goss, deputy chief actuary, Social Security Administration, "Long-Range OASDI Financial Effects of Clawback Proposal for Privatized Individual Accounts."

29. For a more complete analysis of the Shaw plan, see Kijakazi, Kogan, and Greenstein, 2002.

30. Even stronger incentives could arise if the clawback were limited to the level of traditional benefits and the account were large enough so that the clawback would simply eliminate the traditional benefit. In evaluating the actuarial effects of the Shaw plan, the Office of the Chief Actuary took this possibility into account. For further detail, see Goss, Wade, and Chaplain, 2003.

31. These examples were chosen because equity mutual funds currently charge more than 1 percent a year on average, but individual accounts can avail themselves of mechanisms to lower the charges. For details on the relationship between charges and benefits, see Diamond, 2000; and Murthi, Orszag, and Orszag, 2001.

REFERENCES

2003 Annual Report of the Board of Trustees of the Federal Old-Age and Survivors Insurance and Disability Insurance Trust Funds. 2003. March. www.cms.hhs.gov/apps/mcbs.

Burkhauser, R., and Smeeding, T. 1994. Social Security reform: A budget neutral approach to reducing older women's disproportionate risk of poverty. Policy Brief 2/94. Syracuse University Center for Policy Research, Syracuse, NY.

Cohen, L., Steuerle, C. E., and Carasso, A. 2001. Social Security redistribution by education, race, and income: How much and why. Paper presented at the Third Annual Conference of the Retirement Research Consortium, Washington, DC, May 17–18.

Diamond, P. 2000. Administrative costs and equilibrium charges with individual accounts. In J. Shoven, ed., *Administrative Costs and Social Security Privatization.* Chicago: University of Chicago Press.

Diamond, P., and Geanakoplos, J. 2003. Social Security investment in equities. *American Economic Review* 93(4):1047–74.

Diamond, P. A., and Orszag, P. R. 2002. An assessment of the proposals of the President's Commission to Strengthen Social Security. *Contributions to Economic Analysis and Policy* 1(1), art. 10.

Diamond, P. A., and Orszag, P. R. 2003. Reforming the GPO and WEP in Social Security. *Tax Notes,* November 3, pp. 647–49.

Favreault, M. M., Sammartino, F. J., and Steuerle, C. E. 2002. Social Security benefits for spouses and survivors. In M. M. Favreault, F. J. Sammartino, and C. E. Steuerle, eds., *Social Security and the Family.* Washington, D.C.: Urban Institute Press.

Gardner, J., and Orszag, M. 2003. How have older workers responded to scary markets? Watson Wyatt Technical Paper 2003-LS05. June.

Geanakoplos, J., Mitchell, O. S., and Zeldes, S. P. 1998. Would a privatized Social Security really pay a higher rate of return? In R. D. Arnold, M. J. Graetz, and A. H. Munnell, eds., *Framing the Social Security Debate: Values, Politics, and Economics.* Washington, DC: National Academy of Social Insurance.

Goss, S. C., Wade, A. H., and Chaplain, C. 2003. OASDI financial effects of the Social Security Guarantee Plus Act of 2003. Office of the Chief Actuary, Social Security Administration, Washington, DC. January 7.

Gramlich, E. 1998. *Is It Time to Reform Social Security?* Ann Arbor: University of Michigan Press.

Heclo, H. 1998. A political science perspective on Social Security reform. In R. D. Arnold, M. J. Graetz, and A. H. Munnell, eds., *Framing the Social Security Debate: Values, Politics, and Economics.* Washington, DC: National Academy of Social Insurance.

Holden, K., and Zick, C. 1998. Insuring against the consequences of widowhood in a reformed Social Security system. In R. D. Arnold, M. J. Graetz, and A. H. Munnell, eds., *Framing the Social Security Debate: Values, Politics, and Economics,* pp. 157–81. Washington, DC: National Academy of Social Insurance.

Kijakazi, K. 2001. Women's retirement income: The case for improving Supplemental Security Income. Center on Budget and Policy Priorities, Washington, DC. June 8.

Kijakazi, K., Kogan, R., and Greenstein, R. 2002. The Shaw Social Security Proposal: The role of massive general revenue transfers. Center on Budget and Policy Priorities, Washington, DC. September.

Munnell, A. H. 2000. The impact of mandatory Social Security coverage of state and local workers: A Multi-state review. Revised Final Report. AARP, Washington, DC.

Murthi, M., Orszag, J. M., and Orszag, P. R. 2001. Administrative costs under a decentralized approach to individual accounts: Lessons from the United Kingdom. In R. Holzmann and J. Stiglitz, eds., *New Ideas about Old Age Security: Toward Sustainable Pension Systems in the Twenty-first Century.* Washington, DC: World Bank.

Olsen, K., and Hoffmeyer, D. 2001–2. Social Security's special minimum benefit. *Social Security Bulletin* 64(2):1–15.

Paine, T. 1925. Agrarian justice. In W. Van der Weyde, ed., *The Life and Works of Thomas Paine.* New Rochelle, NY: Thomas Paine National Historical Association. Essay originally published in 1797.

President's Commission to Strengthen Social Security. 2001. *Strengthening Social Security and Creating Personal Wealth for All Americans: Final Report of the President's Commission to Strengthen Social Security.* www.csss.gov/reports/Final_report.pdf. December 21.

Reno, V., Mashaw, J., and Gradison, B., eds. 1997. *Disability: Challenges for Social Insurance, Health Care Financing, and Labor Market Policy.* Washington, DC: National Academy of Social Insurance.

Sandell, S. H., Iams, H. M., and Fanaras, D. 1999. The distributional effects of changing the averaging period and minimum benefit provisions. *Social Security Bulletin* 62(2):4–13.

Smith, K., Toder, E., and Iams, H. 2001. Lifetime distributional effects of Social Security retirement benefits. Paper presented at the Third Annual Conference of the Retirement Research Consortium, Washington, DC, May 17–18.

U.S. General Accounting Office. 1990. Social Security: Analysis of a proposal to privatize trust fund reserves. GAO/HRD-91-22. U.S. General Accounting Office, Washington, DC. December 12.

CHAPTER SIXTEEN

Assessing the Returns from the New Medicare Drug Benefit

Bruce Stuart, Ph.D.

After 40 years and several failed attempts, Medicare finally added drug coverage in 2006. But what is the coverage really worth? To economists, the value of a good or service is what the purchaser is willing to pay for it. Congress passed the law, so we can adduce that our representatives collectively believed that the $400 billion in forecast spending over 10 years was worth the cost. (Whether Congress would have passed the law had it been known that the Medicare actuaries were about to raise the price tag to $534 billion is another matter [Pear, 2004].) The Medicare Prescription Drug, Improvement, and Modernization Act of 2003 (MMA) provides value to an assortment of interests. Physicians got a 1.5 percent fee increase on January 1, 2004, instead of the 4.5 percent reduction scheduled under the former law. Rural hospitals also got higher reimbursement rates. Health maintenance organizations (HMOs) with Medicare contracts are now paid about 107 percent of fee-for-service costs, up from 95 percent under prior law. The pharmaceutical industry got a huge new market and avoided price controls. Pharmacists are now official Medicare providers and can, for the first time, directly bill for Medicare-related services. Employers get lucrative subsidies if they maintain "creditable" drug coverage for retirees. So what is left for program recipients? Or, to quote Clara Peller from her famous *Wendy's* ads of the 1980s, "Where's the beef?" The aim of this chapter is to evaluate the transfer and investment returns that beneficiaries can reasonably expect to receive under the Medicare drug benefit.

First is the transfer value of the benefit. Relatively little of the $400 (or $534) billion represents new money available for the purchase of prescription drugs. Most of it reflects federal funds that will substitute for private purchases and other governmental expenditures that would have been made in any event. Some, but by no means all, of the transfer value of the benefit will accrue to Medicare recipients in the form of reduced premiums for prescription coverage and/or lower out-of-pocket payments for drug products.

The second way that the MMA helps beneficiaries is through the return on investment in drug therapies that would not have been undertaken in the absence of the law. Prescription drugs are not desired for their own sake (at least those used for true medical purposes), but rather for the effects they generate in improved health and well being. Every time a drug is administered, the patient is making an investment. The returns may accrue quickly (painkillers) or over a lifetime (treatments for hypertension) and occasionally will be negative (adverse drug reactions). Like financial investments, investments in drug use involve time and risk. Unlike returns from stocks and bonds, these returns are generally not directly measurable in dollars.

The MMA is exceedingly complex, so any assessment of the value of the benefit to program recipients must necessarily be selective. In the next section, I describe the central features of the benefit as implemented in 2006, leaving the longer-term changes in Medicare to other commentators. I then discuss transfer returns under the heading "Who Will Sign Up and Why (or Why Not)?" The underlying assumption in this discussion is that beneficiaries have a reasonably good idea of what their future drug use will cost (at least to the extent that they pay directly). The assumption of foreknowledge is based on a growing body of research showing that drug spending by seniors is highly persistent over time, more so than any other type of health care. Under these conditions, the pure insurance value of coverage (i.e., risk reduction) is much less important to potential customers than the spread between the premium and anticipated spending. Actuaries understand this; it is the reason there were no stand-alone private drug insurance plans in the market before 2006. Although premiums are subsidized under the MMA, not all beneficiaries will gain from it. The behavior of beneficiaries who stand to suffer short-term financial losses if they sign up will ultimately determine how the transfer values of the benefit are distributed.

Next, I discuss the potential investment returns from the Medicare benefit under sections entitled "Will the Benefit Affect the Use of Drugs?" and "Can Pharmaceuticals Pay for Themselves?" For there to be any impact on beneficiary health and well-being, patterns of drug use must change first. There is considerable empirical research suggesting that drug use increases with the generosity of drug coverage. How beneficiaries facing the odd cost-sharing provisions of the Medicare benefit will respond is something else again. Equally challenging is the question of how formulary design and utilization management tools permitted under the MMA will affect beneficiaries' patterns of use. I conclude that both of these drivers have the potential to significantly affect drug use and for that reason we can logically pose the question "To What End"? My emphasis here is on how appropriate drug use can reduce the need, and hence cost, of other health services (or alternatively, how inappropriate drug use can lead to increased expenditures for other health services).

In the final section of the chapter, I summarize my main points and challenge the assumptions on which they rest. I identify a set of key research questions that policymakers should address to assess the early affects of the law. Having waited 40 years to get a drug benefit, beneficiaries have a right to expect that it will do more good than harm. Moreover, if there are signs of harm, Congress should not wait another 40 years to fix them.

Coverage Provisions of the MMA

The drug coverage that beneficiaries obtain under Part D will vary widely depending on both statutory considerations and plan type. The "standard benefit" available to beneficiaries with annual incomes above 150 percent of the federal poverty line (FPL) includes a $250 annual deductible followed by 75 percent coverage of the next $2,000 in spending on covered drugs. At that point, beneficiaries are on their own until their drug spending exceeds $3,600 in total annual out-of-pocket payments (this gap in coverage is commonly referred to as the "donut hole"). Then the plan's catastrophic coverage kicks in with 95 percent coverage until the end of the year. The cycle repeats itself in the new year, albeit with higher cost-sharing thresholds.

Beneficiaries entitled to Medicaid receive a much more generous package, one with no annual premium, deductible, coinsurance, or donut hole. Instead, these enrollees receive all approved drugs with modest copays of $2 for generic and $5 for brand drugs. Medicare beneficiaries with incomes under 100 percent of the FPL and minimal assets are eligible for the same generous benefits. Those with somewhat higher incomes (to 150% of the FPL) and marginally higher assets are eligible for a sliding scale of benefits and premiums that are less generous than those granted to the lowest income beneficiaries but considerably better than the standard benefit.

Ironically, the standard benefit is anything but that. The MMA gives private prescription drug plans (PDPs) and Medicare managed care plans (renamed "Medicare Advantage" [MA]) the alternative of offering the standard Part D benefit or an "actuarially equivalent" benefit package. In 2006, all but a few plans crafted optional approaches, the most common of which eliminated the annual deductible and substituted tiered drug copayments for the 25 percent coinsurance provision in the standard plan. However, just a handful of PDP plans eliminated the donut hole in coverage between $2,250 and $5,100 in total drug spending. A somewhat larger number of MA plans eliminated the donut hole in their 2006 plan offerings.

Like Part B, the new Medicare Part D is voluntary. Beneficiaries are not compelled to enroll, but there are financial penalties for late enrollment. In 2006, beneficiaries had until May 15 to enroll in an approved PDP or MA plan; after that date the monthly premium was set to increase by one percentage point for each month the beneficiary remains outside of the system. This premium penalty is designed to encourage relatively low-risk beneficiaries to join the program even though it might not be in their immediate economic interest to do so. Dual eligible Medicaid beneficiaries have no choice: they must sign up with a private plan if they wish to maintain any drug benefits, or the state will do it for them. Federal matching of state Medicaid expenditures for drugs offered to dual eligibles ceased as of January 1, 2006. States may choose to supplement the low-income coverage these beneficiaries receive from their private drug plans (i.e., pay the copayments or cover off-formulary medications), but these expenditures are not eligible for a federal match. Since January 2006, the three standard Medigap policies with drug coverage (designated as the H, I, and J plans) are no longer available; beneficiaries who wish to maintain private Medicare supplements must purchase two policies, one to cover Part D and the other to supplement Parts A and B. However, retirees with "creditable" employer-sponsored drug coverage (meaning as least as generous as the standard Part D benefit) can keep their current benefits as long as they are still available.

Arguably the most important feature of Part D is that there is no definition of which drugs are actually covered. Private plans that administer the benefit are permitted to limit access to individual medicines through restrictive formularies and utilization management tools such as quantity limits, prior authorization, and step therapy requirements (also known as "fail-first" provisions), wherein beneficiaries are required to undertake a defined course of treatment under one drug before an alternative medication will be authorized. Furthermore, the drug products currently covered under Medicare Part B (mostly chemotherapy and other products that cannot be self-administered by patients) will still be subject to the annual Part B deductible and 20 percent coinsurance. Beneficiary out-of-pocket payments for these medications will not count toward the cost-sharing requirements under the new law, nor will patients be able to count the cost of purchasing drugs outside of the plan's pharmacy network.

Who Will Sign Up and Why (or Why Not)?

How many beneficiaries will ultimately sign up for Part D? Nobody knows. As of late April 2006, approximately 9 million of 15 million beneficiaries who had no prior drug coverage had enrolled. To put this figure in perspective, about 96 percent of individuals entitled to Medicare Part A sign up for Part B. But Part B services are worth far more than the standard drug benefit. In 2004, the actuarial value of Part B coverage was $3,200, for which beneficiaries paid an annual premium of $800 (U.S. Department of Health and Human Services, 2004). The estimated mean value of the Medicare drug benefit is $1,400 with an annual premium for 2006 averaging $383. The difference in net transfer value to beneficiaries is $2,400 versus $1,016. Moreover, unlike Part D, Part B is real insurance. Actuarial studies show that individuals' use of physicians' services (the main Part B benefit) varies widely from year to year. About 15 percent of the variance in physician spending in a given year can be explained by knowing only what beneficiaries spent in the previous year (Newhouse et al., 1989). Medicare beneficiaries sign up for Part B both because it is a good deal and because it protects them from major economic losses associated with unforeseeable medical emergencies. For prescription medications, the variance explained by prior year drug spending is 65 percent or more (Wrobel et al., 2003). To be sure, not all prescription spending can be predicted in advance, but the high persistence in spending from year to year means that most beneficiaries and their advisers will have a reasonably good way to estimate the net value of the new drug coverage for themselves before they sign up.

Shea and colleagues recently estimated take-up rates for a Medicare drug benefit with cost-sharing provisions similar but not identical to those in the new law (Shea, Stuart, and Briesacher, 2003–4). They assumed that only beneficiaries who are made better off by taking the coverage would choose to enroll. Using an iterative simulation model in which premiums reflect the risk profile of those in the pool, a 75 percent premium subsidy would induce fewer than three-quarters of beneficiaries with no current source of drug coverage to sign up. The reason for this is that low spenders never sign up, raising the average premium for everyone else in the pool. As premiums rise, more individuals opt out, and the process continues until an equilibrium point is reached. Could this scenario play out in real life? The following sections describe the implications of the MMA for the beneficiaries according to their pre-MMA drug coverage status, beginning with those who have no coverage whatever.

Beneficiaries with No Drug Coverage

Medicare actuaries have responsibility under the law to estimate a year in advance what monthly per capita cost will be under Part D. The base premium is then set at 25.5 percent of that amount. The average monthly premium for the Medicare benefit in 2006 (about $32) is based on the assumption of nearly universal participation. The break-even point at this premium level is $762 in annual covered drug expenditures ($250 in deductible plus 75 percent of the next $512). Now consider beneficiaries who currently have no drug benefits. Table 16.1 contrasts annual drug spending for those with and without drug coverage in 2000. Almost 38 percent of beneficiaries with no drug coverage that year had annual drug spending below $250, and 65 percent had spending below the break-even point of $762. These fractions will be lower after 2006 because of rising drug costs, but the group as a whole is likely to remain low spenders. Some of these beneficiaries will sign up because the coverage permits purchases of drugs they could not previously afford (see discussion of induced demand below). Others will sign up because of the premium penalties for delayed enrollment. But if sizable numbers of low spenders fail to enroll, then the Medicare actuaries will be forced to compute the next year's premium on a smaller, higher-risk base. If that happens, premiums will rise much more quickly than anticipated and the dynamic described above will begin to unfold.

Table 16.1. *Distribution of Medicare Beneficiaries, by Drug Coverage Status and Annual Drug Spending, 2000*

	Number of Beneficiaries[a] (in millions)	Beneficiaries with Annual Drug Spending in 2000[b]			
		<$250 (%)	$251–2,250 (%)	$2,251–5,100 (%)	>$5,100 (%)
Drug coverage	29.7	20.0	56.9	19.2	4.0
No drug coverage	8.1	37.6	53.1	8.5	0.8

Source: Author computations from the 2000 Medicare Current Beneficiary Survey.
[a]Excludes beneficiaries in institutions.
[b]MCBS spending levels adjusted upward by 17% to account for underreporting.

Low-Income Beneficiaries

Federal officials initially estimated that virtually all beneficiaries eligible for low-income subsidies under Part D would enroll, based on experience under Part B. For Medicaid dual eligibles, this proved to be the case because of automatic random enrollments conducted by the Centers for Medicare and Medicaid Services (CMS) and state agencies in November and December 2005. However, among those who were required to self-enroll, the take-up rates have been much lower than anticipated. Rather than enrollment rates equivalent to those for Part B, the initial take-up in the low-income subsidy program has been closer to the experience in the Medicare savings plan known as QMB (Qualified Medicare Beneficiaries). The QMB program is available to Medicare beneficiaries with annual incomes between the state Medicaid eligibility cutoff and 100 percent of the FPL if they also meet an asset test. The QMB benefit includes payment of the Part B premium and all cost-sharing under both Part A and Part B. The annual actuarial value of this program is more than $2,000, and there is no premium; yet only between 40 percent and 60 percent of eligible persons enroll (Sears, 2003; Reimer and Glied, 2003). Part of the problem is poor outreach, but there is also the stigma of welfare. QMB is administered by state Medicaid programs, and income and asset verification is typically handled by county welfare offices. Eligibility for the Medicare low-income drug benefit is determined in a similar fashion, except that beneficiaries may enroll through Social Security offices as well as welfare departments.

Recipients of Pharmacy Assistance

Medicare beneficiaries enrolled in state pharmacy assistance plans (PAPs) may or may not need to apply for low-income coverage, depending on what actions their states take. State PAPs are allowed to fill in the Part D benefit gaps but are not permitted to automatically enroll recipients as under Medicaid. In other words, if a state wishes to receive the potential savings available by having Medicare pay for the bulk of Part D services, it must figure out how to assure that eligible PAP participants apply (as a backup, states may continue to provide pharmacy assistance to recipients who fail to enroll in Part D, but the cost will be borne wholly from state funds). In a state like Pennsylvania, where PAP applications are processed through the Department of Aging, two separate enrollment procedures would be required. The process is complicated further because many state PAPs require income means tests but have no asset restrictions. The typical state PAP also provides benefits to some recipients with incomes above 150 percent of the federal poverty line, thus making them eligible only for the standard benefit.

Privately Insured People

For all other beneficiaries, the choice to sign up for Part D and if so which plan to select will depend on their alternatives. Table 16.2 shows how the Part D standard benefit compares with the average paid by insurance for beneficiaries with private sources of drug coverage in 2000.

Table 16.2. Drug Expense Paid by Insurance for Medicare Beneficiaries, by Drug Coverage Status and Annual Level of Spending, 2000

	Drug Cost Paid by Insurance			
Drug Coverage	<$250 (%)	$251–2,250 (%)	$2,251–5,100 (%)	$5,100–10,000 (%)
Standard benefit under PL 108-173[a]	0	60	41	51
Medicare beneficiaries with private drug coverage in 2000				
Individually purchased Medigap	23	29	42	[b]
Medicare HMO	37	53	65	[b]
Employer-sponsored	56	73	78	80

Source: Author computations from the 2000 Medicare Current Beneficiary Survey, corrected for underreporting.

[a]Computed at the midpoint of each spending range.

[b]Too few respondents for a reliable estimate.

Medigap Policyholders

For most beneficiaries who previously obtained drug coverage from a private Medigap policy, Part D generally provides improved benefits at lower cost. All of the standard Medigap drug policies had a $250 deductible and 50 percent coinsurance. The best coverage (Plan J) offered some benefits in the range defined by the Part D donut hole, but none above $3,000 in total insured payments. The biggest gain for Medigap policyholders will be dramatically lower premiums. Somewhat better overall coverage plus lower premiums means that Medigap policyholders should come out ahead under Part D.

When Medigap policyholders trade in their old policies for new Part D plans, however, they will either have to buy two policies if they want drug benefits and want to maintain supplemental coverage for Part A and B services, or they will have to enroll in a Medicare Advantage plan. In either case, the drug benefits are unlikely to be significantly more generous than the standard benefit. The catastrophic coverage provisions in the act provide a powerful incentive for plans not to compete on the generosity of their drug coverage. The catastrophic stop loss kicks in at $5,100 *only* for persons who incur $3,600 in total countable out-of-pocket costs for the year. Were a PDP or MA plan to supplement the standard benefit by reducing the coinsurance rate or filling in the donut hole, that would lower enrollees' out-of-pocket payments and push up the stop loss threshold by an equal amount. Plans that take this course of action will forgo federal reinsurance payments, which would otherwise be available to cover the costs of their most expensive enrollees. The rationale for this seemingly odd restriction is that if insurers reduce the cost-sharing of their policyholders, that will lead to increased demand for drugs, which in turn will increase federal outlays under the program. Put another way, if this restriction had not been included in the MMA, Congress would have had to reduce benefits somewhere else in the bill in order to come in under the $400 billion authorization cap.

Medicare HMO Enrollees

Medicare HMOs have been given a new lease on life under the MMA—maybe. The renamed Medicare Advantage program is designed to revamp a declining Medicare managed care market that reached a peak of 17 percent in 1999 and has fallen ever since (Gold and Achman, 2003). The basic problem has been that HMOs needed to offer extra services (principally prescription drugs) or charge lower premiums or lower rates of cost-sharing to induce beneficiaries to join. Even though most plans experienced favorable selection (Mello et al., 2003), their higher administrative costs (primarily marketing) and inability to contract with providers at rates equal to those paid by Medicare made it impossible to make money in many parts of the country.

It appears likely that the combination of higher capitation payments and reduced risk associated with offering drug benefits may increase MA plan participation rates in the future, but in the short run, response after January 2006 was modest at best; in April 2006, 4.9 million beneficiaries (11.7% of the population) had enrolled in MA plans. Part of the reason for the slow pick-up is that CMS statistics indicate that just 17 percent of the value of higher HMO reimbursement rates will go toward enhanced benefits ("Only small part," 2004). Perhaps the most likely scenario is a repeat of what happened after Congress passed the Balanced Budget Act of 1997, which created Medicare+Choice (M+C), the precursor to Medicare Advantage. That law significantly eased market entry by managed care plans. For two years thereafter, plan numbers and beneficiary participation rates rose, only to fall back in the face of flat reimbursement rates. Medicare managed care failed to grow in part because the Health Care Financing Administration (the old name for CMS) kept fee-for-service rates (to which M+C rates were tied) on a tight leash during the late 1990s. Because the new MA capitation rate increases are not spread evenly throughout the country, some regions could see a burst of HMO activity while others see little impact. The longer-run impact is unclear. When scoring the 10-year costs of the MMA, the CBO estimated that only 9 percent of Medicare beneficiaries would enroll on average. The Medicare actuaries assumed 34 percent. They agreed on one thing: Medicare Advantage will not save the Medicare program any money. On the contrary, CBO forecasts that Medicare Advantage will add $14 billion to the program's cost; the Medicare actuaries, based on their much higher MA enrollment forecast, put the added cost at $46 billion.[1]

Retirees

The market for retiree health benefits has been in flux for years. According to the annual Kaiser Family Foundation–Health Research and Educational Trust surveys, the number of large firms offering retiree health benefits fell from 66 percent in 1988 to 38 percent in 2003, and in the latter year only 30 percent offered such benefits to Medicare-eligible retirees (Kaiser Family Foundation, 2003). By contrast, just 10 percent of small firms offer health benefits to any retirees. These are sobering numbers, but it gets worse. A Kaiser-Hewitt survey of large firms, also conducted in 2003, reported that 10 percent of large firms had eliminated retiree health benefits for future retirees in the previous year and 20 percent indicated they were likely to do so in the next three years (Kaiser Family Foundation, 2004). Just 2 percent of the firms surveyed indicated they were likely to drop subsidized health benefits for current retirees, but that was before passage of the MMA.

Congress was clearly worried that the new Medicare drug benefit would accelerate the downward spiral of retiree health benefits in general and prescription coverage in particular. For this reason, the MMA provides a hefty subsidy to employers who maintain retiree drug coverage at least as good as the Part D standard benefit. The CBO estimates the cost of the subsidy at $71 billion over 10 years. But because the subsidy is tax free, the real value of the transfer is closer to $88 billion. These are slippery figures, as CBO itself admits.[2] It all depends on how employers and retirees respond to the incentives in the law. On the one hand, Part D makes it easier for employers to abandon retiree drug coverage after 2006 because their former employees will have the option of obtaining subsidized benefits elsewhere in the market. On the other hand, the subsidy significantly reduces the cost of drug coverage for firms that decide to maintain it. The CBO estimates that as a result of the law, employers will drop drug coverage for 2.7 million retirees, or 17 percent of all beneficiaries enrolled in company-sponsored health plans.[3] Although the affected individuals will have access to Part D coverage, the value of the benefit they get is likely to be significantly less generous than what they stand to lose, as is evident from the statistics shown in Table 16.2.

There is an additional scenario that CBO and other government forecasters have failed to consider because it does not have direct budgetary consequences. There is a distinct possibility that the subsidy will have the unintended consequence of driving good drug benefits out of the retiree market to be replaced by some variant of the Part D standard benefit. The reason for thinking that Gresham's law—that "bad money drives out good"—might apply to the retiree market is that the marginal value of the employer subsidy is maximized when firms offer just the standard benefit or its actuarial equivalent. More generous coverage leverages no additional subsidy. The impact of any such drive to the bottom, should it occur, will likely be concentrated among nonunion and nongovernmental entities, where retiree bargaining power is minimal.

Will the Benefit Affect the Use of Drugs?

The MMA represents such a major change in the way prescription drugs are financed for Medicare beneficiaries that it would be surprising if it did not also change the way beneficiaries use medications. The two major drivers of change are these: demand effects arising from changes in the out-of-pocket cost that beneficiaries will face when filling prescriptions from Part D providers; and supply-side factors relating to drug availability, utilization management efforts, and prescriber information.

The Effects of Demand

Economic theory predicts that when the price of a good drops, consumers will buy more of it. Drug coverage lowers the price to patients, so patients with coverage buy more. There is a virtually universal agreement among economists that this is true. Disagreements arise over the magnitude of the effect, and these tend to hinge on methodological issues and differences in sample frame. The one true randomized controlled experiment of health insurance effects (the RAND Health Insurance Experiment [HIE] of 1974 to 1977) estimated the price elasticity of demand for outpatient drugs at between -0.3 and -0.4 (i.e., that a 10% reduction in price leads to a 3%–4% percent rise in quantity demanded). The RAND HIE excluded persons 65 and older, but various observational studies have produced similar estimates of drug demand elasticity for Medicare beneficiaries (Lillard, Rogowski, and Kingston, 1999; Stuart and Grana, 1998). The CBO used the middle of the range to calculate the demand-inducing impact of the MMA.

Notwithstanding the consistency of research findings, there are three unresolved issues. First, Part D will induce additional demand on behalf of a relatively small group of lower-income but above-poverty-level beneficiaries, and we have limited information about price elasticity for this group. There are studies relating to how very poor elderly people react to small changes in cost-sharing (Stuart and Zacker, 1999) and a growing literature on how middle-income people respond to relatively large changes in copays (Hillerman et al., 1999; Joyce et al., 2002), but nothing directly relevant to the primary beneficiaries of Part D. Will the near poor react to price signals in a similar fashion to the very poor or the nonpoor? According to a new theory of demand for health insurance developed by John Nyman, poor and near poor people cannot afford large out-of-pocket payments, so their observed demand when uninsured provides little information about how they would respond if insured (Nyman, 2003). If Nyman is correct and poor beneficiaries behave like their wealthier brethren when they get drug coverage, then the official estimates of induced demand are too low.

Second, there is neither consistent theoretical prediction nor good empirical literature on which to judge how the Part D donut hole will affect demand for high users. Standard economic theory posits that individuals base consumption decisions on marginal price. Thus, if a person has an insurance policy with 20 percent coinsurance and a $250 deductible, the marginal price is either 100 percent of retail (if anticipated spending is below $250 annually) or 20 percent of retail above that threshold. According to the standard theory, the fact that the average price for someone exceeding the threshold is above the marginal price is irrelevant. Most economists thus believe that gaps in the form of small deductibles have little behavioral impact on the majority of users and simply transfer payment responsibility from insurer to insured. If the standard theory is correct, a donut hole in drug coverage would influence demand behavior only for those beneficiaries who anticipate spending below the stop-loss amount; however, the standard theory is based on an instantaneous time frame and assumes perfect foreknowledge of demand given the marginal price. In reality, the presence of large coverage gaps means many beneficiaries will face full retail prescription prices for extended periods over which they have less than full knowledge ahead of time. How they and their prescribers will respond is an open question that has yet to be addressed by economists or health services researchers.

A final issue is to whom to credit the behavior of retirees who lose value in their drug benefits because employers either drop drug coverage or cut it back to the level of the standard benefit. Because the law of demand cuts both ways, we can safely predict a reduction in the use of drugs for the affected individuals. What will be more difficult, and perhaps impossible to prove, is the extent to which such changes are due to the passage of the MMA rather than to other unrelated factors, including the historical retrenchment in retiree health benefits. This issue has more than philosophic importance because of the numbers involved. Before 2006, one of every two Medicare beneficiaries with drug coverage got it from an employer-sponsored plan. From the standpoint of aggregate demand, even a modest cutback in retiree coverage would swamp the effects of improved coverage for the poor and near poor under Part D.

The Effects of Supply

Three supply-side forces could usher in significant changes in the way Medicare beneficiaries use prescribed medicines under Part D. These include expanded application of restrictive formularies, direct management of prescription drug therapy, and electronic prescribing.

Formularies are simply lists of drugs. Some lists are designed to provide clinical information to physicians and pharmacists about the effects of particular medications; others are designed to restrict or channel availability of drug products to patients. Hospitals have long maintained drug formularies as a way to achieve space and cost efficiencies. For similar reasons, the Department of Veterans Affairs, the Defense Department, and private health maintenance organizations—particularly staff-model HMOs with their own in-house pharmacies—are also longtime users of drug formularies. The widespread application of drug formularies in open-panel health plans and Medicaid programs is a recent phenomenon. The most restrictive formularies are designated as "closed," in that only medications on the list are reimbursable. Open formularies give prescribers and patients more choices within a given therapeutic class of drugs, but those choices are increasingly tied to economic incentives. Tiered copays are a particularly popular method of tying cost to choice of drug, with low copays for cheap generics, higher copays for "approved" branded products, and higher payments still for therapeutically equivalent off-formulary products.

Medicare Part D does not mandate formularies, but the language of the MMA makes it clear that it expects PDPs and MA plans to make use of these cost-saving mechanisms. The law gives plans wide latitude in the development and management of formulary lists. They can be as restrictive as plans wish, as long as products are available in every therapeutic class. Plans must publicize their lists but can change them at will (beneficiaries do not have this option; they must stick with their chosen plan for the whole year regardless of what formulary changes are instituted). Plans are required to have procedures in place to override formulary restrictions when supported by the prescribing physician, but in a departure from current convention, the beneficiary—not the physician—must actually process the appeal. CMS regulates formulary content for certain classes of drugs (e.g., antidepressants), but the law appears to rely on competition as its main quality control: plans that offer unappealing drug lists will presumably fail to attract customers. However, plans that offer a rich menu of drug choices will be punished by low-cost competitors. If the recent history of formulary development in private group health insurance contracts is any guide, Medicare beneficiaries and their doctors can expect to face narrower selections of drug products from Part D providers compared to what they are used to today.

How will formularies affect Medicare beneficiaries' patterns of drug use? A recent survey of more than 12,000 doctors nationwide found that only 13 percent of physicians felt formularies had a positive effect on the quality and efficiency of medical care, whereas 49 percent felt they had a negative effect (Nyman, 2003, p. 222). These results are not surprising; most doctors want prescribing freedom. Research on the effects of formularies on patients is still sparse, but there is a growing consensus that when used in conjunction with economic incentives, as in tiered copay arrangements, patients shift to lower-cost drugs and health plans save money (Joyce et al., 2002). There is some evidence that tiered copays also increase the economic burden on patients (Kamal-Bahl and Briesacher, 2004); however, none of this work has focused on Medicare patients, who may be more vulnerable to drug restrictions.

Usage management programs are a second supply-side factor that may affect beneficiaries' patterns of drug use. In the past, Medicare HMOs have implemented various forms of prior authorization, step therapy, quantity limits, and disease management programs that focus on drug therapy for chronic conditions such as diabetes, heart disease, and asthma. Despite a large literature of case studies hailing the benefits of these programs, there is little hard scientific evidence of their effectiveness. The MMA added a new spin, under the title "Medication Therapy Management Programs" (MTMPs): all approved health plans are required to establish MTMPs for enrollees with multiple chronic conditions and high drug costs. For the first time, pharmacists are to be given a major role to play in actually managing drug therapy for Medicare patients. Maybe that will work.

A third and potentially far-reaching supply-side implication of the MMA is to be found in the provisions relating to electronic prescribing. The law requires that HHS develop and implement electronic order entry standards by September 2009. Earlier versions of the legislation mandated immediate implementation of this technology but were opposed by organized medicine. Medicine won. Beneficiaries will now have to wait several more years to receive the considerable benefits that electronic prescribing has to offer, including error-free transmission of prescription information from physician to pharmacy and improved drug-use review procedures.

Can Pharmaceuticals Pay for Themselves?

There is a widespread belief that giving people good drug benefits will generate savings elsewhere in the health care system. President Bush echoed these sentiments when he signed PL 108-173 into law on December 8, 2003. He said, "Drug coverage under Medicare will allow seniors to replace more expensive surgeries and hospitalizations with less expensive prescription medicine."[4] There are reasons other than the president's promise to focus on potential cost offsets from the Medicare drug benefit. First, cost savings can be directly compared to drug costs, thus providing a common metric for assessing return on the public's investment in the Medicare drug benefit. Second, averted costs are a surrogate for real improvements in health because lower costs reflect the need for fewer resources to manage a patient's condition. Third, if there is a relationship, it should be symmetrical; that is, if improved coverage leads to cost savings, then reduced coverage should raise costs. This last point could be particularly important if, as I suggest above, the loss of generous retiree benefits swamps any improvement in coverage for other beneficiary groups. Fourth, as the Medicare drug benefit unfolds, it will be vitally important to track any compensatory changes in medical spending that may result from PDPs' efforts to drive down drug costs. In a fully integrated health plan, the economic incentive is to optimize total spending by comparing the returns on both drugs and services for which they might be substitutes. PDPs not only lack this incentive; they have no information on hospital and medical spending on behalf of their enrollees.

There is extensive literature on the relationship between drug use and the cost of other health services. By far, the largest number of studies evaluate specific drug products. This is not surprising, because pharmaceutical manufacturers in conjunction with phase III and phase IV clinical trials finance most of the published research on drug effectiveness. Publications showing that new drug products reduce hospitalization and other negative consequences of disease are valued marketing tools for the companies; however, even when reported findings from such studies are technically accurate, it is difficult to generalize them to Medicare. In part, this is due to the selection criteria used to enlist subjects in clinical trials. It is well known that elderly people are usually underrepresented in trials, as are those who may be expected to gain little or be potentially harmed by the drug under review. There is also the problem of publication bias: positive findings are more likely to see print than negative findings. But the most compelling reason why trial data represent a poor basis for measuring cost offsets to drug use is the fact they are available for only a small fraction of the drug products on the market, and then only for the indicated uses for which the drugs have been approved. Thus, even if Medicare beneficiaries with prescription drug coverage had higher use of all of the products shown to be associated with cost offsets, that would not, by itself, guarantee savings for the Medicare program.

The second type of evidence that drug coverage might result in cost offsets comes from a few studies that have found significant adverse events following reductions in coverage. The well-known studies by Soumerai and colleagues that attributed increased nursing home admissions (Soumerai et al., 1991) and acute mental health services (Soumerai et al., 1994) to the imposition of a three-per-month limit on prescriptions in the New Hampshire Medicaid program fall into this category. More recent work by Tamblyn et al. (2001) found evidence that increased cost-sharing for drug products resulted in higher rates of emergency visits and hospitalizations for elderly and poor recipients of Quebec's provincial health insurance program. It is difficult to generalize these findings to the Medicare population because of differences in study samples, data sources, and methodology. Moreover, it is not clear that, just because there are bad effects associated with restricting access to pharmaceuticals for the most vulnerable populations, similar consequences would apply to other beneficiary groups.

Another approach to the question of whether drugs produce cost offsets comes from two studies by Frank Lichtenberg (1996, 2001) that compare Medicare spending for beneficiaries using older and newer drugs. Findings from both a longitudinal and a cross-sectional model indicate that beneficiaries taking newer drugs have lower hospitalization admission rates, length of stay, and surgical interventions compared to those using older therapies. Alternative explanations can plausibly account for Lichtenberg's findings; specifically, the case for savings depends on a strong and untested assumption that new drug introductions are not correlated in time with other non-drug-related influences on inpatient treatment patterns. And even if it is generally true that newer drugs are better, that is not always the case, as was demonstrated in a widely publicized study of antihypertensive medications (Wing et al., 2003).

Only two studies have directly addressed the question of whether Medicare beneficiaries with drug coverage have reduced the use of other health care services. The first is an analysis of Vermont's pharmacy assistance programs by Gillman, Gage, and Mitchell (2003). This CMS-supported analysis examined Medicare spending on inpatient hospital, outpatient hospital, and physician services for low-income Medicare beneficiaries before and after enrolling in the Vermont Health Access Plan (VHAP) or an expanded assistance program known as VScript. The results were compared to changes in Medicare spending for a control group of beneficiaries who had not enrolled in these programs. The study found no evidence of cost offsets associated with either the VHAP or VScript program—in fact, Medicare spending was higher after enrollment for all service types, although the difference declined with time. The study authors attributed these findings to adverse selection (e.g., persons with precipitating events requiring both more Medicare services and more prescription drugs are more likely to enroll), but the inability to control for other relevant factors (such as whether the control group had drug coverage) undoubtedly also played a role. The main lesson from the Vermont study is that unless the coverage-selection decision can be adequately modeled, it will be difficult, if not impossible, to tease out the true effects of drug coverage on Medicare spending.

The second study, by Wrobel et al. (2004), analyzed Medicare Current Beneficiary Survey (MCBS) data from 1996 through 2000 to assess differences in Medicare drug spending for Parts A and B services as a function of beneficiary drug coverage. This study analyzed cross-sectional samples of all beneficiaries, beneficiaries with employer-sponsored supplements with and without drug benefits, and a sample of patients with chronic obstructive pulmonary disease (COPD); some of the COPD sample had drug coverage and others did not. Limited support for the proposition was found only in the COPD sample, where physician services costs were significantly lower among beneficiaries with drug coverage (Stuart et al., 2004). The authors also analyzed longitudinal samples of beneficiaries who either gained or lost drug coverage, and they found no evidence of changes in Medicare spending following the change in drug coverage status.

In sum, while it is clear that appropriate drug use can result in reduced expenditures associated with avoidable hospitalizations and emergency treatments, it requires a major leap of faith to argue, based on the published literature, that Part D drug coverage will save Medicare money in Parts A and B spending. One critical missing link in the causal chain is research showing that drug coverage promotes appropriate medication use. On the one hand, there is some literature suggesting that people with prescription coverage are more likely to receive newer and more expensive drugs (Blustein, 2000; Doshi, Brandt, and Stuart, 2004), which is a key requirement for Medicare cost offsets under Lichtenberg's scenario. On the other hand, there has been no published research addressing the question of whether drug coverage increases the use of inappropriate medications. If it does, the effect would be to moderate or even reverse the cost offsets associated with appropriate use.

Conclusion

So how are we to answer Clara Peller? It depends on who is asking. As far as transfer benefits are concerned, three beneficiary groups appear to be winners under the new Medicare drug benefit. First is the small group of beneficiaries who qualify for low-income coverage, are not Medicaid eligible, and are willing to submit to income and asset verification. Those who are putatively eligible but unwilling to submit to the verification process will only have the standard benefit available.

The second group of probable winners comprises those who previously purchased Medigap policies with drug benefits. Part D coverage is marginally better than that available from the top-end J plan, so there is little gain there. The real transfer returns to this group come in the form of a community-rated premium with a 75 percent subsidy, which is far below prevailing rates in the market before the MMA.

The third group of winners represents beneficiaries enrolled in Medicare Advantage plans. They obtained improved drug coverage and reduced premiums as a result of the Part D subsidy and higher MA capitation rates. If the MA market expands beyond the 11.7 percent currently enrolled, these benefits will be available to other program recipients as well. The question remains whether a one-shot boost will solve the long-term problems that have plagued the Medicare HMO market throughout its history.

The transfer impact of the MMA on Medicaid recipients is more difficult to assess. The early experience in self-enrollment caused havoc for many recipients but appears to have been largely repaired. Most dually eligible people will face somewhat higher copays unless these costs are picked up by the states. Medicaid recipients residing in states with tight restrictions on use might experience easier access to pharmaceutical therapy under the new arrangements. Recipients in states with open Medicaid drug lists will find access to off-formulary medications more difficult; however, given the fact that states have moved aggressively toward restrictive formularies in recent years, one could reasonably predict that future Medicaid recipients would have faced limited drug choices in the absence of the MMA.

For beneficiaries ineligible for low-income subsidies, the MMA offers a mixed future. Perhaps three-quarters of these individuals will incur medication expenses sufficiently high to make voluntary enrollment in a stand-alone PDP pay. If a rejuvenated MA market competes on premiums, additional uninsured beneficiaries may find attractive options available. The rest will either enroll and suffer negative transfers or fail to enroll and suffer future premium penalties. Risk-takers may wait out a decision, betting that Congress will be unable to enforce the premium penalty. If there are substantial numbers of initial holdouts, premium penalties can actually make it harder to achieve a risk-neutral pool. There is nothing concrete about the penalty; Congress can change it at will and presumably would under these circumstances. The MMA even offers a precedent in Section 625, which waives Part B late enrollment penalties for certain military retirees.

Uncertainty also shrouds the future of retiree drug benefits. As noted, one of every two Medicare beneficiaries with prescription coverage before 2006 obtained it from an employer-sponsored plan, so what happens to this market is immensely important to the entire Medicare program. While there seems little question that future retirees will receive less generous prescription coverage than their forebears, it is not at all clear how employer subsidies will shape the trend.

On top of these uncertainties, virtually all Medicare beneficiaries now face the cost of dealing with a much more complex system of financing pharmaceutical therapy. Informing beneficiaries of their options has proven to be a huge challenge, particularly given the bewildering array of plan cost-sharing options and formulary designs. Dislocations and coordination-of-benefit issues are particularly problematical for dual eligibles and low-income beneficiaries of state pharmaceutical assistance plans. There is also a potentially serious quality-of-care issue arising from the separation of drug coverage from other medical benefits. Stand-alone drug plans make no sense from a medical management standpoint. Even if there is good communication between drug plans and medical providers (which is an issue itself), their economic incentives are at odds. Drug plans profit by keeping medication expenses low even if that increases costs elsewhere in the health care system. Moreover, because drug expenditures tend to be highly persistent over time, PDPs have a powerful incentive to cherry pick healthy enrollees (Wrobel et al., 2003). Federal safeguards are supposed to prevent that from happening, but experience under the Medicare+Choice program suggests that the safeguards will be difficult to enforce.

Given the high degree of uncertainty surrounding the drug benefit, prudence calls for careful monitoring of program activities. Evidence on the law's impact on patterns of drug use and possible cost offsets elsewhere in the Medicare program will take a concerted research effort. The framers of PL 108-173 appeared to recognize that need when they included section 1013, which authorized $50 million in FY04 with similar commitments in later years for the Agency for Healthcare Research and Quality (AHRQ) to conduct research on health care outcomes, comparative clinical effectiveness, and appropriateness of health services, with an emphasis on prescription drugs. This auspicious start was short-lived. Congress failed to appropriate any of these funds for FY04, and only $15 million was approved in the FY05 and FY06 budgets. The combination of a benefit of questionable value and a significantly curtailed research effort are ominous signs for the future of Medicare drug coverage.

NOTES

1. Douglass Holtz-Eakin, CBO director, to Jim Nussle, chairman, Committee on the Budget, U.S. House of Representatives, February 2, 2004, www.cbo.gov/ftpdocs/49xx/doc4995/OMBDrugLtr.pdf.
2. Ibid.
3. Holtz-Eakin to Don Nickels, chairman, Committee on the Budget, U.S. Senate, November 20, 2003, www.cbo.gov/ftpdocs/48xx/doc4814/11-20-MedicareLetter2.pdf.
4. President signs Medicare legislation: Remarks by the president at signing of the Medicare Prescription Drug, Improvement, and Modernization Act of 2003, December 8, 2003, www.whitehouse.gov/news/releases/2003/12/20031208_2.html.

REFERENCES

Blustein, J. 2000. Drug coverage and drug purchases by Medicare beneficiaries with hypertension. *Health Affairs* 19(2):219–30.

Doshi, J., Brandt, N., and Stuart, B. 2004. Impact of drug coverage on COX-2 inhibitor use in Medicare. *Health Affairs* 23:1, Web exclusive, February 19. http://content .healthaffairs.org/cgi/content/abstract/hlthaff.w4.94.

Gilman, B., Gage, B., and Mitchell, J. 2003. *Evaluation of Vermont Pharmacy Assistance Programs for Low Income Medicare Beneficiaries.* Final report to the Centers for Medicare and Medicaid Services under contract no. 500-95-0040. Baltimore: CMS.

Gold, M., and Achman, L. 2003. Shifting Medicare choices, 1999–2003. *Monitoring Medicare+ Choice Facts* 8:1.

Hillerman, A., et al. 1999. Financial incentives in drug spending in managed care. *Health Affairs* 18(2):189–200.

Joyce, G., et al. 2002. Employer drug benefit plans and spending on prescription drugs. *Journal of the American Medical Association* 288(14):1733–39.

Kaiser Family Foundation and Health Research and Educational Trust. 2003. Employer health benefits: 2003 annual survey. Kaiser Family Foundation, Menlo Park, CA. www.kff.org/insurance/ehbs2003-abstract.cfm.

Kaiser Family Foundation and Hewitt Associates. 2004. Retiree health benefits now and in the future: Findings from the Kaiser/Hewitt 2003 Survey on Retiree Health Benefits. Kaiser Family Foundation, Menlo Park, CA. www.kff.org/medicare/011404 package.cfm.

Kamal-Bahl, S., and Briesacher, B. 2004. How do incentive-based formularies influence drug selection and spending for hypertension? *Health Affairs* 23(1):227–36.

Lichtenberg, F. 1996. Do (more and better) drugs keep people out of hospitals? *American Economic Review* 86(2):384–88.

Lichtenberg, F. 2001. Are the benefits of newer drugs worth their cost? Evidence from the 1996 MEPS. *Health Affairs* 20(5):241–51.

Lillard, L., Rogowski, J., and Kingston, R. 1999. Insurance coverage for prescription drugs: Effects on use and expenditures in the Medicare population. *Medical Care* 37(9):926–36.

Mello, M., Sterns, S., Norton, E., and Ricketts, T. 2003. Understanding biased selection in Medicare HMOs. *Health Services Research* 38(3):961–92.

Newhouse, J. P., Manning, W. G., Keeler, E. B., and Sloss, E. M. 1989. Adjusting capitation rates using objective health measures and prior utilization. *Health Care Financing Review* 10(3):41–54.

Nyman, J. 2003. *The Theory of Demand for Health Insurance.* Stanford, CA: Stanford University Press.

Only small part of new Medicare HMO money boosts benefits. 2004. *Washington HealthBeat,* February 27.

Pear, R. 2004. Bush's aides put higher price tag on Medicare law. *New York Times,* January 30, p. 1.

Reimer, D., and Glied, S. 2003. What other programs can teach us: Increasing participation in health insurance programs. *American Journal of Public Health* 93:67–74.

Sears, J. 2003. Comparing beneficiaries of the Medicare savings programs with eligible nonparticipants. *Social Security Bulletin* 64(3):76–80.

Shea, D., Stuart, B., and Briesacher, B. 2003–4. Participation and crowd out in a Medicare prescription drug benefit: Simulation estimates. *Health Care Financing Review* 25(2):47–61.

Soumerai, S., et al. 1991. Effects of Medicaid drug payment limits on admissions to hospitals and nursing homes. *New England Journal of Medicine* 325(15):1072–77.

Soumerai, S., et al. 1994. Effects of limiting Medicaid drug reimbursement benefits on use of psychotropic agents and acute mental health services by patients with schizophrenia. *New England Journal of Medicine* 331(10):650–55.

Stuart, B., Doshi, J., Briesacher, B., Wrobel, M., and Baysac, F. 2004. Impact of prescription coverage on hospital and physician costs: A case study of Medicare beneficiaries with chronic obstructive pulmonary disease. *Clinical Therapeutics* 26(1): 1688–99.

Stuart, B., and Grana, J. 1998. Ability to pay and the decision to medicate. *Medical Care* 36(2):202–11.

Stuart, B., and Zacker, C. 1999. Who bears the burden of Medicaid drug copays? *Health Affairs* 18(2):201–12.

Tamblyn, R., et al. 2001. Adverse events associated with prescription drug cost-sharing among poor and elderly persons. *Journal of the American Medical Association* 285(4):421–29.

U.S. Department of Health and Human Services. 2004. *Your Medicare Benefits.* Baltimore: CMS.

Wing, L., Reid, C., Ryan, P., et al. 2003. A comparison of outcomes with angiotensin-converting enzyme inhibitors and diuretics for hypertension in the elderly. *New England Journal of Medicine* 348(7):583–92.

Wrobel, B., Stuart, B., Briesacher, B., and Doshi, J. 2004. *Impact of Prescription Drug Coverage on Medicare Program Expenditures: A Case Study of the UMWA.* Final report to the Centers for Medicare and Medicaid Services under contract no. 500-00-0032.Baltimore: CMS.

Wrobel, M., Doshi, J., Stuart, B., and Briesacher, B. 2003. Predictability of drug expenditures for Medicare beneficiaries. *Health Care Financing Review* 25(2):37–45.

CHAPTER SEVENTEEN

Prescription Drugs and Elders in the Twenty-first Century

Christine E. Bishop, Ph.D.

The Medicare program embodies part of Americans' responsibilities to one another across generations. The Medicare Prescription Drug, Improvement, and Modernization Act of 2003 (MMA) expanded these responsibilities to include a portion of elders' prescription drug spending. This essay considers how any program to expand Medicare to include prescription drugs—not just the one now enacted into law—may affect the distribution of well-being in our society and thus exemplify aspects of intergenerational responsibility. The issues raised here suggest a research agenda to pursue as the new program is implemented. With increased knowledge, policymakers will be able to guide adjustments and expansions that could enhance the program's effectiveness in meeting multiple goals for intergenerational responsibility.

The Effects of a Medicare Prescription Drug Plan

The Medicare prescription drug plan should be evaluated in the broad context of the potential accomplishments of a universal prescription drug program for elders. The goals of a public program covering prescription drugs for elders should include these:

- Protection of retirement income: Medicare prescription drug coverage represents collective payment for a necessity with sharply rising costs and thus can reduce the risks of income insecurity in old age.
- Efficient use of inputs in production of health: Medicare prescription drug coverage can equalize insurance coverage of inputs into care and thus can reduce price distortions that affect the mix of health services that beneficiaries use.
- Improvements in health status: Medicare prescription drug coverage, by paying for needed drugs for beneficiaries previously not accessing them, has the potential to improve average health outcomes, reducing mortality and the incidence and prevalence of disability, and to narrow health disparities.

Protect Retirement Income

Income security in retirement can be threatened by catastrophic health events, particularly for retirees without prescription drug insurance. Under an effective Medicare drug program, the burden of at least some drug costs move from private out-of-pocket payments and privately purchased drug coverage to Medicare, where costs are shared among beneficiaries and across generations. Thus the buying power of retirement income is protected. While Medicare Parts A and B have protected elders' financial security from unexpected costs of inpatient and outpatient medical services, before MMA took effect, Medicare beneficiaries were responsible for purchasing drugs out of pocket or through privately purchased insurance.

From its inception, Medicare has been an important adjunct to Social Security retirement income, because it cushions the impact of adverse health events on disposable income. Paying for prescription drugs, however, was not a major concern in the early days of Medicare, when many elders were just gaining coverage for hospital services.

Prescription drugs were, of course, a critical input into health care 40 and 50 years ago. In 1960, prescription drug expenditures were 10 percent of total health expenditures, with almost all of this amount paid directly by consumers (Figures 17.1 and 17.2). At first glance, this seems like a substantial portion of the health bill that Medicare's founders should have considered for coverage

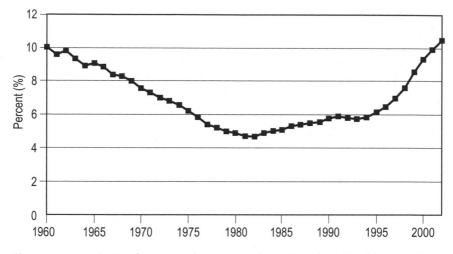

Figure 17.1. Prescription drug expenditures as a proportion of total health expenditures, 1960–2002. *Source:* Centers for Medicare and Medicaid Services, 2004

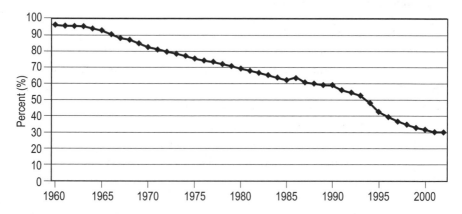

Figure 17.2. Consumer out-of-pocket payment as a proportion of all expenditures on prescription drugs. *Source:* Centers for Medicare and Medicaid Services, 2004

along with hospitalization and physician visits. But two factors kept drugs from being an egregious omission from the list of services to be insured for elders: the nature of the drugs available at that time, which required payments by consumers that were small relative to other health spending; and the fact that Americans younger than 65 also did not have coverage for prescription drugs.

In an era when antibiotics were still hailed as the miraculous wonder drugs they are, expenses for drugs tended to be episodic for individuals. Prescriptions were closely tied to ambulatory care visits, so that the cost of these two aspects of care went together. A patient went to the doctor with a complaint, and the doctor wrote a prescription to deal with it. The patient's total cost for a visit included both the physician's bill and the relatively small price of the remedy he prescribed. Further, the cost of filling a prescription was small in relation to income for most elders. In 1960, annual per capita expenditures for prescription drugs were only $14.39.[1] Early studies indicated that prescription drug use was sensitive not to the price of drugs but to the price of ambulatory care (net of insurance). In the next decades, expenditures for other portions of the health services rose rapidly, as insurance coverage both enabled more use and fostered technological advances. More effective and less invasive procedures and operations found widespread use, driving up total health expenditures. By 1980, total prescription drug spending adjusted for inflation had also risen, but the proportion of total health spending going to drugs had fallen to less than 5 percent.[2]

During this same period, an increasing number of employers added insurance for prescription drugs to the health insurance benefits they offered to working-age and retired Americans. Most state Medicaid programs paid for prescription drugs for their enrollees, and Medicare beneficiaries seeking "gold" level supplemental coverage began buying plans that covered drugs as well as Medicare copays and deductibles. Medicare managed care plans disbursing additional benefits to enrollees under the Medicare payment rules added prescription drug coverage. As a result, the proportion of total prescription drug expenses paid by consumers fell markedly (see Figure 17.2). In effect, standard insurance for working-age insured Americans, and for many Medicare beneficiaries as well, now included drug coverage.

In a cycle familiar in health technology innovation, the pharmaceutical industry responded to this increase in the public's ability to pay for drugs (Goddeeris, 1984; Weisbrod, 1991; Gelijns and Rosenberg, 1994; Danzon and Pauly, 2001, 2002). Pharmaceutical research and development, building on basic scientific advances, provided the health sector with a growing array of prescription drugs to treat chronic conditions and prevent disease. The new drugs were expensive, and many were taken chronically. Thus, the cost of a prescription (say, a 30-day supply of a medicine) was no longer a good indication of the cost of treatment for a disease or condition. Rather than treating a time-limited episode of illness, many drugs are now in effect prescribed for a lifetime. Spending on prescription drugs rose rapidly throughout the 1990s and regained its

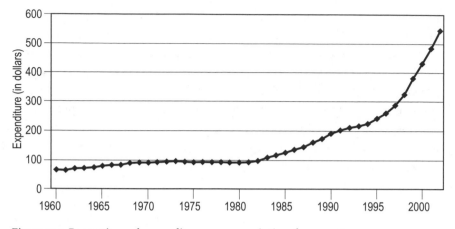

Figure 17.3. Per capita real expenditures on prescription drugs, 1960–2002
Sources: Centers for Medicare and Medicaid Services, 2004; Council of Economic
Advisors, 2004, table B-3, p. 288

10 percent proportion of the total health expenditures sometime in 2001 (see
Figure 17.1). Real per capita expenditures on prescription drugs rose from $68
per person in 1960 (in 2000 dollars) to $548 in 2002 (also in 2000 dollars) (Fig-
ure 17.3).[3] But by this time 70 percent of the total spending was covered by public and private insurance, with only 30 percent paid by consumers out of pocket
(see Figure 17.2).

Older Medicare beneficiaries, already retired, had no way to prepare for the
increased costs that accompanied the increased value of drugs in treating and
preventing disease (Maxwell, Moon, and Segal, 2001). Those who expected to
pay for prescription drugs out of income, on the same basis as food, housing,
and other living expenses, found it increasingly difficult to do so. Of course,
healthy elders have low prescription drug expenses, and wealthy elders are easily able to pay for prescription drugs out of pocket. In 2003, more than half of
all Medicare beneficiaries spent less than $500 out of pocket for prescription
drugs—less than $1.50 per day (Kaiser Family Foundation, 2003, interpolated
from figure 6). This is less than 5 percent of income for the great majority (86%)
of elders with income above $10,000 (U.S. Bureau of the Census, 2004). But al-
most 15 percent of all beneficiaries incurred out-of-pocket expenses of $2,000
or more in 2003 (Kaiser Family Foundation, 2003, figure 6). This amount looms
large for a group with a median household income of $23,787 in 2002 (U.S.
Bureau of the Census, 2004). Because of the high costs incurred by a relatively

small proportion of beneficiaries, the mean total spending for prescription drugs (estimated at $2,322 in 2003) is substantially higher than the median (estimated at about $1,500) (Kaiser Family Foundation, 2003, interpolated from figure 5).

The risk of large uncovered drug expenses posed a threat to income security in retirement that can be dealt with by more complete insurance.[4] But drug insurance premiums must more than cover average expected costs, so elders who purchased prescription drug coverage saw their premiums rise unexpectedly.

Elders without effective drug insurance from former employers, the Veterans Health Administration, or Medicaid had to pay for prescription drugs out of self-purchased insurance or out of current income and assets. They may have been well prepared for the expected expense of prescription drugs of the 1960s or 1970s, but they had no way to foresee the impact of technological change on this portion of their household budgets. The increased liability for drug expenses raised the price of prescription drug insurance, leading elders to drop private coverage if their current drug expenses were less than premiums. Payers for postretirement benefits also felt the pinch and found it difficult to maintain promised coverage for succeeding generations of retirees.

One criticism of a subsidized Medicare drug benefit is that it includes transfer payments from working-age Americans to elders who would otherwise have paid their own drug bills or would have paid for prescription drug insurance from their own funds. But such a benefit also serves as targeted inflation protection for future as well as current retirees, who will face an uncertain need for this especially inflation-prone good at a time when their incomes are fixed. More important is the assurance of access to technological advances that were unknown when many current elders began their retirement planning. Medicare social insurance for prescription drugs can protect today's workers from being denied technological advances that we can barely dream of (Nyman, 2003, 2004). An effective universal prescription drug benefit for elders should increase the probability that retirement income is sufficient to meet necessary living expenses.

Improve the Efficiency and Outcomes of Health Care

In contrast to the transfer effects of pharmaceutical insurance, which shift the burden of payment for an unchanged total from drug-consuming elders to all enrollees and taxpayers without changes in real resource use or benefits, an expansion of Medicare to cover drugs could support two types of real effects:

greater efficiency in the use of health resources to produce the same health benefits and, beyond this, tangible improvements in health outcomes. Another way to see these two effects are as, first, a shift in the mix of health services used to produce health, with more access to prescription drugs enabling lower use of other services (sometimes called offset effects); and, second, improvement in health outcomes, produced through these shifts in use but also brought about by increased use for some elders of this previously inaccessible portion of technology and, ultimately, by technological advances spurred by coverage improvements.

Make Provision of Health Care More Efficient

When an insurance program covers many health services but omits prescription drugs, it is likely that drugs are used less than they should be relative to other health inputs. This is inefficient; when patients and their physicians see low prices for covered services and high prices for drugs, these relative price distortions may lead to overuse of covered services and less-than-optimal approaches to treating and preventing illness. Patients can access the fully insured treatments and interventions they need regardless of cost, while drugs, with less or no coverage, may be underprescribed. Study after study has shown that near-poor uninsured Medicare beneficiaries, who face high out-of-pocket prices for this input into medical care, tend to underfill prescriptions (Safran et al., 2005; Wilson et al., 2005). Underuse of prescription drugs can include not filling prescriptions, owing to cost, and skipping or reducing doses to make prescriptions last longer. Because many of today's drugs are prescribed over the long term to prevent illness and keep chronic conditions under control, patients may not see filling their prescriptions as a life-or-death matter. This less-than-optimal use of prescription drugs likely contributes to poor health outcomes. The resulting acute illness events and chronic conditions require treatment resources and represent a failure to realize potential offsets in the use of acute and long-term care services.

In its advocacy for a Medicare prescription drug benefit, the current administration linked better access to prescription drugs for chronic disease to reduced expenditures for other Medicare and Medicaid services (Bush, 2003). The hope has been that a Medicare prescription drug program will avert other health costs and pay for itself. As noted in Chapter 16 in this volume, by Bruce Stuart, the evidence to date is mixed on whether use of other Medicare services is lower for elders with prescription drug insurance. However, it is important to take income differences into account when evaluating these studies, because effects are likely to be different for different income groups. Upper- and even middle-income individuals can quite easily afford many prescription drug therapies with or without insurance, so insurance provides a meaningful increase in access to prescription drugs only for low-income uninsured elders. Further, a substantial portion of elders insured for prescription drug expenses have chosen to purchase this insurance themselves as part of Medicare supplementation. Many elders who choose to spend premium payments to cover their prescription drugs already have chronic illnesses and conditions and are making a savvy decision in light of their ongoing expected drug costs. This is why analyses of health services use that do not account for this rational self-selection effect are likely to find that elders choosing drug insurance use more rather than fewer Medicare services than elders without drug coverage.

Although Medicare services have been the focus of attention for offsetting costs, long-term care is an important potential source of savings. Prescription drugs that slow the progression and ameliorate the symptoms of chronic illness can avert or slow disability and thus reduce the probability of need for long-term care. States' Pharmacy Assistance Program waiver applications have already made this argument: in promising Medicaid budget neutrality, states have projected that Medicaid expansions to cover near-poor elders for prescription drugs will avert disability and thus will save Medicaid-covered long-term-care costs (Illinois Department of Public Aid, 2001; Wisconsin Department of Health and Family Services, 2002). Preliminary studies suggest that certain conditions associated with functional disabilities are indeed "prescription drug sensitive," so access to drugs should have a payoff in lower nursing home use.[5] A handful of studies detailing the declining rates of disability in the population age 65 and older have linked these trends to improved prevention and treatment of chronic disease, which by definition includes prescription drug therapies (Freedman and Martin, 2000).

Cost offsets due to the impact of prescription drug access on disability could be exceptionally valuable in the years ahead, owing to the increasing number of elders in the populations of the future. By 2030, the U.S. population age 85 and older, the group at highest risk for needing all forms of long-term care, is expected to more than double over its 2000 level, to close to 10 million (U.S. Bureau of the Census, 2005). The time frame for returns on this investment remains in question, however. It may be many years before society reaps the benefits of this offset effect. Further, a Medicare drug benefit alone may not be sufficient to reap potential gains: for many, access to prescription drugs for the prevention or treatment of chronic disease may be necessary before the arbitrary Medicare age of 65 if the full benefit is to be achieved.

Offset savings, whether for acute or long-term care services, may also be generated through future technological change. Just as Medicare coverage of hospital and ambulatory care spurred technological developments targeted to diseases and conditions of elderly people, a Medicare prescription drug program is likely to spur faster development of drugs that prevent and treat diseases of aging. Better coverage of prescription drugs may provide new incentives for cost-reducing technological change rebalanced toward secondary prevention.

It should be noted that the cost of new technology will determine whether it represents a net benefit. While many current new drugs carry a high price tag relative to drugs introduced previously, their price is small relative to the much more expensive hospitalizations, procedures, chronic medical care, and disability-related care they promise to avert. In terms of resource cost, the net payoff may be even larger than it appears, because of the power of the pharmaceutical industry to command high prices. However, future drugs may be much more expensive to develop or produce, yielding diminishing real returns. The power of the pharmaceutical industry to set prices may increase; or it may be reduced by mass purchasing or regulation, changing the net expenditure impact of drug spending. We have no guarantee that future drugs will be developed and priced in such a way that they will continue to support any offset savings, yet insurance is set up to make them accessible by spreading expenditure burdens across the population, regardless of net return.

In summary, an effective universal prescription drug program for elders would reduce the barriers to efficient treatment that occur when one portion of health services is uninsured while others are fully covered. Considering just the substitution of drug therapies for other types of care, this could generate savings on the other health services and long-term care used by elders with less insurance for drugs than for other services.

Improve Health Outcomes and the Quality of Life

As insurance lowers the price for prescription drugs relative to other services, we expect better health outcomes for elders who now face financial barriers to appropriate prescription drug use, as well as cost-offset savings on the other health services they are using instead.[6] Because the costs spent on prescription drugs will not be limited to the savings they generate in other health services, total costs are likely to increase with greater access to prescription drugs. However, because only a portion of Medicare beneficiaries are going without needed drugs, the impact of expanded coverage on both spending and *health* will not be great. As with offsets, this effect is most likely to be seen for beneficiaries who currently are not using prescription drugs because of their cost relative to income.[7] As noted above, many elders are insured for prescription drugs or are able to afford to pay for most prescribed drugs out of pocket. Most state Medicaid programs cover prescription drugs for the very poor; Medicaid waiver and state-funded programs cover the near-poor in a number of states; a substantial number of elders receive drug benefits as part of an employer retirement benefits package; and middle- and high-income elders are able to buy the drugs they need out of savings or monthly income, or prepay expected drug expenses through self-paid insurance. Many beneficiaries without drug insurance coverage buy the drugs their physicians prescribe, even when this means doing without some other important consumer item.

Nevertheless, the potential impact on health of a Medicare prescription drug program may be the effect that most affirms the content of our responsibility across generations because of its potential to reduce health disparities.

The early days of Medicare A and B have something to tell us about the potential of more uniform access to care for reducing health disparities. When Medicare was enacted in 1965, only about half of the population age 65 and older were insured for the costs of hospital services. The oldest and poorest elders were least likely to have hospital coverage, so that elders with the greatest expected need for services faced the highest financial barriers to the use of health services. The result was large disparities in use by age, race, and education, parallel to what we observe with prescription drugs today.

A national hospital insurance program for the aged (Part A of Medicare) and a highly subsidized ambulatory care insurance program (Part B) did something to address these disparities. Although the earliest studies of use under Medicare found persistent differences in the use of medical care between poor and nonpoor, African American and white, oldest old and young elderly people (Davis and Reynolds, 1975), disparities in access to hospital care diminished over time as the health system responded to beneficiaries' enhanced ability to pay for health services.[8] By the 1980s, studies were finding that Medicare spending was not only moving the nation's elders toward a more even distribution of use but also showing up in health averages (Davis and Schoen, 1978; Link et al., 1982a, 1982b; Long and Settle, 1984; Hadley, 1988). Almost 40 years later, the expected additional life span for men reaching age 65 had increased from 12.9 years in 1965 to 15.9 years in 2002, a 27 percent gain; women reaching age 65 in 1965 could expect to live 16.3 more years, but those reaching 65 in 2002 could expect 19.0 more years, a gain of 17 percent.[9] Age-adjusted rates of disability appear to have declined, and they have declined more for African Americans than for whites (Manton and Gu, 2001). The bulk of these improvements may be attributable to changes in behavior (tobacco use, diet) and environment, enhanced by the increasing income and educational attainment of successive elderly cohorts. But the increased access to health services and the new technologies for elders who previously could not fund their own care has also affected health status and longevity (Cutler, 2001).

This is not to say that coverage of Medicare services was enough to eliminate disparities (Gornick et al., 1996; Gornick, 2000, 2003). One source of these disparities is likely access to prescription drugs, because they were not included in Medicare. As pharmaceutical interventions have become more expensive, while an increasing proportion of the population age 65 and older holds insurance coverage for drug therapies, disparities in access to the evolving standard for medical treatment have again widened, reminiscent of disparities in access to hospital and ambulatory care in the early 1960s.

The studies that preview possible effects of Medicare prescription drug insurance on health outcomes examine these issues at two levels: (1) the role of pharmaceuticals in prevention and treatment of specific diseases and conditions and (2) trends in disparities in mortality and disability for population subgroups.

Prescription drug therapies have been developed to address many chronic illnesses and pre-illness conditions. The incorporation of these therapies into medical care surely plays a part not only in declining mortality rates but also in declining disability of elderly people. Prescription drugs are deferring the onset of disabling conditions as well as delaying death. Drugs for hypertension, diabetes, Alzheimer disease, and arthritis are prescribed for individual patients to enable them to live more full lives. At the same time, disability rates are declining (Manton et al., 1997; Manton and Gu, 2001; Freedman et al., 2002, 2004; Spillman, 2004). Although it is difficult to attribute a specific portion of these gains to prescription drugs, at least some of these technological advances surely affect the population statistics for disability.

But health outcome gains are not evenly distributed. Disparities among elderly population groups in mortality and disability are attributable to many causes, and research is just beginning to scratch the surface of the puzzles of health disparities (Geronimus et al., 2001; Seeman et al., 2004). Disparities in health services may be responsible for a relatively small portion of outcome disparities, and even when the focus is on health services, differences in access to care associated with differences in income or insurance are only part of the story (Link et al., 1998). However, differences in access to prescription drugs could be a significant contributor to some disparities in health and disability. In particular, beneficiaries with insurance are more likely to gain access to new technologies (Sharma et al., 2003; Adams et al., 2001; Federman et al., 2001; Doshi et al., 2004). Studies have found that patients with fewer years of education, with lower income, and without drug insurance are less likely to use new prescription drugs (Federman et al., 2001; Brown et al., 2003; Sambamoorthi et al., 2003; Doshi et al., 2004). Provisions of insurance benefit design, including deductibles, copayments, and formularies, affect patient and physician behavior and restrict access to some prescription drugs. Making health services technology, including prescription drugs, more widely accessible represents a commitment to reduce disparities in health services use and, eventually, disparities in health outcomes.

Conclusion

The framework for considering effects of the expansion of Medicare to cover prescription drugs suggests areas for research and evaluation.

With respect to retirement income security, it will be important to understand the effect of Medicare drug coverage on the variability of out-of-pocket health-related expenses, especially for lower-income elders. Contributing to this will be trends for postretirement health insurance coverage of prescription drugs, which could be dismal despite incentives for continuing coverage. After the dust has settled, will there actually be a reduction in the risk that elders will encounter health-related expenses catastrophic relative to their income and assets? A focus on averages could obscure the impact of insurance as protecting a standard of living, especially for low-income elders. It will be useful to monitor changes in the proportion of elders with drug spending greater than a given proportion of discretionary income.

Potential offset effects should be identified and tracked. Again, the most important group to watch is lower-income beneficiaries, who are more likely than higher-income beneficiaries to respond to the out-of-pocket price of prescription drugs.[10] Offsets to be examined should be defined in widening circles: Medicare offset savings are important, but so are offsets to the costs of other public programs, including Medicaid and Veterans Health Administration services. In addition, there may be important offset savings for services whose costs, both monetary and nonmonetary, are borne most heavily by individuals and families, most notably long-term-care services for disability. These may in fact be the most important offset savings of expanded drug coverage.

The potential of the Medicare prescription drug insurance program to fuel overuse of prescription drugs, beyond the point where benefits exceed costs, cannot be overlooked. Clearly these costs must be put up against offset savings and the value of improved health outcomes.

Impacts on health outcomes, and most importantly reductions in disparities in health outcomes, may be the most significant consequence of an effective Medicare prescription drug insurance program. Outcomes are most likely to improve for Medicare beneficiaries who previously were not covered for prescription drug expenses. Studies of outcomes over time, taking many socioeconomic and health utilization factors into account, may provide important insights into the causes of health disparities. It is possible that there will be little net impact on health outcomes arising from the prescription drug provisions of the Medicare Modernization Act, the specific program currently in force. This is due to its potential to reduce coverage for some population groups (Medicaid dual eligibles and retirees covered by employer-sponsored plans) and actually increase barriers to access for certain high-cost users. Once access to preventive prescription drug therapies is available for Medicare beneficiaries, we may observe continuing discrepancies in the health of populations as they become Medicare-eligible, suggesting payoffs for preventive therapies for near-elderly people, especially those at high risk. We should investigate the potential value of the "welcome to middle age" package suggested by Lubitz to fill gaps in access to preventive care for midlife Americans (Lubitz, 2005; Daviglus et al., 2005). Even if economic barriers to access are equalized or reduced, differences in the capacity of various groups to make effective use of access in promoting health outcomes may still remain and will need to be addressed. Research on shifts in health outcome disparities for elders could make use of this natural experiment in changing access and lead us to a better understanding of the links between health services and health.

Over time, expanded markets for chronically administered prescription drugs may drive the direction of technological change toward preventive therapies, eventually providing more of the "high technologies" that Lewis Thomas exhorted us to seek decades ago (Thomas, 1974). The promise of innovations that completely avert disease may ultimately be the greatest benefit of prescription drug insurance for elders.

Acknowledgments

I am grateful to Cindy Thomas, Stan Wallack, and Melissa Morley of the Schneider Institute for Health Policy and Dan Gilden of JEN Associates, Inc., for their insights into the issues raised by this chapter, and to Emily Sandahl for her technical assistance.

NOTES

1. In current (1960) dollars (Centers for Medicare and Medicaid, 2004).

2. Berndt (2001, p. 100) used the phrase "the importance of being unimportant" to explain the indifference of cost-containment policy to drug expenditures until the mid-1990s, but this applies to consumers as well.

3. Real per capita spending is a good indication of the resources flowing into prescription drugs, although some of the most expensive drugs are not purchased at retail.

4. Another source of health-related catastrophic expense, that for long-term care, has not reached this level of public awareness. This suggests that large size and high variability of expenditures for health-related necessities are not enough in themselves to move public policy toward protection of the purchasing power of retirement income. In contrast to prescription drugs, long-term care is not widely covered by private insurance.

5. Unpublished analysis by Daniel Gilden and colleagues, JEN Associates, Inc., Cambridge, MA.

6. But see Freedman and Aykan 2003 for a skeptical view.

7. Within the framework of this comment, these low-access elders are protecting the consumption value of retirement income at the expense of the health benefits they might gain if they purchased needed prescription drugs; in less abstract terms, they are choosing to use their limited income for food, utilities, or rent rather than drugs.

8. For a review, see Gornick, 2003.

9. U.S. Social Security Administration, 2003, table V.A.4, "Cohort Life Expectancies," p. 86.

10. This research must take careful account of self-selection effects of persons needing prescriptions.

REFERENCES

Adams, A. S., Soumerai, S. B., and Ross-Degnan, D. 2001. Use of antihypertensive drugs by Medicare enrollees: Does type of drug coverage matter? *Health Affairs* 20(1):276–86.

Berndt, E. R. 2001. The U.S. pharmaceutical industry: Why major growth in times of cost containment? *Health Affairs* 20(2):100–114.

Brown, A. F., Gross, A. G., Gutierrez, P. R., Jiang, L., Shapiro, M. F., and Mangione, C. M. 2003. Income-related differences in the use of evidence-based therapies in older persons with diabetes mellitus in for-profit managed care. *Journal of the American Geriatrics Society* 51(5):665–70.

Bush, G. W. 2003. President signs Medicare legislation. December 8. www.whitehouse .gov/news/releases/2003/12/print/20031208-2.html.

Centers for Medicare and Medicaid Services. 2004. *National Health Expenditures by Type of Service and Source of Funds: Calendar Years 1960–2002.* www.hcfa.gov/stats/ nhe-oact/ (site discontinued; last accessed March 15, 2004).

Council of Economic Advisors. 2004. *Economic Report of the President.* www.gpoaccess .gov/usbudget/fy05/pdf/2004_erp.pdf.

Cutler, D. M. 2001. Declining disability among the elderly. *Health Affairs* 20(6):11–27.

Danzon, P. M., and Pauly, M. V. 2001. Insurance and new technology: From hospital to drugstore. *Health Affairs* 20(5):86–100.

Danzon, P. M., and Pauly, M. V. 2002. Health insurance and the growth in pharmaceutical expenditures. *Journal of Law and Economics* 45(2):587–613.

Daviglus, M. L., Liu, K., et al. 2005. Cardiovascular risk profile earlier in life and Medicare costs in the last year of life. *Archives of Internal Medicine* 165(9):1028–34.

Davis, K., and Reynolds, R. 1975. Medicare and the utilization of health services by the elderly. *Journal of Human Resources* 10(3):361–77.

Davis, K., and Schoen, C. 1978. *Health and the War on Poverty: A Ten-Year Appraisal.* Washington, DC: Brookings Institution Press.

Doshi, J. A., Brandt, N., and Stuart, B. 2004. The impact of drug coverage on COX-2 inhibitor use in Medicare. *Health Affairs,* www.healthaffairs.org/indexhw.php.

Federman, A. D., Adams, A. S., Ross-Degnan, D., Soumerai, S. B., and Ayanian, J. Z. 2001. Supplemental insurance and use of effective cardiovascular drugs among elderly Medicare beneficiaries with coronary heart disease. *Journal of the American Medical Association* 286(14):1732–39.

Freedman, V. A., and H. Aykan. 2003. Trends in medication use and functioning before retirement age: Are they linked? *Health Affairs* 22(4):154–62.

Freedman, V. A., Crimmins, E., Schoeni, R. F., Spillman, B. C., Aykan, H., Kramarow, E., Land, K., et al. 2004. Resolving inconsistencies in trends in old-age disability: Report from a technical working group. *Demography* 41(3):417–41.

Freedman, V. A., and Martin, L. G. 2000. Contribution of chronic conditions to aggregate changes in old-age functioning. *American Journal of Public Health* 90(11):1755–60.

Freedman, V. A., Martin, L. G., and Schoeni, R. F. 2002. Recent trends in disability and functioning among older adults in the United States: A systematic review. *Journal of the American Medical Association* 288(24):3137–46.

Gelijns, A., and Rosenberg, N. 1994. The dynamics of technological change in medicine. *Health Affairs* 13(3):28–46.

Geronimus, A. T., Bound, J., Waidmann, T. A., Colen, C. G., and Steffick, D. 2001. Inequality in life expectancy, functional status, and active life expectancy across selected black and white populations in the United States. *Demography* 38(2):227–51.

Goddeeris, J. H. 1984. Medical insurance, technological change, and welfare. *Economic Inquiry* 22:56–67.

Gornick, M. E. 2000. Disparities in Medicare services: Potential causes, plausible explanations, and recommendations. *Health Care Financing Review* 21(4):23–43.

Gornick, M. E. 2003. A decade of research on disparities in Medicare utilization: Lessons for the health and health care of vulnerable men. *American Journal of Public Health* 93(5):753–59.

Gornick, M. E., Eggers, P. W., Reilly, T. W., Mentnech, R. M., Fitterman, L. K., Kucken, L. E., and Vladeck, B. C. 1996. Effects of race and income on mortality and use of services among Medicare beneficiaries. *New England Journal of Medicine* 335(11): 791–99.

Hadley, J. 1988. Medicare spending and mortality rates of the elderly. *Inquiry* 25(4):485–93.

Illinois Department of Public Aid. 2001. Medicaid 1115 Research and Demonstration Waiver Application: A pharmaceutical benefit for Illinois' low-income seniors—providing enhanced access to primary care. Illinois Department of Public Aid, Springfield, IL. July 31.

Kaiser Family Foundation. 2003. Medicare and prescription drugs: A chartpack. #6087, June. Kaiser Family Foundation, Menlo Park, CA. www.kff.org/medicare/6087-index .cfm.

Link, B. G., Northridge, M. E., Phelan, J. C., and Ganz, M. L. 1998. Social epidemiology and the fundamental cause concept: On the structuring of effective cancer screens by socioeconomic status. *Milbank Quarterly* 76(3):304–5, 375–402.

Link, C. R., Long, S. H., and Settle, R. F. 1982a. Access to medical care under Medicaid: Differentials by race. *Journal of Health Politics, Policy, and Law* 7(2):345–65.

Link, C. R., Long, S. H., and Settle, R. F. 1982b. Equity and the utilization of health care services by the Medicare elderly. *Journal of Human Resources* 17(2):195–212.

Long, S. H., and Settle, R. F. 1984. Medicare and the disadvantaged elderly: Objectives and outcomes. *Milbank Memorial Fund Quarterly. Health and Society* 62(4):609–56.

Lubitz, J. 2005. Health, technology, and medical care spending. *Health Affairs* 24, suppl. 2: WSR81–85.

Manton, K. G., Corder, L., and Stallard, E. 1997. Chronic disability trends in elderly United States populations: 1982–1994. *Proceedings of the National Academy of Sciences USA* 94(6):2593–98.

Manton, K. G., and Gu, X. 2001. Changes in the prevalence of chronic disability in the United States black and nonblack population above age 65 from 1982 to 1999. *Proceedings of the National Academy of Sciences USA* 98(11):6354–59.

Maxwell, S., Moon, M., and Segal, M. 2001. Growth in Medicare and out-of-pocket spending: Impact on vulnerable beneficiaries. The Commonwealth Fund 430. January. www.cmwf.org/publist/publist2.asp?CategoryID=9 (page discontinued; last accessed March 15, 2004).

Nyman, J. A. 2003. *The Theory of Demand for Health Insurance.* Palo Alto, CA: Stanford University Press.

Nyman, J. A. 2004. Is "moral hazard" inefficient? The policy implications of a new theory. *Health Affairs* 23(5):194–99.

Safran, D. G., Neuman, P., Schoen, C., Kitchman, M. S., Wilson, I. B., Cooper, B., Li, A., et al. 2005. Prescription drug coverage and seniors: Findings from a 2003 national survey. *Health Affairs* Web exclusive, www.healthaffairs.org/indexhw.php.

Sambamoorthi, U., Shea, D., and Crystal, S. 2003. Total and out-of-pocket expenditures for prescription drugs among older persons. *Gerontologist* 43(3):345–59.

Seeman, T. E., Crimmins, E., Huang, M. H., Singer, B., Bucur, A., Gruenewald, T., Berkman, L. F., et al. 2004. Cumulative biological risk and socio-economic differences in mortality: MacArthur Studies of Successful Aging. *Social Science and Medicine* 58(10):1985–97.

Sharma, R., Liu, H., and Wang, Y. 2003. Drug coverage, utilization, and spending by Medicare beneficiaries with heart disease. *Health Care Financing Review* 24(3):139–56.

Spillman, B. C. 2004. Changes in elderly disability rates and the implications for health care utilization and cost. *Milbank Quarterly* 82(1):157–94.

Thomas, L. 1974. *The Lives of a Cell: Notes of a Biology Watcher.* New York: Viking.

U.S. Bureau of the Census. 2003. Age of householder—households by total money income in 2002. In *Current Population Survey, 2003 Annual Social and Economic Supplement,* HINC-02. http://ferret.bls.census.gov/macro/032003/hhinc/new02_001 .htm (site discontinued; last accessed March 15, 2004).

U.S. Bureau of the Census. 2004. Age of householder—households, by total money income in 2003, type of household, race, and Hispanic origin of householder. In *Current Population Survey, 2004 Annual Social and Economic Supplement,* HINC-02, http://pubdb3.census.gov/macro/032004/hhinc/new02_005.htm.

U.S. Bureau of the Census. 2005. *U.S. Interim Projections by Age, Sex, Race, and Hispanic Origin.* www.census.gov/ipc/www/usinterimproj/.

U.S. Social Security Administration. 2003. 2003 annual report of the Board of Trustees of the Federal Old-Age and Survivors Insurance and Disability Insurance Trust Funds. March 17, 2003. www.ssa.gov/OACT/TR/TR03/index.html.

Weisbrod, B. A. 1991. The health care quadrilemma: An essay on technological change, insurance, quality of care, and cost containment. *Journal of Economic Literature* 29:523–52.

Wilson, I. B., Rogers, W. H., Chang, H., and Safran, D. G. 2005. Cost-related skipping of medications and other treatments among Medicare beneficiaries between 1998 and 2000: Results of a national study. *Journal of General Internal Medicine* 20(8):715–20.

Wisconsin Department of Health and Family Services. 2002. Medicaid 1115 Research and Demonstration Waiver Application: A pharmaceutical benefit for low-income Wisconsin seniors. Madison, WI. March 29. http://cms.gov/medicaid/1115/wi03045 .pdf (page discontinued; last accessed March 14, 2004).

Index

Page numbers in *italics* refer to figures and tables.